PRACTICAL HORSE NUTRITION

DISCLAIMER

It is hoped that the principles of Horse Nutrition as explained in this book are applicable to the readers' interests. However, it MUST BE mentioned that feeding and nutrition is only one aspect of getting a horse to perform adequately. Parasite control, growth and conditioning of the horse before 4 years of age, current training programme and ability of horse, rider and groom are equally important in obtaining desired results from the horse.

As all these application are beyond the daily control of the author, no responsibility whatsoever, is accepted for any result which MAY eventuate as a consequence of the implementation of any recommendation in this book.

PRACTICAL HORSE NUTRITION

by

R. H. KERRIGAN
B.Sc. Agr. M.A.I.A.S. M.A.A.A.C.

First published in 1986 by
R. H. Kerrigan
"Marooan"
Lochinvar via Maitland NSW 2320

Second Edition 1989

Designed and Typeset Wilderness Publications Pty Ltd,
Wollombi Road, Cessnock, N.S.W. 2325
Printed at Griffin Press Limited, Adelaide, South Australia

ISBN 1 86252 327 4

DEDICATION

This book is dedicated to the many students who have participated in my horse lectures over the years.

Their active interest and discussion on many matters relating to the feeding of horses has allowed the refinement of my lecture notes and their presentation in this book.

The feeding methods detailed in this publication have stood the test of practice and time. Results, obtained by horse owners, using the principles of nutrition outlined in this book, have produced results, in many horse disciplines, varying from racehorses and eventers to the pleasure horse.

It is hoped that you the reader will be able to achieve similar success.

"MAROOAN"
LOCHINVAR
via MAITLAND
N.S.W.
AUSTRALIA

CONTENTS

APPRECIATION FIRST EDITION

This book is written for the average horse owner and trainer, and is similar to the approach used in the presentation of nutritional lectures to large numbers of horse owners, of varying interests, over many years.

This approach has stood the test of time and acceptance and whilst the methodology may not be acceptable to the academic or the theoretical nutritionist, practical detail is what horse feeding is all about. There is little use having theorectical systems which the practical person is unable to understand.

The text has been compiled with continual and constant references to many recognised and recent scientific and academic publications. However, as this book has a decided practical approach, there is no listing of references pertaining to any comment or remark. Such approach would tend to clutter up the, hopefully, easy reading style.

A list of the various references and or scientific articles and publications used in the compilation of this book is listed at the end for those who desire further reading.

All horse people, be they University and College Students, Veterinary Surgeons and Animal Nutritionists, Race Horse and Trotting Trainers, or the one horse owner, should be able to benefit in some way from the contents of this publication.

I am indebted to the following people who kindly and critically read the first draft of this book and who offered comment,where appropriate.

Andrew Holmes, B.V.Sc., Stewart Holmes, B.V.Sc., and Ian Gollan, B.V.Sc. of Maitland N.S.W., John Morgan, B.V.Sc., of Scone N.S.W., Laurie Daube, B.V.Sc. of Adelaide, S.A., Lesley Dowey of Arabesque Stud North, Richmond N.S.W., and Jill Rymill formerly of Mostly Books, Adelaide, S.A.

The author wishes to record his sincere appreciation to these people, and in doing so accepts any responsibility for the complete contents of the book.

Photographs, apart from those taken by the author, were kindly supplied by Michael Perrot, Andrew Holmes B.V.Sc, Ivan Caples B.V.Sc., John Stewart B.V.Sc., Marcus Oldham College, Geelong, Lesley Dowey and Ian Tudor.

Diagrams were carefully drawn by David Dial,

Editing by Christine Berry and Barbara Gordon

Finally, my thanks to my wife Margaret and daughters, Jo-anne, Susan and Vicki who through our combined specific interest in performance horses, made me realise the need to research understand the principles of horse nutrition for optimum performance.

R.H.KERRIGAN

AUGUST 1986

SECOND EDITION

This book attempts to translate any available scientific result into the every day horse feeding situation, a problem which will continually confront horse feeders, due to the varied nature of horse activities.

The past few years has also seen a tremendous increase in our knowledge of the practical applications of HORSE NUTRITION. There is no possible way that scientific experiments, by their nature of design and analysis, and by the restricted facilities and funding available for such experiments throughout the world, are able to duplicate EVERY HORSE FEEDING SITUATION.

This second edition reflects the practical interpretations most of those changes of which the author is aware.

Most of the scientific papers, published over the past four years, on any aspect of HORSE NUTRITION, have been researched. Whilst some scientific research, by its very nature, tends to produce results under specifically controlled conditions, much of the information and results provided, can be translated in practical horse feeding terms. Some information contained in this book is also from current scientific experiments, still in progress and the results yet to be published. The permission of those researchers to use this information, after discussion as to its relevance, is appreciated.

R.H.KERRIGAN

SEPTEMBER 1989.

INTRODUCTION

IF ONLY HORSES COULD TALK.

They would probably tell most of us that the feeds we were using were unpalatable, unwanted or simply causing some type of pain or internal problem. Whilst we, as humans, are able to determine our own likes and dislikes as to the food we eat, we prepare horse rations with, at times, complete disregard for the nutrient and palatability requirements of the horse.

Feeding horses, for a considerable period of time, has been considered an ART more than a SCIENCE. The experience of the "old hands" has been passed down from generation to generation with the result that one of the main attributes of a successful horse handler has been to know when a horse is "doing well" and to adjust the feeding schedule accordingly. Whilst the past system of feeding horses has undoubtedly produced results for those concerned, there has been little scientific approach to the subject.

This was generally for the following reasons:

1. In most instances little concern has been shown re the cost of feeding. If someone said they were getting good results from a particular feed then this often started a fashion which spread amongst other horsepeople, without any regard to the content of the various basic rations that each person was feeding. Free advice from successful feeders and/or trainers was readily applied, without regard to the individual circumstances of each horse.
2. Little scientific evidence was available concerning the nutritional requirements of horses and most horse feeding practices as a result, were based on experience.
3. Whilst over the past few years, there has been research work carried out on horses producing results which have some practical application, these results appear to have been "lost" in the scientific literature and/or the proceedings of various professional conferences or are presented in a form which has little relevance to the practical horse feeding situation.

The basic aim of this publication is to attempt to simplify the information currently available and to present the data, and any possible practical implications, in a manner so that it may be understood by the ordinary horse owner. Hopefully the information in this book will not only help the horse feeder to understand what feeds are all about but will also allow the feeding of less expensive rations for the same end result.

Not only should this be of value to the horse feeder but the general health and performance of the horse should benefit also.

Section One

Technical Aspects

1. DIGESTION BY HORSES AND COWS

Cattle and horses eat the same type of feed. Pasture, grass, grain, chaff etc. can all be eaten by both types of animal, however the similarities between the horse and the cow end at their mouth.

The digestive tracts of the two species are vastly different in the way in which feed is broken down and absorbed into the blood stream. It is important to understand the differences and their effect on the growth and performance of horses in particular.

The following Table compares digestive tracts of the horse and the cow.

	HORSE	COW
Average Live Weight	450 kg.	450 kg.
Average Food Consumption per day - Dry matter	10 kg.	12 kg.
Average Stomach Capacity	16 kg.	180 kg.
Stomach Capacity as % of Total Digestive Tract	8%	70%
Small Intestine Capacity	52 kg.	62 kg.
Large Intestine Capacity	112 kg.	36 kg.
Total Capacity of Digestive Tract	180 kg	278 kg.

.These figures show very clearly that the front end of the digestive tract is the most important in cattle nutrition, whilst the rear end of the digestive tract is most important in horse nutrition.

More importantly, the horse does not possess the large rumen or fermenting vat for CELLULOSE or FIBRE (the outer covering of plant cells) digestion, that enables the cow to eat quickly and to digest poor quality feeds, without affecting the cow's health.

In comparison to the cow of the same live weight, the average weight of DIGESTA, (feed) in the horse's digestive tract is only about 65% of that weight which the average cow contains. The small size of the horses' stomach, in particular, requires that continual and small quantities of good quality feed are needed to ensure satisfactory feed digestion and continued good health of the horse. This feature of the horse's digestive system has been developed over millions of years with the evolution of the horse where grazing occupied up to 20 hours/ day or 83% of the horse's time. Modern feeding methods should allow for any horse to have access to feed all the time, that is how nature designed the horse to function.

Cattle belong to the RUMINANT group of grass eaters. Simply put, cattle have four stomachs whilst the horse is a MONOGASTRIC and has only one stomach.

The different stomach sizes and digestive actions mean that the horse:

DIAGRAMMATIC REPRESENTATION OF DIGESTIVE TRACTS' CAPACITIES

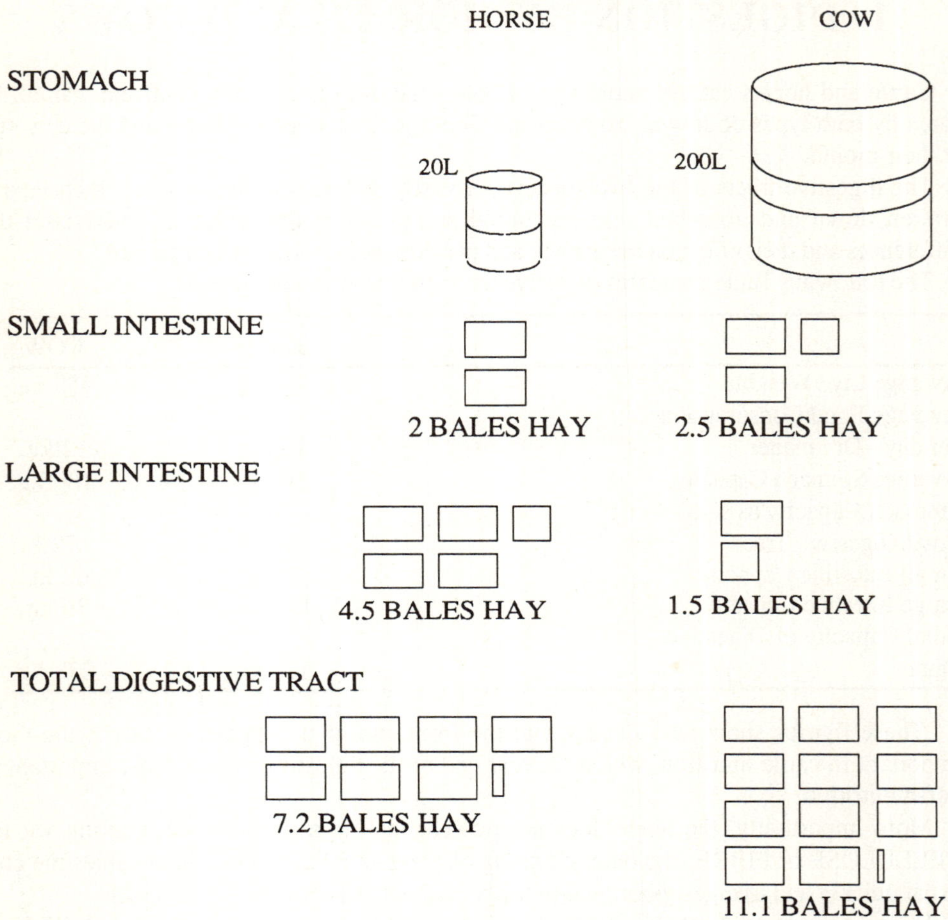

Cattle for same size and same appetite hold 50% more feed in digestive tract than horses. The digesta or feedstuffs pass through the horse in one-third or 33% of the time the same quantity of food passes through the cow.

1. is not capable of rumination or chewing the cud.
2. cannot belch or vomit, except in extreme cases of gastric dilation,which is very rare and indicative of a very sick horse.
3. has a much faster rate of food passage from the stomach to the large intestine than in cattle.
4. has feed digestion processes in the intestinal tract which resemble those digestion processes in the human, where feed is predominantly absorbed in the small and large intestine. In the cow or ruminant, fermentation of the feed in the rumen

allows food digestion to take place more readily in the small intestine as well as the fourth stomach, instead of the large intestine.

COW

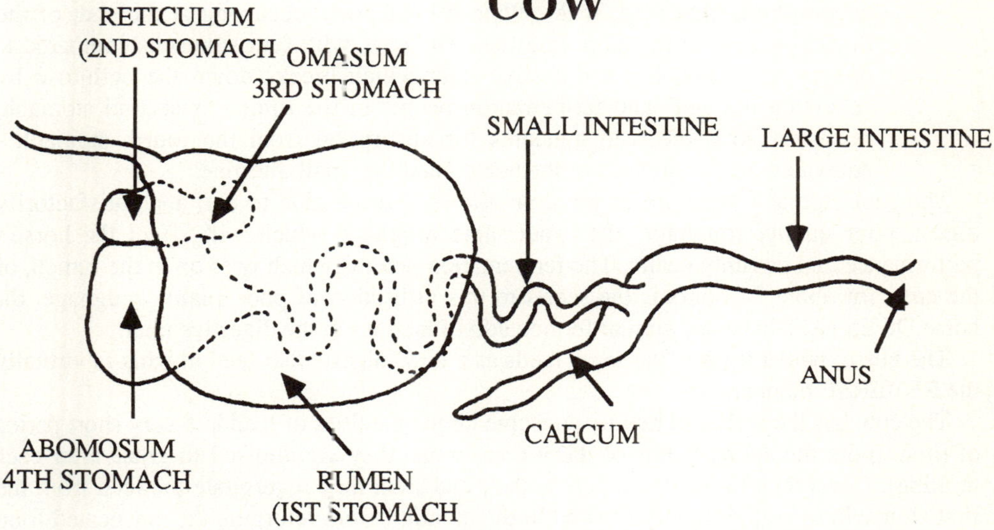

DIGESTIVE TRACTS

HORSE

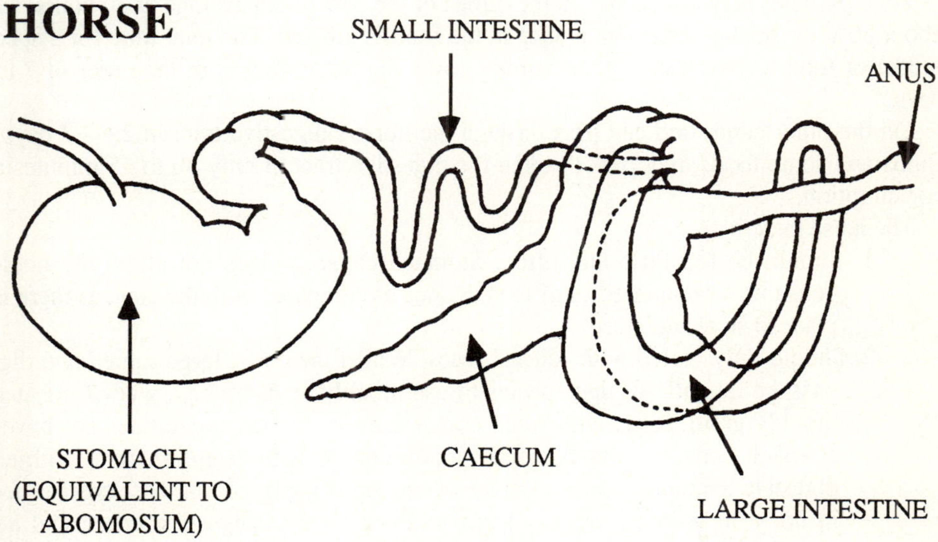

5. possesses bacteria and other micro-organisms in the large intestine which decompose and break down the cellulose in the digestive tract and which are, in general, identical to the micro-organisms in the second stomach or rumen of the cow.
6. the horse's digestive system is designed to utilise feed in the single stomach and small intestine by the action of saliva and digestive juices and enzymes decomposing that feed, with cellulose breakdown occurring at the end, of the digestive tract, in the large intestine. The cow, with four stomachs compared to one in the horse, has a digestive tract which breaks down the cellulose by "chewing the cud" and fermentation occurs in the rumen or second stomach, releasing ALL the feed nutrients for absorption from the fourth stomach - equivalent to the stomach of the horse - and the small intestine.

The four stomach structure of the cow allows it to be able to eat, and satisfactorily digest, poor quality roughage, the exact same roughage which will affect the horse's performance and possibly health. The fermentation process which goes on in the rumen, of the cow, for about 24 hours is the secret to this utilisation of poor quality roughage, the horse DOES NOT have any similar fermentation functions in the digestive tract.

The horse, whilst it takes the same feeds as a cow, digests that feed in what is virtually the REVERSE manner.

The cow has the ability to rapidly consume large quantities of feed in a very short period of time, (note the eating habits of dairy cows when they are allowed to graze after each milking). Cows then ruminate, or "chew their cud", i.e. they regurgitate the feed from the first stomach, to be thoroughly chewed in the mouth, before returning the masticated food particles back to the second stomach or rumen. Here the fermentation process takes place, where cellulose decomposing micro-organisms attack the food particles even further and break them down, so that absorption of the individual food nutrients can take place further down the digestive tract in the small and large intestine.

Food particles may be retained in the rumen of the cow for an average of 80 hours, where about 80% of the digestible dry matter in the food is utilised. The total time for a specific intake of food to pass through the normal cow's digestive tract is of the order of 7 to 10 days.

On the other hand food can pass through the horse's digestive tract in 2.5 - 3 days and fluids and some foods may pass through the digestive tract in only 30 to 45 minutes after consumption.

The horse therefore:

1. Should be fed little and often. Stomach capacity does not allow the horse to consume large quantities of feed at once as compared with the cow, as there is no place to store such feed.
2. Should only be fed with "clean" feeds. Whilst the cow's large rumen and digesta passage rate allows that species to use mouldy or damp hay, weevil infested or mouldy grain, feeds with weed contamination etc. the horse does not have the stomach capacity, gut bacterial population or feed retention time within the digestive tract to use such possible second grade feeds. Use of these types of feeds, in horse nutrition, generally leads to some form of digestive upset, and hence should be avoided at all costs.

2. HORSE FEED COMPONENTS

All horse feeds are made up of the following parts:

1. WATER
2. CELLULOSE or FIBRE
3. PROTEIN
4. ENERGY as CARBOHYDRATE
5. ENERGY as VOLATILE FATTY ACIDS
6. ENERGY as FAT
7. MINERALS
8. VITAMINS
9. ELECTROLYTES

Horse feeds are simply various mixtures of one or more of the above components. Long past are the days when we had little idea of what was contained in horse feeds. Technical and scientific advances are such that information is now available of the part that each feed component plays in horse nutrition, and we now also know, based on records of chemical analysis, what individual feed components the various horse feeds contain. If there are no recorded details of the composition, of a particular feed, then modern technology allows such information to be obtained in a very short period of time.

It is now possible to formulate or mix horse feeds so as to supply the individual horse's exact technical daily needs, in relation to age, weight, expected growth rate, pregnancy, lactation and the activity of the horse and the type of work or performance expected of each animal.

It is also possible to look at the cost of horse feeding and to formulate "least cost" feeds. A "LEAST COST" ration is one which is supplying the horse with all the daily nutrient needs, at the lowest cost. With horse feeding costs, increasing all the time and representing a significant part of the weekly cost of maintaining a horse, any reduction in feeding costs, whilst maintaining the same technical standards in the ration has to be of value to a horse feeder.

Horses have colloquially been known as "chaff bandits" or "hay burners" for some period of time. If by a little application of the principles outlined in this book you are able to achieve the same results by using less "hay" or better "hay", then you will get increased performance from your horse, and will, most likely, be financially rewarded for your effort.

The PRINCIPLES OF HORSE FEEDING are very different from those of feeding other animals. Most animals, cattle, sheep, pigs, poultry, etc. when given more food than they require for "normal" maintenance needs, i.e. to keep themselves alive, will use that extra food to produce meat, fat, milk, wool, etc. Horses, however, were never designed by nature to use feed, in excess of maintenance requirements, in the production of meat, milk, fat etc.

Horses were designed, by natural evolution, to use excess feed for exercise, excess feed being held in reserve, within the horse's body, to allow fast and rapid escape from predators, escape being the horse's natural defence mechanism.

If we OVERFEED horses in relation to their actual requirements, especially if the horse has NO WAY in which it can use or BURN UP the excess feed, we generally end up, dependent on the level of overfeeding, with a horse that can be difficult to control or one which actually gets sick from too much feed and not enough exercise.

Modern horse management practices, where we "HARD FEED" horses confined in stables or small yards, without adequate exercise, are CONTRARY to how nature designed the horse to function.

Not only will feeding a horse, in excess of its daily needs, cost more in feed bills, but it can also lead to extra cost in terms of veterinary attention to cure the man-made problem, plus loss of use of an affected horse until the animal has fully recovered from the overfeeding problem.

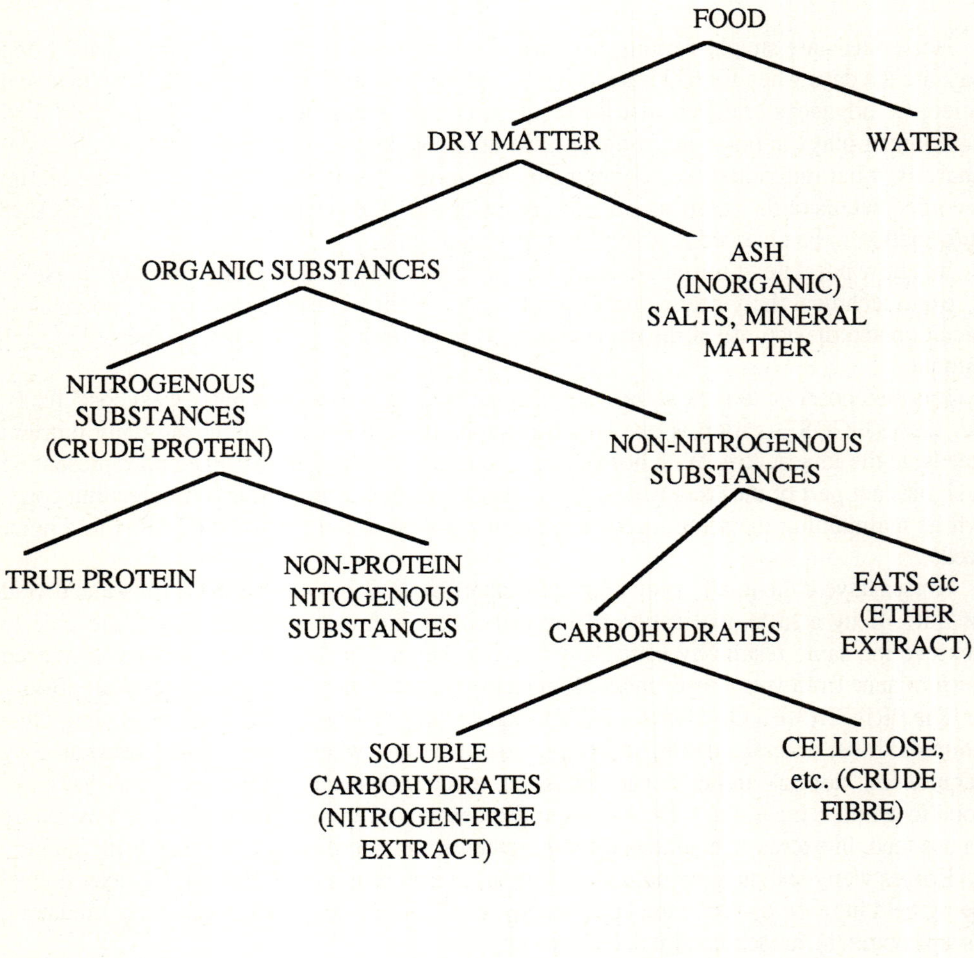

3. WATER AND FAECES

Water is an essential component of horse feeds.

Firstly, WATER is required for plant growth to ensure that vegetative material can be satisfactorily produced for the use of horses to eat.

Secondly WATER is involved with satisfactory operation of ALL the microscopic body cells of the horse by maintaining, in conjunction with ELECTROLYTES, maximum body cell TURGIDITY allowing continual OSMOSIS to take place and thirdly WATER is most important in the digestion of the fibre or cellulose fraction of the feed in the large intestine.

Body cell TURGIDITY is explained, in simple terms, by blowing up a balloon. At some stage, the balloon will become fully stretched eliminating any lines or creases which were previously present in the wall of the balloon. The balloon is now fully turgid. Allow some air to escape from the balloon, and lines and creases will appear in the outer wall, exactly the same as appears in the cell walls, due to a reduction in internal pressure. This creasing of the cell walls reduces overall wall contact and hence reduces the process whereby the individual feed constituents in the blood, pass into the separate microscopic body cells and the waste products of cell function pass out, again to be carried by the blood to the livers and kidneys for excretion, via the urine, out of the horse. OSMOSIS, the movement of nutrients across the cells walls by means of a pressure gradient, will only function effectively if ALL THE WALLS of the individual body cells are in contact with each other. This CONTINUAL CELL WALL contact requires the horse to have access to adequate amounts of WATER, as well as ELECTROLYTES.

Thirdly, horses require WATER for a number of body functions.

1. transfer of nutrients and water products around the body, insufficient water for this purpose causes DEHYDRATION.
2. food digestion.
3. production of sweat to cool the horse.
4. milk production.

REDUCED BODY WATER CONTENT results in REDUCED DRY MATTER INTAKE which, in turn, leads to REDUCED PERFORMANCE.

INCREASED ENERGY NEEDS FROM WORK OR PERFORMANCE INCREASES THE NEED FOR WATER.

An active animal can die of thirst when it has lost about 15% of its body weight, as water. For a normal thoroughbred, about 450 kg (1000 lbs) this means a loss of only 67 kg. or 67 litres (18 gallons) of water in the form of body weight before death may occur.

Water is also a most important component of SWEAT, which is used by the horse as a temperature regulating mechanism, to reduce body temperature, during periods of active exercise. Horses have been known to lose as much as 30 litres or more of sweat, most of which is water, and the balance being electrolytes, in some forms of physical horse activity.

Water is available to the horse mainly from two sources. Firstly the water content on feed and secondly drinking water. Green feed contains varying levels of water, dependent on the stage of growth. Young actively growing pasture may contain up to 85% water and be able to provide the horse with ALL its immediate water needs. Pasture of such high water content may, in fact, need to be supplemented with hay to "BULK UP" and slow down the digesta passage. Average green pasture would have a water content of about 60-65%, whilst dry mature pasture 40% or less. After making allowance for the water content in the feed, the horse will "top up" its water requirements from any available supply of drinking water.

Water intake is directly correlated or determined by the water content of the feed being eaten. Stabled horses, on HARD FEED, will be eating a ration, containing about 12% water. The water intake of such horses will amount to be between 2 and 4 litres/kg DRY MATTER of feed eaten.

Translated to practical terms this should mean that the average thoroughbred should drink or consume between 18 and 50 litres/day (4.75 to 13.2 gallons/day), dependent on activity to maintain optimum water levels in its body.

Water consumption of horses has been shown to rise by about 1% for every 1 degree CENTIGRADE rise in temperature above 15 degrees C. WORK and PERFORMANCE can increase water consumption by up to 300%, due to increased body activity and loss by sweat. Likewise, a high yielding lactating mare may produce the equivalent of 12 litres or more of water/day in the milk.

The performance of a horse can be reduced by a water intake which is only 3-4% below optimum levels, causing PARTIAL DEHYDRATION, probably undetected by the horse person's eye, noticeable only if measuring daily water intake. Such slight but important reductions in daily water intake affect the ability of the body cells in the horse to absorb food components and excrete waste product, by the process known as OSMOSIS. Electrolytes play a vital role in this and the whole matter is discussed in detail in the Chapter on ELECTROLYTES.

Water intake depends on:

1. Whether the horse is still growing, or mature, i.e. over four years of age.
2. Extent and degree of work or exertion, affects sweating
3. Increase or decrease in daily temperature, also affects sweating.
4. Whether peak performance levels and incorrect nutritional composition leads to electrolyte imbalance - this in itself can lead to a reduced water intake below an optimum level. (refer chapter on electrolytes).
5. lactation.

Every time a horse eats, the digestive system secretes large volumes of FLUID, based on water, to activate and complete the digestive process and absorption of the available feed components. Cellulose or fibre digestion, in the large intestine of the horse, requires considerable amounts of water, so as to function correctly. It has been estimated that a 450kg horse is required to absorb some 75-80 litres of fluid/day, from the digestive tract, a volume which is about three times the amount of blood PLASMA in the same horse. By far, the greater percentage of this fluid being absorbed from the large intestine is water, and the absorption of this water, to-gether with the absorption of ELECTROLYTES from the large intestine is vitally bound up with the production of VOLATILE FATTY ACIDS from cellulose breakdown.

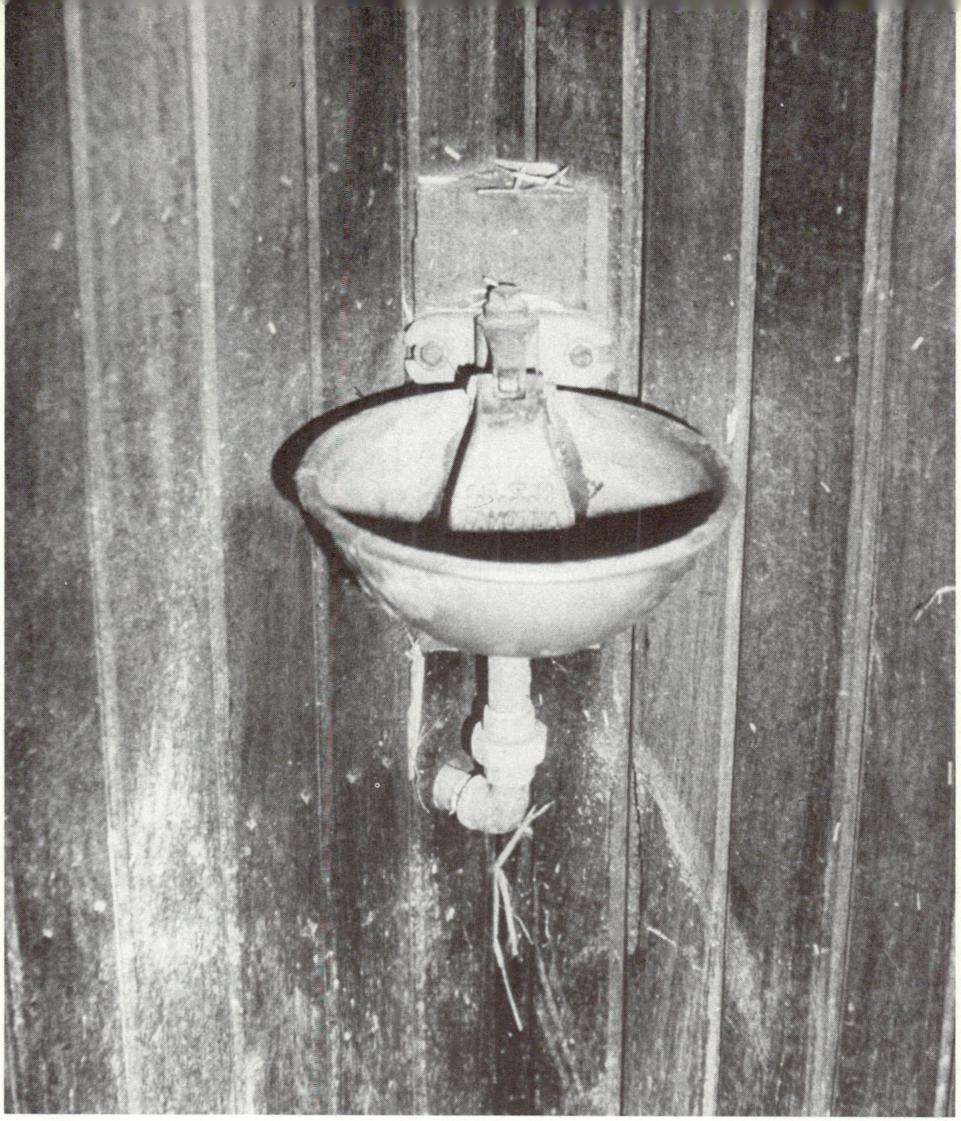

Automatic waterers do not allow accurate measurement of daily water intake.

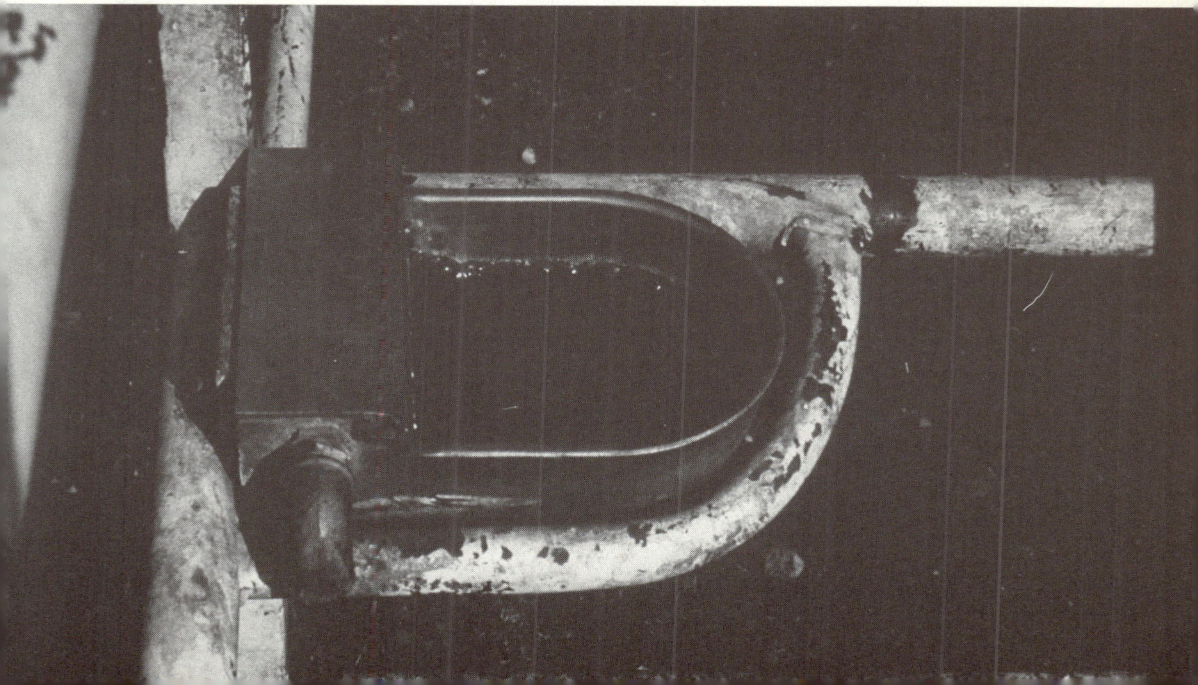

After this digestive process is completed, the rest of the horse's body reclaims this fluid, from within the digestive tract. The volume of fluid which moves in and out of the digestive tract, at and after each feed, can imposes strains on the horses' fluid movement system, to the extent, that if excess fluid remains in the digestive tract after feed absorption has been completed, there is a good chance that the horse will develop DIARRHOEA. If on the other hand, the water balance of the horse is such that too much water is removed from the digestive tract, especially the large intestine after feeding, IMPACTION COLIC can occur.

Horses are able to drink water at a fairly rapid rate, between 500 ml and 1 litre/minute in animals which have not suffered any water restriction beforehand.

By far the greater percentage of horses, when given restricted feeds, as in a stabled situation, will always drink in conjunction with the intake of food and rarely at other times. Part of the reason for this is probably for SALIVA production,as most HARD FEEDS only contain 10-12% moisture.

Studies of the drinking patterns of horses, restricted to stalls but adequately exercised, have shown that WATER DEFICIENCY can occur in a horse from any one of the following:-

1 - physical lack of availability

2 - an increase in sodium concentration within the body

3 - a decrease in blood plasma volume

and that the horse is able to correct for any such deficiency in body water content when given free access to water.

Horses, subject to intensive exercise and hard work, sometimes fail to drink, even when it is obvious from sweat and other fluid loss that the horse requires water. This problem is a function of the ELECTROLYTE loss in the sweat and if the horse is being fed the correct electrolytes for the activity, the problem will no longer exist.

Partial dehydration of racehorses, due to insufficient water intake, has been diagnosed as a major problem in the thoroughbred industry in Australia, and can occur when water loss is only about 2% or slightly more of body weight. Visual examination for PARTIAL DEHYDRATION, including the use of the PINCH TEST can only detect dehydration after about 6% loss has occurred in body weight. There is probably a lot of horses, working and competing at less than optimum performance, due to undetected PARTIAL DEHYDRATION, at levels of less than 6%.

This continuing daily need for water, especially in relation to energy use, is in marked contrast to possible losses of PROTEIN and FAT. The horse can lose all its body FAT and 50% of its body PROTEIN before it will become adversely affected. The loss of less than 6% of body water will, on the other hand affect the horses' performance.

Experienced racehorse and performance horse trainers use a horse water intake on a daily basis as a critical means of assessing just how a horse is "doing".

There are extremely wide daily variations in individual horse's water intakes. The average daily water intake is estimated to be in the range of 2.5 to 4% of body weight. The important point is to ensure that the daily water intake of the individual horse does not vary very much and is reasonably constant.

Horses "off colour" or horses about to show some reduction in performance, or horses getting some type of internal infection or disease, will nearly always reduce their water intake 24 to 36 hours before the horse shows visible signs of a problem.

Watering of horses individually by bucket, whilst it may be labour intensive, and daily recording of the individual horse's water intake will allow the trainer to note when a reduction in water consumption occurs and take immediate measures to clarify the situation. The use of automatic waterers in training stables does NOT presently allow measurement of individual horses' water intake and these trainers are losing the advantage of a very simple and practical way of monitoring individually each horses health.

Some racing stables, which water with buckets, have difficulty in getting thoroughbreds in full training to drink more than 20 litres per day. It would appear that these horses are in a state of mild dehydration and, as such, it is most unlikely that they will perform to the best of their ability. These horses are normally in full training and it is most likely that an electrolyte imbalance, or a specific Vitamin B problem, is occurring. This subject especially as it applies to performance horses will be discussed in more detail in a later part of this book.

Problems can also occur with the taste or palatability of water from various sources. Water taste and quality can vary tremendously, dependent on whether water supply is from town supply, farm dams, bores, running streams or rain water collected in tanks. The addition of fluoride to some water supplies can further complicate the water palatability problem.

For those who travel with horses to various places with differing water supplies, the use of small quantities of one or more of the following, molasses, sugar, vinegar, epsom salts, cinnamon oil and electrolytes in the drinking water, all the time, appears to overcome the water intake problem, resulting from palatability. The amount of any of the above flavouring agents to be used in each bucket of water has to be determined for each individual horse by trial and error, but all have been used successfully in the past. With some water supplies and or some horses, none of these tricks work, so water has to be carried when travelling.

Time of watering a horse can be of considerable importance in some situations. With performance horses, especially endurance and eventing horses, WATER can be provided at any rest point in whatever quantity the horse wishes to drink, PROVIDED THAT HORSE IS TO CONTINUE with the same level of physical exercise after the drink as before. If however, the horse has completed its activity, water, in any quantity, should NOT be provided for at least 45-60 minutes after cessation of that activity. A short sip is sufficient but to let the horse drink to satisfaction is a recipe for disaster, refer CHAPTER on NUTRITIONAL DISORDERS. The Americans described the need NOT TO WATER performance horses, until they have cooled down as "R and R", REST and ROUGHAGE.

FAECES INSPECTION

FAECES, or EXCRETA or MANURE, is the residue of the feed, principally fibre and cellulose, which is unable to be used by the horse for nutritional purposes. FAECES of a healthy horse consists of undigested residues of plant material, predominantly cellulose and lignin, residues of gastric juices, bile, pancreatic secretions etc., debris from the lining of the digestive tract, and products from the micro-organisms present in the large intestine, plus WATER. An average 450 kg thoroughbred on an average diet produces about 13-18 kg (30-40 lbs) faeces/day.

In association with the use of water measurement intake as a means of monitoring horse's health, the astute horse feeder will also take continual note of the consistency of the horses' faeces, despite the obvious human dislike and resistance to such a practice and quickly note any change in either colour, appearance or consistency. Even the slightest changes in the colour and or appearance of the FAECES is indicative of something unusual happening inside the horse, whilst the presence of DIARRHOEA is a definite indication that the horse has problems which need urgent attention.

PRESENCE OF WHOLE GRAIN

1. feeding too much grain for the horses' needs.
2. feeding grain which has not been de-hulled and you are seeing the indigestible grains hulls coming out, this is natural.
3. increasing grain content in the ration too rapidly and not allowing the digestive enzymes and micro-organisms in the digestive tract time to adjust their populations to the changed feed.
4. the horse may not be chewing the grain due to teeth problems.

FAECAL COLOUR

Colour of FAECES will vary in the range of brown to khaki green to a mid green, dependent on the colour of what goes in the mouth,and the colour of the bile, a digestive fluid secreted by the liver. The horse on fresh green feed will have a greener colour to the faeces than the horse on old hay and grain, where the faeces will be a browner colour.

Obvious colour changes include :-

1. darker colours, sometimes even to black, will be expected where grazing legumes provide a reasonable proportion of the feed, requiring extra bile to be produced to digest the extra protein in the legumes.
2. Red and or Black will probably indicate the presence of blood in the faeces.
3. Light green is probably an indication of diarrhoea, caused by microbial infection.
4. Light brown and or yellow is an indication of diarrhoea caused by a nutritional problem.

FAECAL ODOUR

1. SPOILED MEAT smell is from rotting protein, indicating the horse has too much protein in the diet in relation to its daily needs.
2. STALE BISCUIT smell comes from a diet with too much energy, especially carbohydrate, in the ration.
3. ROTTEN PUTREFIED MEAT smell is probably diarrhoea, caused by either bacterial infection and or internal parasites.

FAECAL MOISTURE.

1. LACK OF VISIBLE SHINE indicates some level of DEHYDRATION is present.
2. EXCESS SHINE, especially in the form of strings or drops of excess mucous on the outer surface, caused by some type of internal infection or parasites.
3. VERY LIQUID, actually runs out of the horse, a positive sign of DIARRHOEA.
4. VERY HARD either dehydration or metabolic disturbance which causes the horse to absorb all the water in the feed before the digesta reaches the large intestine.

SAND

Ingestion of SAND is common in some areas, particularly where the horses are grazing very short pasture, growing on sandy soils. Too much sand, in the digestive tract, produces the condition known as SAND COLIC. If the horses' diet contains sufficient water, sand will often be passed in the faeces, with little problem. In other circumstances, up to 20 or so kgs of SAND can accumulate in the large intestine, initially blocking, and eventually rupturing the digestive tract.

Presence of sand in the faeces can be determined by placing some faeces in a jar, covering with water, shaking well and allowing to stand over night. Any noticeable amounts of sand will appear in the bottom of the jar and allowing for normal ingestion of dirt, any excess quantities should provide a warning to change feeding practices and or paddocks.

INTERNAL PARASITES.

FAECAL INSPECTION is not a very reliable method of assessing the internal parasite burden of your horse, even about 48 hours after the administration of an anthelmintic.

One of the important points in internal parasite control is:-

THE SMALLER THE WORM THE MORE DANGEROUS IT IS TO THE HORSE.

As a result, the small microscopic immature forms of worms, some of which can do tremendous damage, to the horse are invisible to the naked eye. Secondly, unless you happen to look at FAECES, immediately after passing from the horse, those worms on the outside of the faeces will dehydrate and disappear rapidly, and those inside the faeces will also disappear as the manure dries out.

There are some exceptions to this general rule. BOTS take some time to desiccate and dry out, TAPEWORMS readily seen are not considered very dangerous to the horse and the LARGE ROUNDWORM, some 150-200mm (6-8 inches) long which can cause problems in foals, by completely blocking the digestive tract,will remain visible for a couple of days after passing out in the faeces.

Whilst FAECES INSPECTION may be difficult with horses that gain access to pasture for most or all of their time, simply because if two or more horses graze together, how do you know which horse produced what faeces, it is relatively easy for faeces observation to take place in stabled situations. As these are the places where horse training and feeding costs are the greatest, any change in faeces colour and or texture as well as consistency can be used, in conjunction with water intake, as a diagnostic tool to allow early notification of impending problems.

To carefully assess the horses' faeces consistency and also the horses'urinary output, astute trainers in fully stabled situations always use straw as a stable bedding. Whilst straw may be initially more expensive than shavings and other bedding materials, the practical facts are that faeces and urine affected straw can be visually assessed by virtually untrained staff during daily stable cleaning routines and any change in output noted, giving the trainer an early warning sign as to the horse's health.

Some trainers have their stablehands note daily, in a shorthand system, on blackboards, strategically placed at the front of each the stable, each horse's faecal texture and colour, as well as urinary output, in relation to the amount of straw removed and/or replaced each day.

Unfortunately shavings and other similar materials tend to absorb urine, in particular, and generally cannot be removed as one intact piece of contaminated bedding at a time. This makes for inaccurate and difficult measurement of urine and faecal output by most stable staff.

Performance horse trainers not using straw as a bedding material for stabled horses are missing a valuable aid in monitoring horses' health.

FAECES EATING

COPROPHAGY is the name given to the habit of some animals to eat the faeces of other animals of the same species. Whilst some people may find this practice offensive, it is a common occurrence amongst foals but rarely observed amongst older horses.

One very detailed study revealed that the practice of FAECES EATING or COPROPHAGY was very common amongst foals from one week to nineteen weeks of age, with the greatest frequency occurring in the first 8 weeks.

The foals tended to eat the faeces of their mothers, but, in some instances, were observed eating their own faeces, those of the stallion or those of another mare.

The fact that most of the faeces ingested by foals are from its mother has led to the suggestion that PHEROMONES, specific horse smells and or odours, signal to the foal,the presence in the faeces of certain acids which the foal may need to assist in the functioning of the immunological defence mechanism, which protects the foal against disease. COPROPHAGY has also been suggested as being desirable to increase growth and sexual development within the foal, to provide some feed nutrients,and to allow introduction of the cellulose digesting bacteria to the large intestine.

SALIVA

Saliva production is an important part of feed utilisation by the horse.

Saliva has three functions:

1. to moisten the food, making it slippery to help swallowing
2. starts the digestive process as saliva contains a low level of enzyme which starts the breakdown of the cellulose in the feed, allowing absorption of food components to commence in the horse's stomach.
3. it corrects the food to a neutral or slightly alkaline value, known as pH, so that the feed can be absorbed more readily further down the digestive tract,in the small and large intestines.

Fit horses produce up to 30 litres (7 gallons) of SALIVA per day, dependent on the weight of the horse, the type of work being undertaken and whether the feed is all young pasture with a high water content, or consists of grains, chaff etc. with about one quarter the water content of young actively growing pasture.

4. FIBRE

FIBRE, also known as CELLULOSE, is the outer cell wall covering and binding material that keeps plant cells intact. All plant material, green feed, hays, grains and products derived from plant cells such as bran, pollard, oil meals etc, all contain cellulose of various forms.

Cellulose, or fibre, consists of a group of related compounds which are somewhat similar to starch (carbohydrate or energy), but which are generally resistant to breakdown in the animals' digestive tract, unless acted upon by micro-organisms as in the rumen of the cow, or by digestive enzymes, as in the saliva and stomach of the horse, and micro-organisms in the large intestine of the horse.

The CELLULOSE content of the plant CHANGES as the plant grows and matures.

Young actively growing plants are lush and very soft. Grasses, in particular, in the early stages of growth, tend to fall over and are unable to maintain an upright stance. These plants generally have individual plant cell walls of HEMI-CELLULOSE, which is too soft to allow the plant cells to build one on top of each other, as in bricks in a wall. HEMI-CELLULOSE is digested with comparative ease by horses, sometimes too readily leading to "feed scours". Horses on this type of pasture may even have to be supplementary fed with hay, simply to slow down the rate of feed breakdown and passage through the digestive tract.

As a plant continues to grow, it normally increases in height with the HEMI-CELLULOSE changing to CELLULOSE.

This is a basic plant growth process as the increase in the cellulose content allows the plants to stand erect. Cellulose allows the individual plant cells to sit one on top of each other, as with the brick wall, and allows the plant to gain in height. If hemi-cellulose did not change to cellulose, the plants would most likely fall over and reduced plant growth and production would occur as the effect of sunlight on total plant growth would be reduced, due to a shading effect of some plant tissue lying on top of other plant tissue.

At the end of the growing season for each plant species when the plant matures and sets seed or grain, CELLULOSE in the stem, in particular, turns to LIGNIN. LIGNIN is much stronger than cellulose and therefore much thicker, because the stem is being asked to support a somewhat heavy seed head for a sufficient length of time, so that the seed may mature allowing the plant to reproduce itself in the next season. Whilst LIGNIN is stronger than CELLULOSE, it is also LESS digestible in the horse, and, as such, any energy reserves in the lignin may not be available to the horse for nutritional purposes.

Plants of the LEGUME family, namely clovers, lucerne (alfalfa) and medics DO NOT contain as high a lignin content as do plants of the GRASS family and this is one of the reasons why lucerne, a member of the legume family, is so preferred as a horse feed.

The effect of CELLULOSE and its related compounds on horse nutrition are important in two ways:

A. the younger and more actively growing the feed, the more digestible is the cellulose compounds. As feeds mature, increase in cellulose levels and later lignin levels lead to less utilization of the total feed by the animal.

B. The cow with its four stomachs is able, by the fermentation process, to break down cellulose to readily assimilated food nutrients which can be absorbed further down the digestive tract.

Whilst the enzymes contained in the SALIVA and secretions from the stomach cause the plant cells to separate and allow partial breakdown of the CELLULOSE in the initial parts of the digestive tract of the horse, by far the greater proportion of CELLULOSE breakdown and utilisation in the horse DOES NOT occur until the feed reaches the large intestine and its allied organ, the caecum.

CELLULOSE OR FIBRE BREAKDOWN

CELLULOSE has to be ruptured and broken down, inside the digestive tract of the horse, so as to allow release, from within each individual plant cell of all available feed components, PROTEIN, ENERGY, VITAMIN, MINERALS and ELECTROLYTES. If cellulose breakdown DID NOT OCCUR within the stomach and small intestine of the horse, NONE of the feed components present in the plant cells would be available to the horse, other than ELECTROLYTES, most of which are bound within the cell walls and ENERGY in the form of VOLATILE FATTY ACIDS, both of which are produced by bacterial action on the cellulose in the large intestine.

Practically, CELLULOSE breakdown by horses, within the digestive tract, depends on the type of feed being eaten and water intake of the horse.

GRAZING

When horses derive all their nutrient requirements from pasture, grazing management should attempt, as far as possible, to ensure that the pasture being grazed is in the active growth stage and standing upright. This is the stage of plant growth where all the outer plant cell material is CELLULOSE. Under normal seasonal conditions, this CELLULOSE phase of plant growth will occupy the greatest part of the life of the growing plant.

If the pasture has to be grazed when the plants are young, succulent and fresh, most of the outer plant cell walls will be HEMI-CELLULOSE, extremely digestible and will probably pass through the horse much faster than normal and some of the food components will be lost in faeces as the digestive tract will not have enough time to extract these components during the digesta passage. It may well be desirable, in this situation, to feed hay on a freely available, supplementary basis so as to slow down the rate of digesta passage. This period of plant growth will be very short in terms of the life of the plant and will always occur at the start of the growing period.

Once flowering and seeding commences, LIGNIN production commences, with grasses always containing higher LIGNIN levels than legumes. If the pasture species composition is mixed with both grasses and legumes present, the reduced amount of LIGNIN in the legumes will counter balance the larger quantities in the grasses and will be adequate for most horse not doing much work. If the pasture composition is grass only, then the level of LIGNIN will probably be sufficient to have an effect on nutrient utilisation.

HAY AND CHAFF

Feed only good quality hay of chaff, preferably made before the plant has come into flower and certainly made before the plant has set seed or produced grain. This will ensure a hay or chaff with little or nil lignin content, as the plant has not had to support a seed head. The practice of feeding oaten or wheaten hay or chaff, made when the seed is in the "DOUGH" stage or later, will involve feeding large quantities of LIGNIN to the horse with a consequent adverse effect on overall nutrient utilisation and subsequently horse performance.

GRAINS

1. DEHULLED GRAIN

This is not a very common term in horse feeding but simply means that the HULL or outer covering of the grain, especially OATS and BARLEY, has been removed before sale of whole grain as feed. DEHULLED GRAIN normally is not physically modified in any other way

2. FEEDING WHOLE GRAIN

Feeding whole grain to horses can be quite effective, if the horse does not have to continually perform at medium to high levels of activity. Some people become very concerned for their horse, when what appears to be whole grain appears in the faeces.

If feeding whole grain to a horse, attention to the following points will be of help.

A - Remember that the CELLULOSE is predominantly broken down by the micro-organisms which inhabit the large intestine. There are numerous types of these micro-organisms, some of which break down CELLULOSE and some which do not. If the horse has been on a low CELLULOSE diet, BEFORE introduction of whole grain, such as lush green pasture, the number and level of activity of the CELLULOSE acting micro-organisms will be low. Immediate introduction of the whole grain into the horses' diet will stimulate an increase in the number of these CELLULOSE destroying micro-organisms, but not overnight. It will take at least 3 weeks, after changes in feeds, for any noticeable change to occur in micro-organism numbers.

B - On this basis alone, one can expect some whole grain to be passed by the horse for about three weeks after commencement of feeding, individual horse variations excepted.

C - The initial weights of whole grain fed, and rate of weekly or monthly increase, can have a significant impact on rate of excretion of whole grain. If whole grain feeding is started at about 1KG/day (450kg horse) and increased at the rate of about 0.5 kgs/day on a weekly basis until the desired amount is reached, then, with all but the unusual horse, no problems should occur. Feed at a higher initial rate or increase at a faster rate and whole grain will probably appear in the faeces while ever the MICRO-ORGANISMS in the large intestine are trying to increase in numbers to handle the increased whole grain being fed.

D -Some people mistake the presence of seed hulls from the grain in the faeces as being whole grain. The seed hulls, or outer protective covering of each individual grain, are most indigestible and are always removed in any process which physically alters the grain. Some samples of feed grains however are direct from the farm and will have the hulls still attached, when purchased for feeding.

3. CLIPPING GRAIN

Both oats and barley have an extension on the top of the grain, known as an AWN. This spike like projection is all CELLULOSE, desirable for the growth of the plant but unnecessary for feeding horses. CLIPPING involves physically removing these awns or long projections from the tip of the oat of barley grain. Removal of the AWN will reduce the cellulose intake of the grain component of the ration by about 10%, but WILL NOT increase the decomposition of the remaining cellulose within the horse's digestive tract.

4. BOILING GRAINS

Physically adding water to and boiling grains, before feeding, splits the outer grain coat, which contains cellulose and possibly lignin, and releases what is left of the more digestible starches and related carbohydrates to be assimilated in the stomach and small intestine. The other effect of BOILING GRAINS is to partially or completely destroy some of the feed constituents, especially the vitamins present as well as cause a down grading of the energy component of the white interior of the grain, known as the ENDOSPERM. In human nutrition, no one eats boiled flour. Wheat flour is very similar to the endosperm of oats, barley etc. and boiling of those grains will have the same destructive effect as boiling flour. As well, boiling grain takes time, the resultant feeds are not easy to handle and, in summer weather, is an excellent attraction for flies.

5. SOAKING GRAINS

Instead of adding water to grain and boiling the combined mixture of grain and water, SOAKING GRAIN is sometimes practiced. SOAKING can be done in either of two ways.

A - The addition of boiling water to the grain a short time before feeding WILL soften the outer CELLULOSE coat of the grains, without exposing the contents of the ENDOSPERM to possible oxidation by exposure to the air. Simply cover the required amount of grain with boiling water about 0.5 to 1 hour before feeding, and add to the ration when cool. This approach to assisting CELLULOSE breakdown inside the horse is much more preferable to BOILING GRAINS and also takes a lot less time and effort.

B - cover the grain with cold water and allow to soak for 12 to 24 hours. This softens the grain which swells by taking up water, and the wet product is sometimes ROLLED before feeding.

Research trials show that SOAKING GRAIN does not provide any marked improvement in digestion when compared to other methods of CELLULOSE treatment.

6. CRACKING GRAIN

This practice involves physically breaking the outer coating of the grain, consisting mainly of the cellulose type compounds to produce small pieces of broken grain with exposed endosperm. This broken grain will enable the horse to digest the more soluble carbohydrates at the start of the digestive tract. Cracked grain, exposed to the air for any length of time before feeding, will suffer breakdown of some food components in the ENDOSPERM or white internal "flour" due to oxidation. If cracked grain is a preferred feed, it should be cracked and stored on a daily basis and not purchased in large bags and stored for any length of time before use.

DIAGRAMS ILLUSTRATING VARIOUS METHODS OF PREPARING GRAINS FOR HORSE FEEDING.

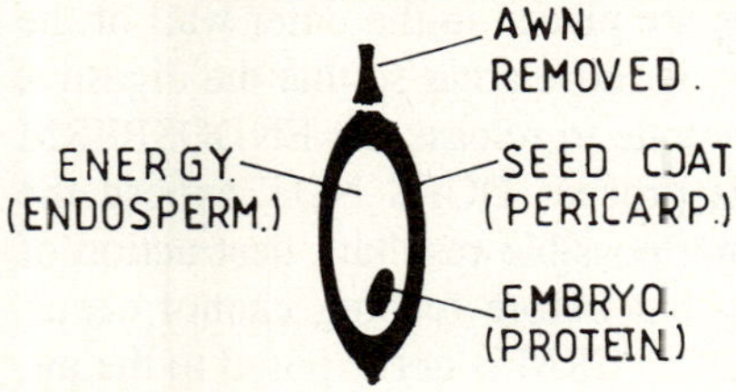

CLIPPED OATS OR BARLEY AWN ONLY REMOVED—INCREASES AVAILABLE ENERGY IN GRAIN BY 8—10% BY REMOVAL OF CELLULOSE IN AWN.

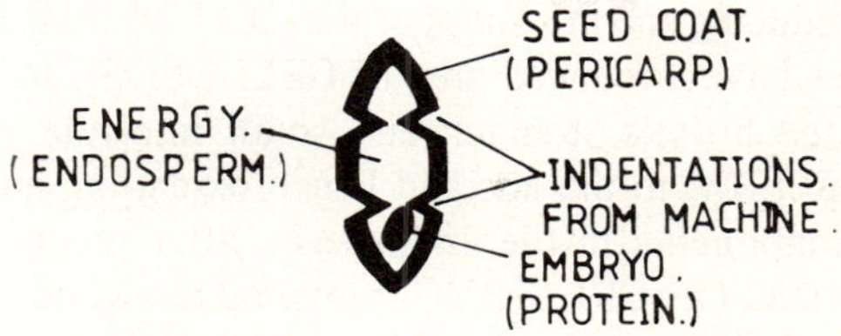

CRUSHED OR CRIMPED—DEPRESSIONS MADE IN SEED COAT—ALLOW DIGESTIVE JUICES TO PENETRATE EASIER—NO LOSS OF NUTRIENTS DUE TO OXIDATION.

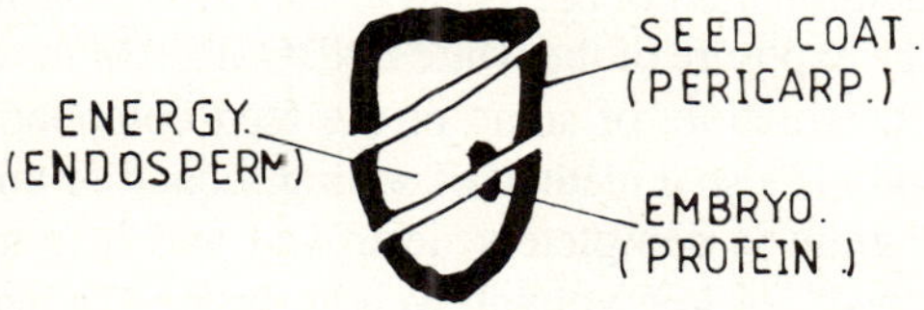

CRACKED CORN—BREAKS SEED COAT—MAKES ENDOSPERM MORE READILY AVAILABLE TO DIGESTIVE JUICES—BUT ALSO LOSS OF NUTRIENTS CAN OCCUR AS OXYGEN (AIR) CAN REACH ENDOSPERM.

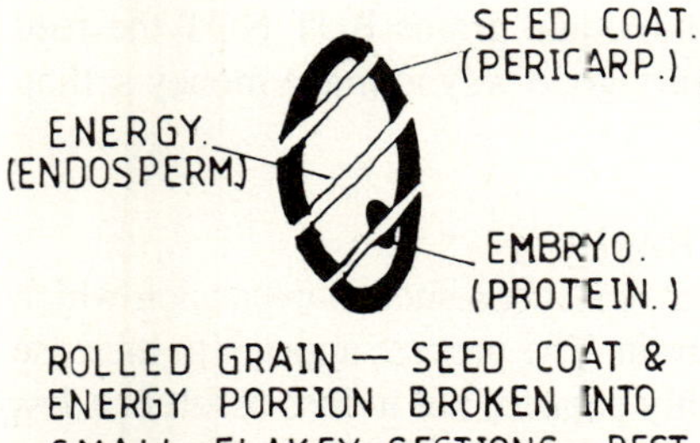

ROLLED GRAIN—SEED COAT & ENERGY PORTION BROKEN INTO SMALL FLAKEY SECTIONS—BEST FOR DIGESTION BUT MUST BE DONE DAILY OTHERWISE EXPOSURE OF ENDOSPERM TO AIR WILL CAUSE LOSS (OXIDATION) OF FOOD NUTRIENTS.

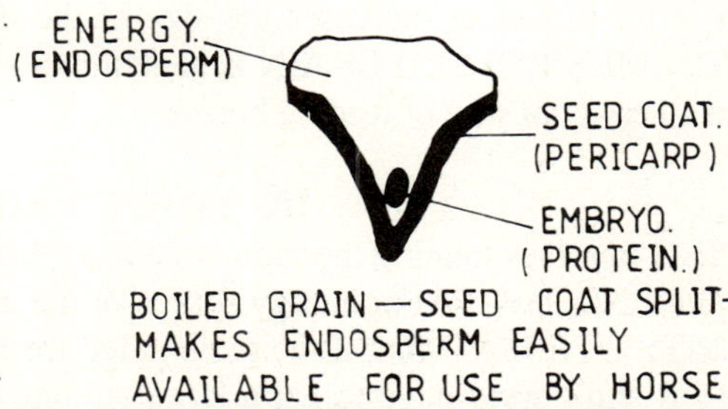

BOILED GRAIN—SEED COAT SPLIT—MAKES ENDOSPERM EASILY AVAILABLE FOR USE BY HORSE. BUT BEWARE! BOILING MAY DESTROY OTHER FOOD NUTRIENTS IN THE GRAIN.

7. CRIMPING or CRUSHED GRAIN

This procedure involves passing the grain, especially oats and barley, through a roller mill, carefully adjusted so that indentations or grooves are placed in the outer wall of the grain, reducing the thickness of the CELLULOSE layer in those areas so that the digestive enzymes have a reduced area of CELLULOSE to penetrate to release the ENDOSPERM inside the horse's stomach and small intestine. This process DOES NOT expose the ENDOSPERM to the air, and hence oxidation, and any possible resultant destruction of food components in the endosperm, after processing but before feeding cannot occur. CRIMPING OR CRUSHING, provided the white ENDOSPERM is not exposed to the air, is the preferred method of making CELLULOSE more readily digested by the horse.

8. ROLLED GRAIN

This occurs when the outer shell of the grain is actually broken. The remaining grain has a "flattened" appearance and the white ENDOSPERM is exposed and very noticeable. ROLLING is generally carried out in the same machine which CRUSHES or CRIMPS, the difference being, that to ROLL the grain, the machine is set with the rollers much closer to-gether. It is quite possible for an inefficient operator to produce ROLLED rather than CRUSHED grain because attention has not been paid to the correct machine settings for the particular sample of grain. The exposure of the white ENDOSPERM in rolled grain can lead to oxidation, and therefore destruction, of some of the feed components in the exposed endosperm. ROLLING of grain is also a method of selling second or third grade grain, the physical appearance of the grain is completely destroyed and it is not possible to tell whether the grain was "pinched", of low volume weight, hence low endosperm and high cellulose content and therefore of considerably reduced value for horse feeding.

9. STEAMED AND ROLLED GRAIN

This process was originally devised to kill any possible weed seeds which may be present in the grain. In this process, the grain is initially passed through steam, for about 3 to 5 minutes, taking up water and then rolled. The product is usually sold on the basis that the steaming of the grain will improve digestibility. The process is generally used on very poor quality grain, normally oats and barley, grain which is so "pinched, having low volume weight and hence low energy content that it could not be sold as whole grain. The addition of steam, prior to rolling,increases the size of the individual grains BUT NOT the feed value. STEAMED ROLLED GRAIN is generally a very good way to make money selling water and a very poor way of feeding horses.

10. POPPED GRAIN

POPPING involves treating the grain with a dry heat, causing a sudden expansion which ruptures the ENDOSPERM or energy source of the grain. The process appears to increase the ENERGY UTILISATION, if the grain is fed freshly popped, but it does result in a low density feed and horses have to eat a large volume of POPPED GRAIN to get any feed value. For this reason, of low volume weights, POPPED GRAIN is sometimes rolled to increase volume weight.

11. MICRONIZED GRAIN

Very similar to POPPED GRAIN, except the source of the heat is from INFRA-RED energy.

12. PUFFED PELLETS

The production methods used to produce PUFFED PELLETS are very similar to that used to produce POPPED GRAIN. PUFFED PELLETS, whilst not necessarily being used to increase the digestibility of CELLULOSE in the ration, does allow the incorporation into the ration of less digestible sources of cellulose or fibre. PUFFED PELLETS are made by extruding the already pelleted feed with steam under pressure which expands the feed to about twice the normal volume by producing air pockets inside. The practice of "PUFFING" or expanding feed volume has been used for some considerable time in the human and dog food industries and the feeding of PUFFED PELLETS to horses is one way of slowing down the rate of feed intake of fast eaters and reducing the possible occurrence of colic and other potential problems.

Whilst technically, the above techniques are theoretically desirable to allow the horse to utilise food components more efficiently by enabling faster breakdown of CELLULOSE and or by reducing the amount of cellulose in the diet, it should be noted that these techniques are really only applicable to horses which are in continual work or training. These horses are the ones who generally have a problem in getting enough food nutrients into their digestive tract, especially energy, to replace the food nutrients used in work. The average horse, doing little exercise or work does not require feeds physically treated, as above, to assist CELLULOSE breakdown.

Feeding of excess energy to horses which are not in training or working hard, generally leads to digestive upsets and problems such as founder, tying up, colic etc. It is most inadvisable for feeding of horses. with low work loads, to look at boiling grain, cracking or crimping or rolling or any of the other techniques, as not only does the grain generally cost more but it may also cost more in veterinary fees and lost horse use if the grain or energy component is not worked out of the horse on a regular basis.

5. PROTEIN

PROTEIN is responsible for the formation, growth and maintenance of ALL BODY TISSUES and makes up about 22% of the FAT FREE components of the mature horse and about 80% of the horse if the fat and the water contents are not considered. Protein must be present in adequate and correct proportions in all horse diets, otherwise all the different body tissues WILL NOT form, grow or be maintained at optimum rates, BONE, for instance, contains 20% PROTEIN. In addition, Protein level in the ration controls the use of all the other food components and too little or too much protein in the feed can have quite dramatic effects on the horse.

PROTEINS present in the feed as AMINO ACIDS are absorbed by the horse in the small intestine, and in addition, a small amount of protein production will take place in the large intestine as a result of the decomposition of cellulose or fibre.

PROTEINS consist of twenty four AMINO ACIDS. These are complex substances, based on Nitrogen, and generally have Sulphur as the next major component. Horses are able to make most of the AMINO ACIDS from the other feed components, within their digestive tract, and in terms of present knowledge, there are 10 AMINO ACIDS which cannot be made in the digestive tract and therefore are required to be supplied to the horse in the feed.

These 10 ESSENTIAL AMINO ACIDS are:

ARGININE	LYSINE	METHIONINE,
TRYPTOPHAN	HISTIDINE	ISOLEUCINE,
LEUCINE	PHENYLALANINE	THREONINE,
	VALINE.	

METHIONINE can be partially replaced in the diet by CYSTINE, a non essential amino acid, and PHENYLALANINE by TYROSINE, another non essential amino acid. Both CYSTINE and TYROSINE are present in most horse feeds.

PROTEIN QUALITY, that is, the presence in the protein component of the ration of the 10 essential amino-acids, is important in feeding horses. High quality proteins, sometimes described as containing the FULL AMINO ACID PROFILE, for horse feeding are recognised as containing the ten essential amino acids detailed above.

Such high quality protein is generally found only in feeds of animal origin - e.g. fish meal, skim milk, meat meal etc. or in good MIXED PASTURE with some form of legume component, and hays made from such pastures, and in SOYBEAN MEAL and CANOLA MEAL.

All other common horse feeds are generally LACKING in one or more of the ten essential AMINO ACIDS and hence are not balanced from the horses' requirements.

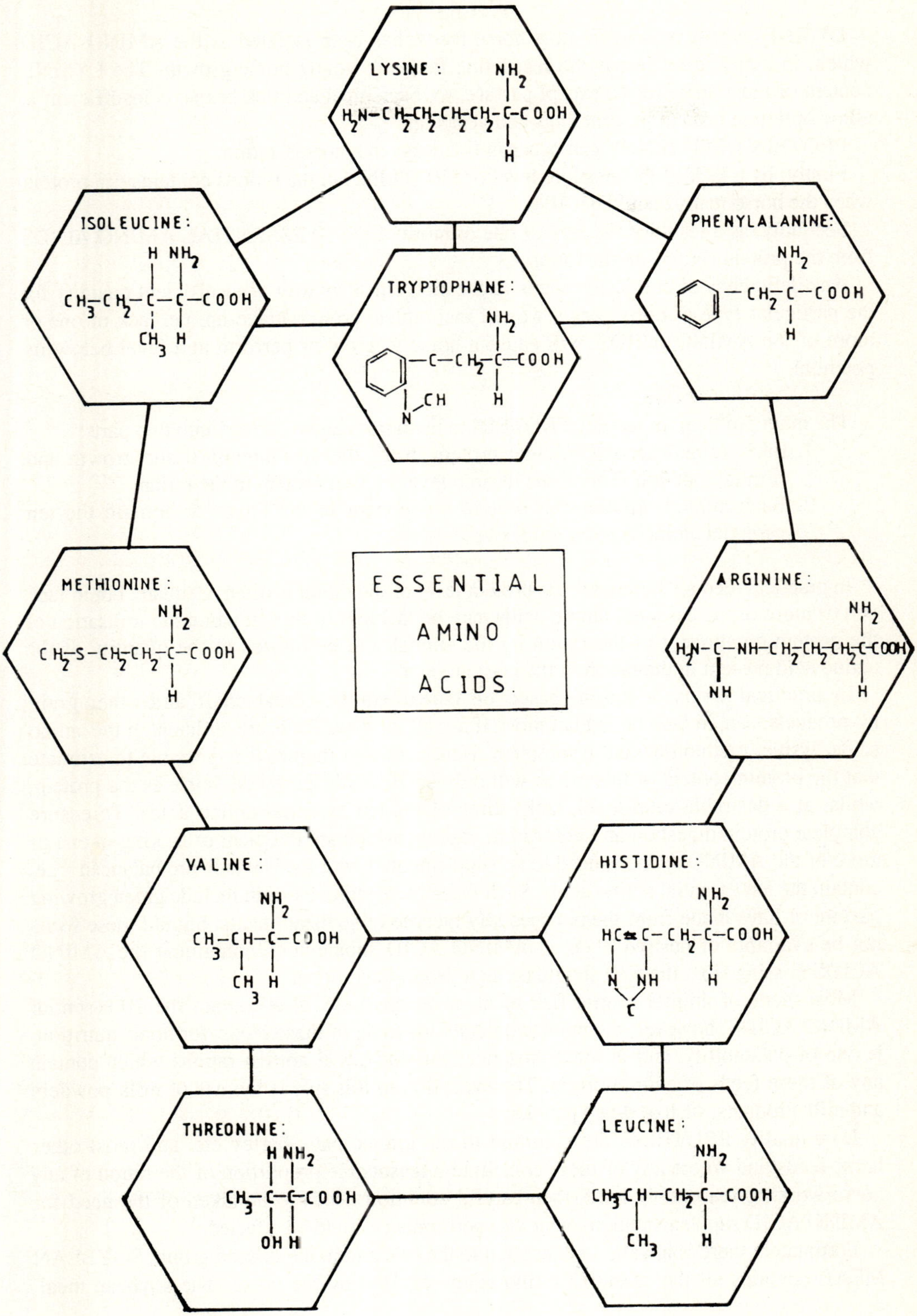
ESSENTIAL AMINO ACIDS.
LYSINE :
ISOLEUCINE :
PHENYLALANINE :
TRYPTOPHANE :
METHIONINE :
ARGININE :
VALINE :
HISTIDINE :
THREONINE :
LEUCINE :

LYSINE, whilst present in most horse feeds, has been isolated as the AMINO-ACID which, in many instances, is the restricting factor in young horse growth. The LYSINE content of most horse feeds, except pasture, soybean meal and tick beans, is insufficient to allow optimum growth in weanlings and yearlings.

PROTEIN DEFICIENCY can occur in two ways in a horses' ration.

Firstly, by a lack of the absolute level of PROTEIN, i.e. the rations contains 6% protein when the horse really should get 10%.

Secondly, as a result of the lack of one or more of the 10 ESSENTIAL AMINO ACIDS from the protein sources in the ration.

Any deficiency of complete protein in the diet, either by way of insufficient quantity for the particular type of horse, or by way of incomplete protein make-up, i.e. lack of one or more of the AMINO ACIDS, will cause a horse to grow or perform at a level below its potential.

The main problem, in feeding PROTEIN to the horse can be divided into two parts:

1. Each animal needs sufficient protein in the diet to maintain tissue growth and normal function. This is the desired level of total protein in the ration.
2. Each animal requires the protein component in the ration to contain the ten essential amino-acids listed above.

In practical feeding situations, the protein level of the ration is often adequate, but in fact, one or more of the essential amino acids may be lacking. In this situation the utilisation of the protein component of the ration by the animal will be limited to the quantity of the amino acid present in the ration in the least amount.

In practical terms, a ration, based on cereal grains, cereal chaff and other grain by-products, can, in fact, be fed but most, if not all, of these feeds are deficient in the amino acids, lysine, methionine and tryptophan. Hence, rule of thumb, it is possible to estimate that the protein content of this ration will only be 70% utilised by the horse as the protein, whilst at a desirable total level, lacks three of the ten essential amino acids. To ensure complete protein digestion and absorption, rations, which are deficient or lacking in one or more of the AMINO ACIDS, need to be supplemented with feeds which are balanced - i.e. contain the ten essential amino acids. Such feeds of vegetative origin include green growing pasture or hays made from them, especially lucerne or soybean meals. Should these feeds not be available or desired, then an AMINO ACID supplement, containing the AMINO ACIDS missing from the feed should be included in the rations.

Most feeds of animal origin, fish meal, meat meal etc. also contain the 10 essential AMINO ACIDS, however, the main problem with some of these feeds, for horse nutrition, is one of palatability, and in many instances the horse will not eat rations which contain any of these feeds of animal origin. The exception to this rule is the use of milk powders and milk products, such as whey powder.

Low quality PROTEINS are common in the grains, oats, barley etc. and most other horse feeds and where any of these constitute a reasonable proportion of the ration of any horse working reasonably hard, then careful attention needs to be taken of the need for AMINO ACID supplementation, otherwise performance could be affected.

Fortunately there is always an exception to the rule and in the oilseed group, SOYBEAN MEAL contains all the essential amino acids required by the horse. The soybean meal, however, must be made by the extruded process as this destroys the anti-nutritional factors present in the raw soybean.

PROTEIN PRODUCTION IN THE LARGE INTESTINE

Some protein is produced within the large intestine and caecum of the horse by action of the micro-organisms on the cellulose residue which produce not only VOLATILE FATTY ACIDS but also PROTEIN. The amount of protein produced has been determined at about 12% only of the NET supply of PROTEIN to the horse, an amount which has little effect on both the required ration protein levels and correct amino-acid balance.

The addition of small amounts of live YEAST to the diet of horses has produced up to 10% more NITROGEN retention in the horse on the same ration, as compared to horses without added yeast. The added yeast appears to increase and or activate the microbial population of the large intestine and increases the ability to extract nitrogen from within the cellulose or fibre of the cell walls.

NON PROTEIN NITROGEN

NON PROTEIN NITROGEN, sometimes know as artificial NITROGEN, specifically in the form of UREA, MAY be used as a PROTEIN source in the horse, to replace some of the natural protein in the feed. Horses have been fed up to 50% of their expected protein requirements, as UREA, with no adverse effects. PROTEIN, which can be assimilated, and used by the horse, is produced by the action of the UREA with the fibre or cellulose content of the ration, within the large intestine. For this to be effective, highly fermentable dietary fibre is essential, in other words feed, with a cellulose content, which is soft, good quality grazing and or hay and certainly with no seed present. The chances of killing the horse from UREA POISONING is however very high UNLESS THE UREA is thoroughly and completely mixed in the horse rations. This thorough mixing of urea, depends solely on operator competence and this is often difficult to achieve in commercial feed mixing operations. It is too late when the horse has died of UREA poisoning, which can be fast and silent.

PROTEIN REQUIREMENTS FOR MAINTENANCE

PROTEIN is continually required to keep the body systems of the horse operating, even when the horse is resting and at a constant body weight.

PROTEIN REQUIREMENTS FOR GROWTH

Adequate PROTEIN levels in the daily ration are essential for growth. If there is any deficiency of the PROTEIN levels, or in young horses, under 4 years of age, any lack of any of the essential AMINO ACIDS, growth will be restricted, no matter what the levels of the other feeds components are in the ration. Protein requirements for growth are some 15% higher than protein requirements for maintenance.

PROTEIN REQUIREMENTS FOR WORK

Work or exercise as experienced in competition causes increased demands on the protein requirements of the horse. However these demands have not been carefully evaluated, possibly because of the many different types of exercise and work which various horses perform.

It is known, from enzyme level changes obtained from blood test results, that muscle damage does occur in some horses during exercise and PROTEIN would be required to allow those damaged muscles to repair themselves. Nitrogen is also lost through sweat and this nitrogen has to be provided by PROTEIN breakdown.

The extra PROTEIN requirements of work or exercise are satisfied by the extra DRY MATTER which the horse normally consumes as opposed to the DRY MATTER intake at rest and not by any large increase in the actual percentage protein, in the ration.

PROTEIN REQUIREMENTS FOR PREGNANCY

In the first 8 months of pregnancy, the PROTEIN requirements of the mare are similar to that of the adult dry horses. In the last three months of pregnancy, when foetal size increases considerably, PROTEIN requirements of the pregnant mare rise some 33%, to supply the extra protein needs of the rapidly growing foetus.

PROTEIN REQUIREMENTS FOR LACTATION

The PROTEIN content of milk is at its highest level immediately after birth and then slowly decreases as lactation progresses. In addition the amount of PROTEIN available to the lactating mare also determines the amount of milk produced.

In terms of ration level, PROTEIN values for lactating mares should be about 50-60% higher than for the same mare when dry.

PROTEIN DEFICIENCY

It is very difficult for most people to diagnose a protein deficiency in horses. Symptoms include decreased growth and development in young horses and in mature animals, reduced food intake, body tissue loss, poor hair coat, and reduced hoof growth. In common with most nutritional disorders, protein deficiency can be complicated by simple things like worm infestations, external skin conditions such as lice etc., bacterial and viral infections, and possible deficiencies of other nutritional components.

If any one, or all, of the above problems do not exist, a protein deficiency will cause decreased food intake, rough hair coat, REDUCED growth and performance. From a management angle, this will probably be observed by the practical horse feeder as an initial reduction in appetite, to be followed later by an observed reduction in expected growth and performance.

In pregnant mares, about 66% of the total products of conception, foetus plus associated tissues and fluids, are material with a very high content of protein and 20% of the body weight of the foal, at birth is protein. Mare's milk also contains, on average, a protein level of about 3.1%.

A decrease in milk production will occur in lactating mares, even to the stage where mares will dry up, ceasing to produce milk to feed their foal, and hence affecting foal growth, in order to conserve the remaining body protein reserves to allow the survival of the mare. Mature horses will lose weight, and stallions and mares, at mating, could well have reduced fertility levels to the extent that conception may not be possible. However once the possible protein problem has been evaluated, correction could be either late in the breeding season when conception may take place, leading to a late foal or alternatively the mating

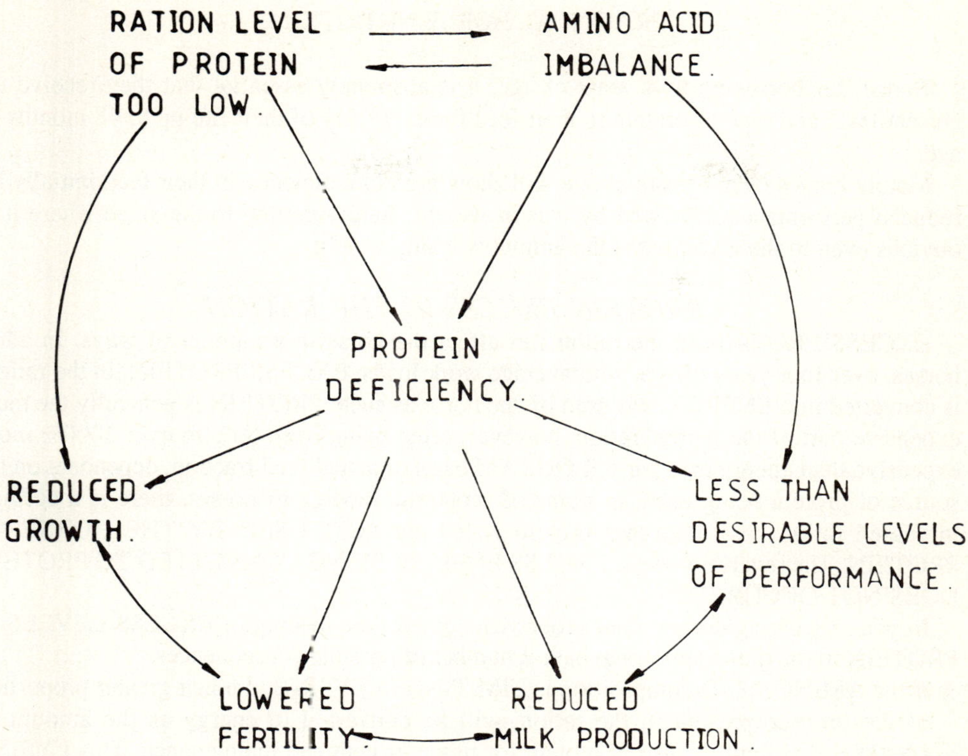

RATION PROTEIN PROBLEMS.

Protein deficiency SYMPTOMS are not easy to diagnose and or correct, and if a cure or correction of the problem is possible, there is often long lasting and PERMANENT adverse effects from a period of reduced protein intake.

REDUCED GROWTH cannot be completely corrected. It is not possible to increase ration PROTEIN levels above normal levels, after a period of reduced protein intake, and expect the horse to fully recover. GROWTH of a young horse, to 4 years of age, is a continuous process and it is not possible to turn the clock back to correct a problem which occurred in the past. Once the horse has reached 4 years of age, it is possible for some form of PROTEIN compensation feeding to take place, but at this stage the horse has a fully developed skeleton and is fully grown, and the PROTEIN in the ration is only needed for TISSUE MAINTENANCE and REPAIR.

Hence, for horses up to 4 years of age, it is absolutely essential that they receive the correct level and type of protein in their feed for every day of their life up to 48 months of age.

Mature horses over 4 years of age will show protein deficiency in their feed initially by reduced performance, followed by loss of weight, finally getting to the stage where it is obvious even to the layman that the animal is losing weight.

PROTEIN EXCESS IN THE RATION

EXCESS PROTEIN in the ration can affect the horse in a number of ways. In adult horses, over four years of age, with average work loads, EXCESS PROTEIN, in the ration, is converted into ENERGY and used by the horse as such. PROTEIN is generally the most expensive part of the horses' ration, however, often being from 50% to over 3000% more expensive than energy on a per KILOGRAM basis of actual feed fraction, dependent on the source of protein being used. In terms of economic feeding of horses, there is a definite increased ration cost, if excess protein is fed and NOT USED BY THE HORSE AS PROTEIN. The reverse process, EXCESS ENERGY BEING CONVERTED TO PROTEIN DOES NOT OCCUR.

In young growing horses, under four years of age, the feeding of EXCESS LEVELS of PROTEIN in the ration appears to have a number of possible consequences.

1. If the AMINO ACID composition is LIMITING in LYSINE, a much greater proportion of the protein, present in the ration, will be converted to energy as the amount of LYSINE will limit the use of protein for tissue growth and maintenance. This LYSINE LIMITATION may well restrict growth, even though the apparent CRUDE PROTEIN level is correct.
2. if the LYSINE LEVEL of the ration, for young growing horses is adequate, EXCESS PROTEIN in the ration will probably cause no adverse effect on growth, PROVIDED THE ENERGY LEVEL in the ration is constant. FOALS, weaned at 4 months of age and then fed a ration containing some 22% crude protein for 12 months, about 57% above the normal expected level of 14%, showed no adverse effects, including no effect on the CALCIUM metabolism and skeletal development of the foal.
3. If the LYSINE LEVELS of the ration, for young growing horses are again adequate, young foals, where both the PROTEIN and ENERGY levels of the ration were INCREASED to-gether, suffered increased daily losses of both CALCIUM and PHOSPHORUS, which could be of concern on diets where the levels of both minerals were marginal. The foals were FED PROTEIN and ENERGY, at various levels up to about 30% above expected requirements.

EXCESS levels of PROTEIN in the ration of young horses have also been incriminated as being partly responsible for the developmental problems of EPIPHYSITIS and OSTEOCHRONDOSIS. There is also some credence given to the need to increase the levels of COPPER and ZINC in the rations of young growing horses fed high levels of protein.

As the average practical horse feeder is not going to be so scientific as to be able to increase PROTEIN level in the feed without altering ENERGY LEVEL, most will be increasing levels of both in the feed, even if unknowingly doing so, then care should be taken with feeding young growing horses, when increasing the protein level of the ration, as there is the possibility of increasing CALCIUM and PHOSPHORUS excretion, leading to possible bone and skeletal problems.

EXCESS LEVELS of PROTEIN in the ration of performance horses, or horses which have to work reasonably hard, appears to have no beneficial effect and, in fact, may have ADVERSE effects. It is known that EXCESS LEVELS of PROTEIN in the rations of performance horses can cause an increase in blood ammonia concentrations, increased sweating and therefore ELECTROLYTE demands, early fatigue in endurance horses and decreased speed in thoroughbreds. In all type of horses, there will be an increase in URINE VOLUME as the body attempts to excrete the excess protein and this, in turn, leads to greater thirst and therefore greater water intake, which, in turn, will probably have an effect on the ELECTROLYTE levels in the horse.

EFFECT OF EXERCISE ON PROTEIN REQUIREMENTS.

EXERCISE or WORK does increase the daily requirement of PROTEIN by the horse. The increase in daily requirements is however generally met by the increased amount of feed which the horse eats when working, as opposed to the same horse at rest.

Mature horses undergo changes in the manner in which they use the protein content of the ration, in response to long term low level exercise. Changes occur in the way in which the body muscle uses protein with increased nitrogen, derived from protein, being lost in sweat as part of the cooling process of the horse.

If a horse is eating about 9 kg D.M.(DRY MATTER) of feed at rest and that feed contains about 8% protein, the horse will be receiving about 720 grams protein/day. If, however, that horse is required to work reasonably hard, the daily feed consumption may well increase by 100% to 18 kg D.M./day and at the same time, whilst protein level in the ration is remaining constant, the actual daily intake of protein will have doubled to 1440 grams

Provided nature horses, at rest, are receiving adequate levels of quality protein in their ration, the additional DRY MATTER intake which will occur when the horse starts to exercise will provide the animal with additional protein needs.

There is no need to increase the protein level of working horses, above the recommended base figure, it is however necessary to ensure that the recognised base figures are correct and that the protein is balanced for all essential AMINO ACIDS.

If the amount of PROTEIN in the ration is held constant, by feeding the same weight of a specified ration each day, increasing exercise will produce significant changes in the amino acid and protein metabolism of the horse. A specific experiment measured this effect where a number of horses were worked on a treadmill at a trot, over a 14 day period, for sufficient length of time each day until gait inco-ordination occurred.

The effect of exercise on horses fed a constant level of protein from normal feed was :-

1. a significant increase in blood plasma volume, up some 30% on pre-exercise level and this remained at an increased level, some 18%, even after exercise had ceased
2. the increase in amino acid levels and hence protein levels of some 27% above the values at the start of the research meant that protein synthesis of some description was taking place within the horse, most likely within the large intestine.
3. At the end of the second week of exercise the levels of amino acids, and hence protein, had decreased to below the initial starting levels, about 12% less indicating that the protein level of the ration, at a constant weight of feed intake per day was not sufficient to provide the horse with all the protein required to maintain the rate of exercise.

6. ENERGY

The energy component of the horse's ration is the FUEL for maintenance and activity or work undertaken by that horse.

ENERGY REQUIREMENTS OF THE HORSE

ENERGY REQUIREMENTS OF ANY HORSE can be subdivided as follows.

A. MAINTENANCE REQUIREMENTS

MAINTENANCE REQUIREMENTS are defined as the energy being necessary to keep the horse in a state of constant body weight and metabolism. All horses need some form of energy to maintain the continual operation of the individual body cells. The horse is a living animal whose body cells even when the horse is in the resting state are operating, be it a much reduced level.

B. GROWTH REQUIREMENTS

Any horse which has reached SKELETAL maturity, commonly accepted as being about 4 years of age, has just progressed through a phase, where there is a continual increase in the number of body cells, as the horse grows from a foal to an adult, often a weight increase in thoroughbred horses of about 400kg or so over a 48 month period, the greater percentage of which occurs in the first 12 months after birth. This growing horse has a continual need for ENERGY to be supplied, not only, to maintain the function of the existing body cells but also to take part in the production of the new body cells as growth progresses.

C. WORK REQUIREMENTS

Work, exercise, performance or any activity which a horse exhibits, OVER AND ABOVE the activity of resting will require additional ENERGY. This ENERGY is similar to petrol in a fuel tank of a motor car. The more exercise or works the horse does, the more ENERGY is required in the ration to allow the muscle cells to function properly. As with the petrol in the fuel tank of the motor car, this energy is stored within the horse and released to the muscles cells, as required.

The most interesting point regarding ENERGY use, by a horse, relates to the history of the evolution of the horse over time. In previous times, when all horses ran wild, the main defence of the horse was flight, the ability to gallop away from any predator, faster than the predator could move. Nature has designed the horse, over millions of years, to use ENERGY as a means of producing ACTION. Selection of the horse, by man, has encouraged this ability of the horse to use ENERGY, in the feed, for action. In most other animals, which eat the same physical types of feed as the horse, the cow, sheep goat etc., nature has designed, and man has selected, the animals to use additional energy requirements in the diet to produce meat, milk or wool etc. Only in very few instances in the world, are horses selected for meat and or milk production.

THE PRACTICAL PROBLEM WITH FEEDING ENERGY TO A HORSE IS THAT ANY ENERGY FED, IN EXCESS OF THAT NEEDED FOR GROWTH AND MAINTENANCE, HAS TO BE USED BY THE HORSE AS A FUEL FOR EXERCISE AND ACTIVITY.

Overfeeding energy, and restricting exercise, to any horse is a sure way to get problems, which are discussed in detail in later sections of this book.

D. PREGNANCY REQUIREMENTS

The additional requirements of PREGNANCY for increased energy needs, of the mare, are virtually exactly the same as a non pregnant grown horse up to and including the first 8 months of pregnancy. From the ninth month until parturition, when the foal grows considerably in size, energy requirements of the pregnant mare can increase by about 20% to ensure satisfactory growth of the unborn foetus.

E. LACTATION REQUIREMENTS.

Milk production has large energy needs. Any person who has any experience with dairy cows will realise, that for maximum milk production, feed large amounts of energy in the form of grain. The lactating mare has energy requirements some 50% greater than a dry mare and it is obvious that one of the main reasons why foal growth is less than desirable is that the mares are not fed enough energy in the ration to be able to produce the milk which the foal requires. An excellent example of underfeeding.

EACH OF THESE FIVE CATEGORIES OF PHYSIOLOGICAL ENERGY REQUIREMENTS OF THE INDIVIDUAL HORSE can then be further affected and or influenced by the following.

1. live weight
2. average daily temperature
3. temperament of the horse
4. weight and ability of rider and or driver.
5. level of fatigue.
6. internal parasite burden or worm population
7. weight of daily feeds in relation to horse gut fill needs

1. LIVE WEIGHT

ENERGY needs are based on the live weight of the horse. A pony at 13 hands of 250 kgs. will naturally need less energy than a thoroughbred of 16 hands and weighing, say 450 kgs. This is an obvious but actual example of one of the basic factors determining energy needs. The number of times that quiet children's ponies have been given rations which would suit a racehorse in full training are many. Such a small pony is being fed energy levels well in excess of its needs, on a live weight basis, and also in regard to the amount of work it is doing, no wonder people get uncontrollable and or sick ponies.

2. AVERAGE DAILY TEMPERATURE

Any decrease in daily temperature will require the feeding of more energy to a horse as a greater amount of the energy being fed will be used by the horse to keep itself warm.

Similarly, increasing temperatures, especially over 34 degrees C, as can occur in some places in summer time will require a reduction in energy levels in the feed.

3. TEMPERAMENT OF THE HORSE

Horses which sweat readily are usually nervous horses and the external signs of sweating mean that the horse is, in fact, using or burning up energy in the sweating process. Informed punters will never bet on a racehorse or trotter which is sweating whilst the horse is in the enclosure before it goes onto the track. Tradition has it that these horses will have used some or all of their energy up in the sweating process BEFORE they even start the race.

Unfortunately horse temperament is often moulded and formed by the person responsible for breaking the horse in. Temperament may also be moulded by the attitude of the people responsible for the daily care of the animal. This book is not intended to explore the vast subject of horse psychology and horse handling, except to say that the change of stable and/or people attending to some temperamental horses has often led to vast improvement in the horse's temperament and consequently in the horse's performance.

The problems of horses which sweat profusely and use up energy before a race or performance, will generally NOT be corrected by feeding extra energy to replace that which is "sweated out". Feeding extra energy will probably only make the condition worse.

Horses, with such conditions, are being affected by either specific electrolyte problems, communication problems with humans, generally always the humans fault, as someone does not know enough about horses to be able to recognise the problems of horse communication and psychology.

4. WEIGHT AND ABILITY OF RIDER AND OR DRIVER

The effect of the driver of a harness horse, on ENERGY requirements of the horse will not be nearly as great as the effect of the rider.

In harness horses, the animal is not carrying additional weight upon its back, weight which sometimes completely upsets the balance of the horse. The harness horse is actually pushing into a collar which in turn pulls a vehicle of some description. The harness horse is still able to maintain its natural balance, at any gait, and as such will have reasonably consistent energy use patterns, in relationship to its work loads. The main problem with harness drivers and horse energy use will be when the horse is asked to work harder than the exercise level it has been trained and conditioned for, causing the onset of FATIGUE and possibly EXHAUSTION.

For ridden horses, the ability of the rider, especially BALANCE and SOFT HANDS, can have considerable effect on the efficiency of ENERGY USE. The horse is so designed that, with no rider on its back, some 60% or thereabouts of its normal weight falls on the forelegs and, in movement, has combined actions of neck, body and legs which allow for the most efficient movement and energy use.

When a rider mounts a horse, the ideal riding position(s) are such as to allow the horse to maintain the weight distribution patterns, as shown in the riderless state. Adoption by the rider, in the saddle, of this correct body position or posture, known as BALANCE, will still allow 60% of the COMBINED WEIGHT OF HORSE and RIDER to fall on the front legs and the horse will attain the highest level of efficiency in performance and energy use.

If the rider is unable to adopt positions in the saddle which DO NOT allow the combined weight distribution of horse and rider to place 60% of the total weight on the forelegs, at all gaits or paces, then the horse will become UNBALANCED, will not be able to perform as desired and will use MORE ENERGY than is necessary to perform a particular task.

CORRECT RIDING POSITION, THE RIDER COMBINING WITH THE HORSE TO BECOME BALANCED AND THE RIDER NOT FIGHTING AGAINST THE HORSE ARE NECESSARY FOR EFFICIENT ENERGY USE.

5. LEVEL OF FATIGUE

The level of FATIGUE, or the inability of the muscles and the body to function normally, can affect energy use by the horse. FATIGUE will occur in any horse, at a much faster rate if the horse has NOT been conditioned and or trained adequately for the task to be performed. Training and conditioning programmes for horses encourages the muscle tissues, in particular, to become more efficient users of ENERGY. FATIGUE can occur, in a horse, which contains reasonable levels of energy in the body, but which CANNOT be used effectively, by the muscles as they have not been conditioned to use that energy under the physiological conditions, existing in the race or event.

FATIGUE is due to either or both the following:-

1. lack of energy reserves in the horse, caused by insufficient energy in the previous rations, fed to the horse.
2. inability of the muscles to use energy reserves in the horse, due to lack of training and or conditioning of the muscles for the particular work.

6. INTERNAL PARASITES

Worms or internal parasites inside horses compete directly with the horse for the food components. In horses, with heavy worm burdens you need to feed the horse, as well as the worms. In horses which have lost weight or physical condition, due to heavy worm infestations, it is obvious that the worms are taking from the horse more than is being eaten each day and the worms, not the horse are winning the battle for the feed components.

This "LOSING BATTLE" will affect the amount of energy available to the horse. Very simply, worms reduce the available food nutrients, especially energy that the horse can get out of any ration. You neither make money nor derive personal pleasure from horse worms. Every horse should be properly and thoroughly drenched at frequent intervals, dependent on each horses' expected work output and the manner in which each horse is fed or grazed.

7. WEIGHT OF FEED AND GUT FILL

Nature designed horses to eat most of the time, from 16 to 20 hours/day. Apart from eating, the average healthy horse spends about half an hour per day lying down, and the balance of the time resting but standing up. The horse's digestive system, with its extremely small stomach in relation to the total capacity of the digestive tract, makes it essential that food should be continually eaten to maintain digesta flow through the complete length of the digestive tract.

If the rate of digesta flow is not continual and gut fill is not reasonably consistent, then the horse is liable to suffer from one or more of the known nutritional disorders and probably from some unknown ones as well.

A normal 450 kg. horse, at rest, is expected to have a daily dry matter feed intake of about 10 kgs. with a range from 6.70 kg. to 11.70 kgs.

This horse at rest or doing light work only has an energy need which when translated back to practical terms is in the order of 4.60 kgs. of starch or its equivalent, or 46% energy in the feed.

Such energy could be provided by 10 kgs. of good quality lucerne hay which will also give adequate gut fill and movement.

This same quantity of energy could also be supplied by 5.8 kgs. of corn (maize). However, this quantity of maize does not provide enough total dry matter to allow the horse to maintain normal gut fill.

Similarly, with the same 450 kg. horse in the peak of training, energy requirements could rise so high that it is just not physically possible to get the horse to eat enough high quality high energy feed to satisfy its daily energy needs. Special feeding techniques are being used to get the extra energy into the horse. Refer to later sections of this book.

Excess energy fed to the horse, over and above its daily needs, generally end up causing nutritional disorders, leading to sick horses, veterinary bills and long periods of recovery.

ENERGY is available to the horse in three different forms.

ENERGY AS CARBOHYDRATE

The CARBOHYDRATE type energy is contained within the cellulose walls of the individual plant cells, in the substance called the ENDOSPERM. Endosperm is readily seen in grain as the white interior, of all but the yellow maize and other coloured grains, under the hard seed coat. The most practical example of ENDOSPERM is FLOUR, used to make bread. Flour is the ENDOSPERM of wheat.

The ENDOSPERM of growing plants, and other horse feeds, is not so easily seen simply because the endosperm is spread throughout numerous microscopic individual plant cells and not collected to-gether in one large visual amount, as in grain. The practical reason for the presence of noticeable quantities of ENDOSPERM in grains, is simply that this is the ENERGY source for the germinating seed (grain), allowing it to survive during the period when the first tips of the young plant are pushing up through the soil and before they have penetrated the soil surface where energy requirements of the plant are taken over by PHOTOSYNTHESIS or the action sunlight on green plant tissue. If grains (seeds) did not contain ENDOSPERM (CARBOHYDRATE type energy), they would not be able to penetrate the soil surface and commence to produce continual amounts of plant material by the action of sunlight on chlorophyll, known as PHOTOSYNTHESIS.

The CARBOHYDRATE type energy is made available to the horse by breakdown of the cellulose in the digestive tract and release of the internal plant cell contents, including ENDOSPERM, for modification by the digestive juices and enzymes, within the stomach and small intestine. CARBOHYDRATE type energy CAN ONLY be absorbed, by the horse, within the small intestine and is digested within minutes of being reduced to a form which can be taken up in the blood stream.

The various methods used to treat grain so as to increase the rate of cellulose or fibre rupture in the stomach, and hence early release of CARBOHYDRATE type energy, are discussed in full in the chapter on FIBRE.

Any CARBOHYDRATE TYPE ENERGY NOT ABSORBED into the horse's bloodstream by the end of the small intestine, is excreted with the faeces, as the large intestine DOES NOT POSSESS the ability to absorb this form of ENERGY.

Feeding horses with medium to high work loads and hence medium to high energy needs, especially those horses in training or performing work, requires the use of feeds which allow rapid breakdown of the cell walls so that the PROTEIN and the CARBOHYDRATE type energy can be absorbed by the horse in the stomach and small intestine - i.e. before the food undergoes cellulose breakdown in the large intestine.

Once a horse starts to perform work, energy needs to be absorbed in the small intestine, in particular, and hence the need to consider, what most horse people call FEED QUALITY, in performance horses. In practical terms this means feed containing less cellulose or cellulose or fibre which is soft in appearance and allowing rapid breakdown and release of the readily digestible sources of energy.

CARBOHYDRATE use in the horse basically converts starch and the sugar type compounds, which form energy, into simple glucose. Glucose in then absorbed by the digestive tract into the blood stream and then carried to the various parts of the horse's body where as the related compound GLYCOGEN, it is responsible for maintenance of the horse and for muscle function.

GLYCOGEN IS MUSCLE FUEL.

The amount of GLYCOGEN used by the horse for muscle energy production is controlled by the release of INSULIN, produced in the PANCREAS. Different training programmes of Thoroughbred racehorses have been shown to have different effects on the way in which GLUCOSE moves through the various parts of the horse to finally provide muscle energy, clearly indicating that nutritional needs of energy can change, within the same horse, at different stages of a training programme.

ENERGY AS VOLATILE FATTY ACIDS

VOLATILE FATTY ACIDS, abbreviated to V.F.A., are compounds which are produced in the large intestine by the action of the bacteria, and their associated enzymes, on decomposing and digesting the CELLULOSE or fibre. These VOLATILE FATTY ACIDS are absorbed directly by the large intestine and used by the horse as an energy source.

VOLATILE FATTY ACIDS, as a source of energy, are able to supply a horse, at rest or doing very little work, with most of its' daily energy needs. A horse, which is fed HAY only, will probably get from 40 to 80% of its daily energy requirements from VOLATILE FATTY ACIDS.

As far as performance horses are concerned, i.e. any horse which is doing sufficient work to sweat at the completion of that work, the energy obtained from VOLATILE FATTY ACIDS will be supplying a lesser percentage of the horse's daily needs as the production of VOLATILE FATTY ACIDS from the cellulose or fibre does not increase, in either amount or speed of increase at the same rate as the increase in the energy demands of the horse, associated with increasing work output.

VOLATILE FATTY ACIDS are absorbed into the blood stream of the horse in a manner similar to the absorption of GLUCOSE but VOLATILE FATTY ACIDS are not changed to GLUCOSE but used, in the form produced by cellulose digestion, by the various parts of the horse. These volatile fatty acids are also responsible, under some conditions, for certain nutritional disorders. These will be discussed in detail later in this book.

The production of VOLATILE FATTY ACIDS, from cellulose breakdown in the large intestine, is also responsible for the absorption of ELECTROLYTES from the large intestine. The ELECTROLYTES are generally held within the cell walls which need to be broken down by microbial digestion, within the large intestine, to allow release into the digesta for absorption.

ENERGY AS FAT

The term FATS, in horse feeding, is identical to the terms LIPIDS and OILS. There are slight differences in chemical composition, such that FATS are generally solid at room temperature, whilst OILS are always liquid at room temperature but as far as horse nutrition is concerned, the term FATS includes both and relates to organic compounds which are insoluble or do not dissolve in water.

FATS contain many compounds including four unsaturated fatty acids, which are required by the horse, OLEIC ACID, LINOLENIC ACID, ARACHIDONIC ACID and LINOLEIC ACID. The needs of the horse for any of these essential fats is not at all clear but the addition of small amounts (0.5%) LINOLEIC Acid to the ration may be of value.

Pasture and allied green feeds contain very low levels of FATS, often less than 0.5% of the DRY MATTER content, and most of those FATS present in pasture are of the UNSATURATED type.

FATS have FIVE functions in the horse.

In very small quantities, at amounts which can be supplied by the natural low FAT levels of feeds of vegetative or plant origin, FATS are important;-

1. in combination with PROTEIN in body cell wall structure.
2. vitally important in the structure of hormones of the PROSTAGLANDIN group, involved in the control of a number of body functions.
3. low levels of FATS in the bloodstream act as the transport mechanism around the horse's body for the FAT SOLUBLE VITAMINS A, D, E and K.
4. Internal body FATS act as a storage depot for the FAT SOLUBLE VITAMINS A, D, E and K, if excessive levels, of these vitamins are fed to the horse.
5. The FAT components of feeds are another source of ENERGY. 1 kg. of fat will in fact produce the equivalent of 2.25 kg. of energy in the horse. Fats, therefore in horse nutrition, are a CONCENTRATED form of energy.

As a potential source of ENERGY in the horse, FATS have to be eventually converted into a source which can be used by the muscle cells and the effectiveness of the use of this ENERGY, derived from the decomposition of FATS, is affected by the level of VITAMIN E available to the horse.

In theory, the average horse contains enough reserves of FAT in its body to supply sufficient energy for about 5 days of average exercise. In practice, this does not happen as there are a considerable number of other components in the horse's body which will be depleted well before 5 days activity been completed.

FATS are added to horse feeds in two types.

1. ANIMAL FATS derived by the rendering of tallow from cattle sheep, pigs and poultry, commonly used in the cheaper horse feeds.
2. VEGETABLE OILS derived from seeds of plants, commonly called OILSEEDS, namely SOYBEAN, SUNFLOWER, LINSEED, COTTONSEED, RAPE or CANOLA, generally more expensive than animal fats and only used either as an additive to the more expensive feeds or as a single specific product, e.g. extruded soybean meal.

The horse's requirements for ESSENTIAL FATTY ACIDS for normal body processes are capable of being supplied from normal everyday plant material, which contains about 0.5% FAT, and FAT SUPPLEMENTATION of the fed is not required for these normal body requirements.

Where the supplementation of horse's rations with FAT MAY be of value is:-

1. as a source of concentrated energy, it is necessary to clarify whether in fact FAT added to a ration will be a suitable source of energy for a particular horse.
2. to improve palatability and reduce possible dust problems
3. adds a "shine" to the rations which impresses the feeder, looks better but may have the opposite effect on the horse.

The level of feeding FATS in horse rations is currently one of considerable debate.

If the objective is to simply put a shine on the horse's coat, and possibly encourage shedding of the winter coat faster in the spring, the best method is to add one tablespoon, about 45 grams of vegetable cooking oil or sunflower seed/horse/day to the feed.

If FATS are required for ENERGY producing purposes, consideration needs to be taken of the type of activity the horse is being asked to do. Any horse being asked to do short very active exercise DOES NOT require fat in the ration, the horse is simply not working for a sufficient length of time to be able to use fats to produce energy. If however the horse is being asked to do long consistent exercise then FATS in the ration may be a source of energy.

MAXIMUM current recommended feeding levels of FAT are no greater than 15% of the DRY MATTER or 30% of total ration weight which in terms of vegetable cooking oil comes back at 1.5 litres/horse/day. Over about 0.5 litres/horse/day, practical palatability problems will be encountered in feeding fats to horses, especially if the FATS are added to the ration too quickly.

ONE OF THE PROBLEMS WITH THE INCORPORATION OF FATS IN HORSE FEEDS IS OXIDATION.

OXIDATION involves the destruction of the fat by oxygen, in the air, and oxidised FATS tend to go rancid, producing an offensive taste and or smell.

If FATS are to be used as a supplement for horses, they should be mixed with the feed, immediately prior to feeding, to avoid any possible RANCIDITY problems.

Oil seed based meals produced by the extrusion process contain very little fat. The extrusion process basically expels the oil or fat component from the seed. The oil component then is used for the manufacture of margarine and other products and the residue left is then treated to produce oil seed meals, e.g. soybean, sunflower, linseed meals etc.

Soybean seeds, not subject to any form of oil extraction and treated with heat under pressure for a short period of time, less than a minute, will contain the fat component and in fact this form of horse feed can contain 18-20% fat as opposed to soybean meal which generally only contains about 1-2% fat.

Whilst it is possible to feed untreated and unprocessed sunflower, corn and other oil containing grains to horses, do not under any circumstances feed untreated soybean. Soybean must be heat treated before being fed to horses to destroy certain substances contained in the raw grain which can affect the uptake of other nutrients in the horse.

DO NOT FEED ANY QUANTITY OF OILSEEDS or similar fat containing compounds to horses where coat colour is an important. PALOMINOS, DUNS etc. fed any level of fat containing feeds can get darkened coats which may take up to 6 months to lighten in colour once the feeding of the fat containing compounds has ceased.

ENERGY USE IN THE HORSE

CARBOHYDRATE TYPE ENERGY is broken down within the digestive tract into GLUCOSE and a number of VOLATILE FATTY ACIDS. These breakdown products are absorbed, from the small intestine, in the case of GLUCOSE, and the large intestine in the case of the VOLATILE FATTY ACIDS, into the blood stream and carried to the liver. Within the liver, GLUCOSE and some of the VOLATILE FATTY ACIDS are changed to GLYCOGEN, sometimes called LIVER STARCH, which is then carried by the blood to the muscles cells. The remaining VOLATILE FATTY ACIDS are converted to FAT within the liver.

FAT TYPE ENERGY is absorbed, into the bloodstream, from the digestive tract in the small intestine in the presence of BILE, essential for FAT and FAT SOLUBLE VITAMIN absorption. The FAT is then transported, as such, in the bloodstream to various FAT depots where it is stored in the horse's body, until required.

The priorities of ENERGY use in the active horse is as follows:-

1. initial energy is supplied from the relatively small energy store of A.T.P. (adenosine triphosphate) and C.P. (creatinine phosphate) within the muscle cells, probably for no longer than for the initial 10 or 12 seconds of activity.
2. the next source of energy is the GLYCOGEN, held within the muscles and the liver, when the muscles are operating in an ANAEROBIC environment, providing energy for about 10-20 minutes after depletion of the original A.T.P. and C.K. energy supplies and the FATS when the muscle systems are operating in the AEROBIC phase, which can occur from about 20 minutes on into exercise after depletion of the CARBOHYDRATE energy reserves.

Circulating GLUCOSE, within the blood stream, is not a significant source for AEROBICALLY working muscle.

Both CARBOHYDRATE and FATS are broken down to GLYCOGEN which is then changed to A.T.P. ADENOSINE TRIPHOSPHATE which is the energy compound used by the muscle cells but which cannot be stored in any significant quantity in the horse.

The determination of whether FAT will be needed by the horse as a source of ENERGY is made by a complex biological process inside the horse involving amount of CARBOHYDRATE ENERGY AVAILABLE, amount of stored FAT available and the ENERGY needs of the horse at the time.

FAT which is required for ENERGY sources, is released from the FAT depots and undergoes a complex chemical process which simply hydrolyses the FAT, (breaks the fat down by a reaction with water), to produce GLYCEROL and FREE FATTY ACIDS. The GLYCEROL can be readily converted to GLUCOSE then to GLYCOGEN for muscle cell energy requirements, whilst the FREE FATTY ACIDS are broken down further into compounds, similar to glycogen which can be used for energy supply.

The conversion of CARBOHYDRATE to MUSCLE ENERGY can be carried out IN THE ABSENCE OF OXYGEN, or the ANAEROBIC MUSCLE ACTIVITY phase, that

phase of physical activity which constitutes about the first two minutes or so of activity at a pace estimated to exceed 320 metres/minute (fast canter).

The conversion of FAT to MUSCLE ENERGY, however, requires large amounts of OXYGEN to allow the process to work which means that at paces or speed over 320 metres/minute, FAT is of NO VALUE as a source of ENERGY for a performance horse, except in ENDURANCE RIDING. At speeds less than 320 metres/minute (fast trot, medium canter or less), MUSCLE activity in the horse is by AEROBIC means or in the presence of oxygen and FAT can be satisfactorily converted into muscle energy.

From a practical viewpoint, any horse which performs at a reasonably fast pace for two minutes or less, should not have FAT in the rations as a source of energy. This would include most racehorses and standardbreds, showjumpers, cutting and campdrafting horses. The use of FATS as an energy source in these types of horses will decrease performance.

Any horse which works for longer than two minutes, and especially at a slower pace, as with ENDURANCE HORSES are able to effectively use FAT as an ENERGY source.

There is no specific cut off or change over levels where the horse will cease using one type of energy and change immediately to the use of the other type of energy. There will be in all horses a period of transition where some energy will come form CARBOHYDRATE sources and some from FAT sources, that period of gradual change over dependant on previous training programme, speed of exercise at the time and the length of time since the exercise commenced.

Any horse which has a training programme where the muscles are well conditioned, to use energy, in the presence of OXYGEN, will reach its ANAEROBIC threshold for energy use at a higher speed than an unfit or out of conditioned horse, in other words correct training procedures NEED TO BE INTEGRATED WITH correct feeding techniques to enable the best results from the horse.

In one particular study with Arabian horses ridden some 60 k's, where FAT, in the form of CORN OIL, was fed prior to the ride as 8% of the ration, the horses required 15% less feed and performance was considered not to be affected.

LACTATE or LACTIC ACID is the normal end product resulting from the use of GLYCOGEN in the muscles and the A.T.P. for energy use. The level of LACTIC ACID, in the blood, increases considerably when the rate of travel of the horse is at or exceeds a medium to fast canter or faster. The horse is naturally able to handle the disposal of this waste product LACTIC ACID when at rest. The problem with the performance horse is that the build up in LACTIC ACID occurs at much faster rates than the product can be excreted from the horse. One way to allow the horse to be able to handle greater amounts of LACTIC ACID, whilst working, is to ensure the horse's training programme is intensive enough to condition the muscles and the other body organs to the demands of exercise of the level expected. Horses which have trained and conditioned correctly will have about 50% less LACTIC ACID accumulation during and after exercise than will horses which have not been conditioned or classed as unfit. Virtually all performance horses, with very high LACTIC ACID levels immediately on the completion of strenuous exercise will, in approximately 2 hours of rest, have LACTIC ACID levels which have returned to normal.

Only about 25% of the ENERGY in the ration of any horse is used for the PRODUCTION OF MUSCLE ENERGY. The balance of the ENERGY fed is used to generate HEAT, most of which is used as part of the process of the digestion of FIBRE and CELLULOSE in the large intestine and the balance is used to as part of the overall body processes, especially in exercise or active work.

ENERGY BALANCE

NEGATIVE ENERGY BALANCE occurs when the horse is using more energy/day than it is receiving in its feed or from stored body reserves. NEGATIVE ENERGY BALANCE can be visually seen as the horse is losing body weight and will suffer a change in muscle shape and conformation. This situation will occur when the horse has already exhausted its internal body fat reserves, due to a prolonged period of being fed rations with a lower energy level than required for work and exercise and is still being fed a ration where energy levels are still not high enough to provide for normal body maintenance and exercise or work needs.

POSITIVE ENERGY BALANCE occurs when the horse is receiving more energy/day in its feed than it is using in physical activity.

POSITIVE ENERGY BALANCE occurs in two phases.

1. when the energy supply in the feed exceeds the horse's daily needs, but the horse is NOT GAINING IN WEIGHT but rather building up its internal fat storage depots.
2. when the energy supply in the feed exceeds the horse's daily needs, the internal fat depots have been built up and the horse then commences to lay down excess fat inside the muscles, causing an increase in body condition and or conformation which can be visually assessed.

Most horse owners determine the energy needs of their horses by appearance. A horse in NEGATIVE ENERGY BALANCE will be losing weight, a horse in POSITIVE ENERGY BALANCE will appear to stay in the same physical condition for some time whilst the internal fat deposits are laid down and then once these internal body fat depots are at "full capacity", the laying down of internal muscle fat will show as increasing body condition, increasing muscle bulk and weight gain.

LACK OF ENERGY IN THE RATION

Lack of sufficient energy in the horse's feed will lead to a decrease or reduction in the horse's expected performance. ENERGY is the body fuel and, if there is not sufficient "fuel in the tank" or ENERGY in the feed to satisfy the horse's needs, then something will suffer.

In young growing horses, generally under two years of age, lack of energy in the ration will cause REDUCED GROWTH. The reduction will probably NOT be detected by the naked eye and even if picked up using regular weighings from scales, there are many other reasons, one could think of as being, able to cause the same possible reduction in growth rate.

In young horses, both growing and working hard, insufficient energy in the ration will probably affect both growth and performance. Two year old thoroughbreds and standard breds in training have very specific nutritional needs, including energy levels in the rations, as these horses are still growing whilst being required to perform at what would be accepted as a heavy work load for a mature horse which has ceased skeletal growth.

In mature horses, insufficient energy in the ration will lead to less than required performances and if ration energy levels are very low, loss of body weight as the horse draws upon muscle tissue to provide energy for body maintenance when that energy should come from feed.

Insufficient energy in the ration of pregnant mares generally does not affect the growth of the foal. The mare will draw upon her own energy reserves in the muscles and internal fat depots to make up any energy deficiency which occurs in the ration and to protect the developing foetus. In the lactating mare, lack of energy in the feed will cause reduced milk production and may even cause the mare to cease milk production completely, either occurrence likely to affect the growth of the foal.

IN PRACTICAL HORSE FEEDING SITUATIONS, THE EFFECT OF LACK OF ENERGY ON A HORSE'S GROWTH AND OR PERFORMANCE SHOULD RARELY OCCUR, PROVIDED THE FEEDER HAS A KNOWLEDGE OF THE ENERGY NEEDS OF THE HORSE, THE ENERGY CONTENTS OF THE FEEDS AND HOW THAT RELATES TO THE TRAINING PROGRAMME.

The reason for this statement is very simple.

Most horse feeds contain sufficient energy to maintain any horse in reasonable condition. After all horses were eating most of these feeds and doing very nicely, before man invented all sorts of ways of measuring energy and trying to justify in scientific terms what the horse has been doing for years.

The horse has the ability to take energy from feeds at the times of high energy intake and store some of that energy in the muscles and internal fat depots, the horse "muscles up", puts on weight and generally improves in condition. When energy levels in the daily feed intake falls below what the horse requires and is able to extract from the feed, the horse will then draw upon the energy reserves in the muscles and fat depots to satisfy its energy requirements, visually losing condition and weight as the muscles get smaller with release of energy producing compounds from the muscle tissue.

EXCESS ENERGY IN A HORSE RATION

The main problem with the supply of ENERGY to horses is one of OVERFEEDING or supplying TOO MUCH ENERGY, in the ration, in relation to the horse's needs.

The level of ENERGY FED needs to be SUFFICIENT TO ALLOW THE HORSE TO DO WHAT is required, i.e. grow, perform, lactate etc. but not high enough to cause the horse any problems from EXCESS ENERGY IN THE DIET.

Excess CARBOHYDRATE type ENERGY can be retained within the horse, as GLYCOGEN, being stored in the liver and or the muscles or else converted into FAT as part of the horse's internal fat deposits. EXCESS FAT, in the ration, remains as FAT in the internal fat depots. Once stored inside the horse, ENERGY can only be used for muscle activity, work and or performance.

If the amount of energy stored as FAT, reaches a situation of "saturation", i.e. the horse is receiving more energy/day in the ration than it is using in body maintenance and exercise, - POSITIVE ENERGY BALANCE,- the horse is unable to convert any more CARBOHYDRATE energy to fat or to store any additional FAT in the ration as FAT in the horse, the feeding of additional ENERGY, in either form has to be released from the horse somehow. This release generally occurs in a manner which can cause any one of the energy related NUTRITIONAL DISORDERS, such as FOUNDER, TYING UP, METABOLIC BONE DISEASES in growing horses and or COLIC.

HORSES ARE UNABLE TO WITHSTAND THE BUILD-UP OF CONTINUAL BODY ENERGY RESERVES, WITHOUT ADEQUATE EXERCISE TO USE THAT ENERGY IN THE MUSCLES.

All the above comments are made in the context of any increase in the ENERGY content of the ration being made in isolation, the ration levels of all the other feed components remaining steady.

Often in horses, when the level of one feed component is changed in a ration, there are often changes in the level of other feed components. Data does exist which shows that if both the ENERGY and PROTEIN levels of the rations of young growing horse are increased above normal levels, there can be an increased excretion, from the body of young growing horse, of both CALCIUM and PHOSPHORUS.

THE FEEDING OF ENERGY LEVELS IN EXCESS OF THE HORSE'S DAILY NEEDS AND STORAGE ABILITY IS DANGEROUS.

Most commercial animals, cattle, sheep, pigs, poultry etc., are fed ENERGY levels in the rations well in excess of that ENERGY required for BODY MAINTENANCE and GROWTH. This AVAILABLE ENERGY, that energy above BODY MAINTENANCE requirements, is used for production purposes, to produce more meat, milk, wool etc. In all of these, instances feeding of excess energy, over and above maintenance needs, produces a product which can be related to a direct commercial and financial gain to the owner of the animal.

All these "commercial animals" also have digestive and physiological systems, considerably different from the horse, which allow the cow or pig or poultry to be able to effectively use quite large amounts of energy in the diet, WITHOUT THE ANIMAL DEVELOPING PROBLEMS.

Part of this reason is the differences between the ways, the various species of animals uses feeds, developed by natural selection over million of years and part by selection, by man, commonly called BREEDING, of strains of these animals which can effectively utilise extra energy, over and above maintenance levels, provided in the feed. Meat chickens have been developed which are able to convert larger than normal amounts of energy in the rations into chicken meat. However, the birds were at their physiological limit as the heart, in particular, was not able to pump sufficient blood around the bird to keep it alive, in the event of the slightest noise or fright. This is but one actual example of the possibility of breeding for the efficient use of energy in domestic animals.

None of these domestic animals possessed RAPID MOVEMENT or FLIGHT as their main weapon of defence and survival in the wild. Horns were common on most early breeds of cattle and sheep and pig tusks are still are formidable defensive weapon.

The feeding of EXCESS ENERGY LEVELS in the rations of LACTATING MARES has been shown to have no effect on the constituents of the milk, milk energy levels included, in fact, caused the mare to put on body weight and to improve in condition.

ENERGY

Energy levels in rations being fed to lactating mares should be sufficient to keep the mare in reasonable body condition, she can adapt her lactating energy requirements from adjustments in body weight.

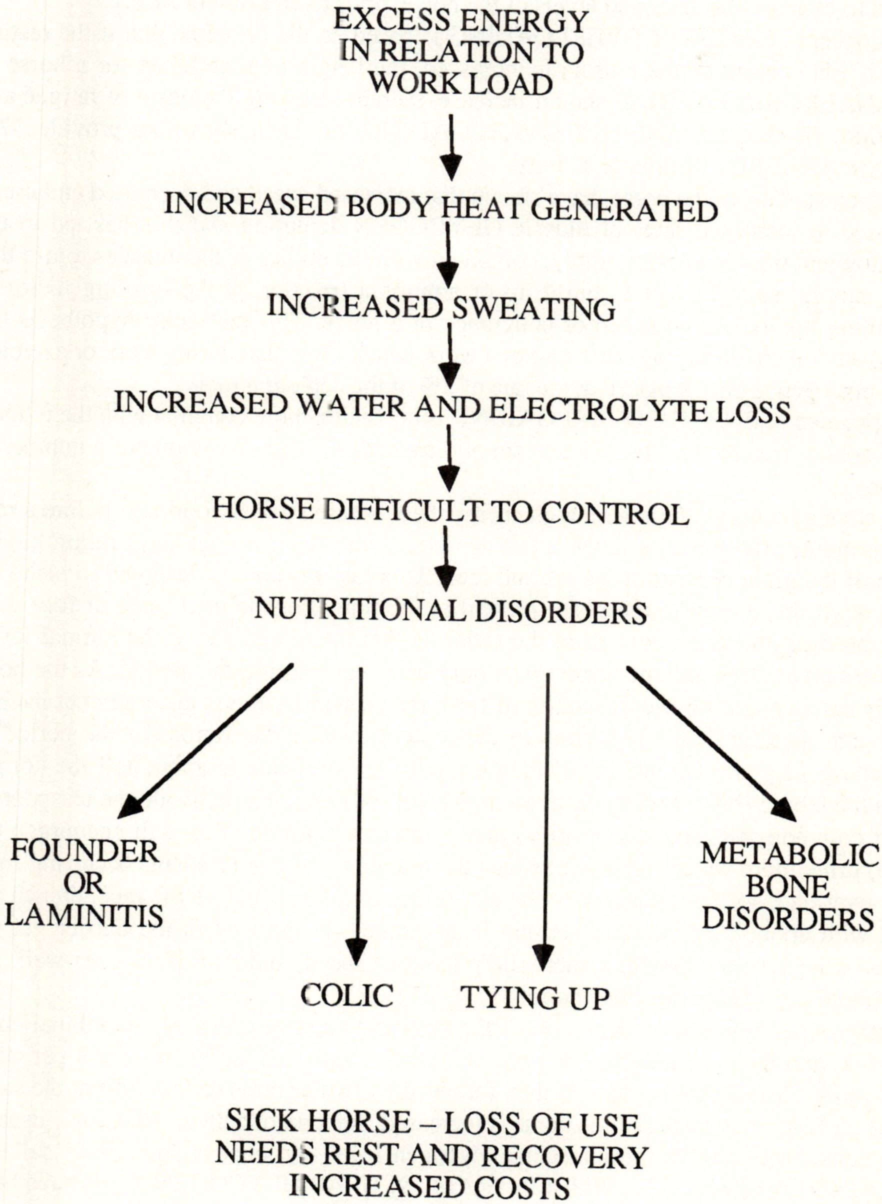

ENERGY OVERLOADING

ENERGY OVERLOADING is also known in various parts as GLYCOGEN OVERLOADING, GLYCOGEN PACKING, GLYCOGEN DEPLETION and SUPERCOMPENSATION, and all the terms refer to any practice or feeding change which attempts to increase the glycogen levels of the horse, prior to an event or race.

The concept of ENERGY OVERLOADING is based on the principle that if the resting GLYCOGEN content of the muscle is increased, the length of time taken for a horse to reach ANAEROBIC FATIGUE should increase, thereby delaying the onset of fatigue and exhaustion. In humans, ENERGY OVERLOADING has been shown to provide 37% increase in ANAEROBIC muscle activity.

Research studies, in the horse, have shown that increased speed and decreased endurance are related to increased rates of muscle GLYCOGEN depletion and this has led to the suggestion that muscle energy supply, combined with the ability of the muscles to use that energy supply, and not lactate build up or ammonia toxicity, is the limiting factor in determining the maximum speed or endurance of a horse. This particular hypothesis has been assisted in credibility by other research work which show that during work or exercise, muscle glycogen is only replaced at the rate of 2% of the depletion rate.

The practice of ENERGY OVERLOADING is becoming more common with the trainers of race horses, pacers etc. The practice simply involves the use of any one of a number of strategies.

One strategy involves horses on high energy diets, where three or four days before a race or performance, the horse is given a fast workout, with the previous days ration having about half the grain content of the normal feed. This fast workout is designed to make the horse use all the energy in the body, present at the time. For the next three or four days before the race, the grain content in the ration is then increased above the normal level, sometimes up to 20%, and the horse given only light work during this period. As the horse can only eat a certain physical quantity of feed, the protein source is generally cut back in weight, and there is then a reduction in the protein level of the ration for the period of 'overfeeding' of grain. On the day of the race, cut back the grain to about half the normal level in the feed. Whilst feeding the extra high levels of grain, mix in about one teaspoonful each of common salt (sodium chloride) and potassium chloride. This will encourage the horse to drink more water and hence reduce the likelihood of any problems occurring from energy overload, such as ty-ing up, colic etc. About four hours before the race, drench the animal with about 100 grams of sodium bicarbonate. On the way to the barrier get the rider/driver to give the animal a short sharp burst of speed, and then if all goes well, the horse should run a faster race than normal.

Another strategy involves depletion of the muscle energy reserves by a combination of hard work, and diets containing low protein, carbohydrate and fat levels over a period of several days. This depletion phase is then followed by two or three days of rest at the same time the carbohydrate intake of the horse is increased, sometimes called "repletion", usually with a consequent rise in intramuscular glycogen level, by what is sometimes called a "REBOUND OVERSHOOT". Whilst INTRAMUSCULAR GLYCOGEN levels have been increased, no improvement in performance has been demonstrated.

Problems encountered with ENERGY OVERLOADING include:-

1. increased intracellular water retention, due to high muscular glycogen concentrations.

2. the possibility of increased dehydration.
3. the system of ENERGY OVERLOADING WILL ONLY WORK in those horses whose training and conditioning programmes has been designed to get the muscle fibres to store and metabolize glycogen rapidly. If this does not happen, ENERGY OVERLOADING is more likely to produce TYING UP than increased performance.

This practice would need to be adopted with caution, especially with horses already on high energy rations. To those interested in trying the technique, a strong word of caution is offered. The training and conditioning programme of the horse is all important but this is a book on feeding horses, not training horses, so those aspects of training necessary to get the muscles to store and use glycogen faster than normal will NOT be covered. Be careful and change slowly, otherwise all sorts of problems may result.

As far as CORRECT ENERGY USE in the horse is concerned, two major problems are faced.

1. DEFINITION OF EXACT ENERGY NEEDS
2. DEFINITION OF WORK LOAD OF THE HORSE

In the pleasure horse industry, led in or in hand classes, pony club, hacks etc., there is considerable difficulty in defining in absolute terms just what is required from the horse. The aims of the feeder of these types of horses can all be quantified in general terms, e.g. to win ribbons, to have a quiet, well behaved horse, to have a horse looking nice but it is difficult, if not impossible to get these descriptive terms into numerical figures, which somehow can be related to the THEORETICAL METHODS OF MEASURING ENERGY LEVELS OF HORSE FEEDS.

In the performance horse industries, the aim is for the horse to go faster and or stronger. Thoroughbred racing horses, standardbreds, endurance horses, eventers etc. are all required to be able to perform to a TIME RESTRICTED limit, in other words the winner is generally the horse with the fastest time.

With these types of horses, there is some numerical measurement of the level of activity and, therefore, the possibility of relating ENERGY INTAKE on a mathematical basis to actual and expected performance.

Since the level of ENERGY FED controls the amount of work produced, all other factors being at optimum levels, the horse, in these types of activities, is being asked to become more efficient in using ENERGY than both its predecessors and all the other horses in the race or competition. Man, in selecting for improved athletic performance which involves greater speed, is changing HOPEFULLY, the horse's ability to use energy.

Emphasis is placed on HOPEFULLY because the ability of the horse to perform better is NOT COMPLETELY RELATED to increasing energy levels in the ration.

EFFICIENT ENERGY USE IN THE PERFORMANCE HORSE IS RELATED TO AND AFFECTED BY:

1. LEVELS OF ALL OTHER FOOD COMPONENTS IN THE RATION, there are some 40 or more of these in total including PROTEIN, MINERALS , VITAMINS ETC. If any one of these is NOT PRESENT IN THE CORRECT AMOUNT RELATIVE TO

THE AMOUNT OF ENERGY BEING FED then something can and usually will go wrong, even if it is only slightly less than desirable performance.

2. EFFICIENT ENERGY USE is VITALLY TIED IN with training programmes which develop the abilities of the muscles, in particular and the other body systems in general, to use energy more efficiently. If additional energy levels in rations are NOT related to increased and or improved training schedules, then the horse will not be able to use the additional energy effectively.

ENERGY in a horse's ration which is in EXCESS of the horse's needs will be responsible for one or more of the following:-

1. the production of additional muscle and associated tissue, commonly called FATTENING. Unlike other animals which eat and exist on vegetative material, the horse does not produce large amounts of what people commonly recognise as FAT. The horse will, when increasing MUSCLE SIZE, lay down FAT within the muscle, but rarely on the outside of the muscles as in sheep and cattle. Horses are also able to lay fat down inside the abdomen within and around the digestive tract and other organs. When one uses the phrase TO FATTEN A HORSE, what is really meant is to build more muscle on that horse.
2. TEMPERAMENT AND BEHAVIOUR of the horse will be affected. This will be especially so in the horse which is overfed energy and confined to a small yard or stable where the horse is unable to exercise adequately and use or "BURN UP" the surplus energy it does not require. In most instances, the horse will behave EXACTLY as required at home, in familiar surroundings. Take that horse out to a show or event, in strange surroundings among other horses and it will most likely misbehave, play up and do all sorts of things, unheard of at home. On many occasions, the pony club horse or the hack has performed as required at home but "BLOWN UP" or misbehaved when taken out. Instead of trying a new and harsher bit, changing other gear and changing training techniques etc., a reduction in the energy level of the ration is probably all that is required. The horse is being OVERFED ENERGY in relation to its workload.
3. Development of any one of the problems, commonly called NUTRITIONAL DISORDERS, problems which result in the horse from the OVERFEEDING OF ENERGY in relation to workload and the other feed components in the ration. These problems include LAMINITIS or FOUNDER, COLIC, TYING UP, OSTEOCHRONDOSIS and HYPERLIPAEMIA.

Refer to the separate chapter on NUTRITIONAL DISORDERS for a full description of these particular problems

Often horses are NOT PERFORMING to expectation, due to either INSUFFICIENT ENERGY or TOO MUCH ENERGY in the ration relative to their work requirements. The feeders then, instead of correcting the problem of energy content in the ration, resort to the feeding of one of the many supplements on the market in the search for some form of "miracle cure". Energy is the only feed, apart from protein, that will allow the horse to perform better and bucketfuls or injections of additional supplements to horses on energy diets, unsuitable for the horse's needs, will not make any difference to the horse's performance.

7. MINERALS

A strong well developed and properly maintained skeletal system is important to an animal. Minerals are essential for the construction of the horse's skeleton and, more importantly, for the maintenance of the skeletal and other body functions throughout the horses' life. Various individual minerals are involved in the function enzyme production, energy transfer, vitamins, hormones and some amino acids.

Electrolytes, required in very small but continuous amounts in the horse for many vital body functions include four minerals.

Abundant scientific evidence exists as to the average quantities of each mineral that horses at various stages of growth and performance require. Knowledge is now also becoming available of the effects of mineral OVERDOSE in horses. In most instances, it is becoming apparent that overfeeding of mineral supplements may be undesirable. Some minerals, fed in excess of the normally accepted levels, may interfere with the absorption of other minerals or vitamins, or, themselves, may individually produce toxic symptoms in the horse. The administration of excessive levels of minerals to a horse can also upset the ELECTROLYTE balance and usage, adversely affecting muscle activity and performance. Some of these symptoms produced by over feeding minerals, may be at a sub-clinical level, i.e. no external symptoms are visible, but the horse reacts by sub-standard performance.

Excess ration levels, or oversupplementation, of the following minerals are known to adversely affect the horse, some in quite dramatic and dangerous ways:- PHOSPHORUS, IRON, ZINC, MANGANESE, COPPER, IODINE, SELENIUM and FLUORINE.

The term MINERAL refers to a particular family of inorganic compounds, and does not solely cover CALCIUM and PHOSPHORUS as assumed by some people. CALCIUM and PHOSPHORUS, whilst very important minerals, in horse nutrition, are only two of some sixteen minerals which need to be considered when feeding horses.

SOIL FERTILITY AND MINERALS IN HORSE FEEDS

The individual mineral content of the soil will determine the amount of each individual mineral present in grazing pasture as well as in any product which comes from a plant (grains and seeds) which has grown in that soil. Such plant derived feeds will include GRAINS, OILSEED MEALS, CHAFFS, GRAIN BY PRODUCTS such as BRAN, POLLARD, WHEAT MIDDLINGS etc.

The mineral content of such feeds, when fed to horses WILL ONLY contain the minerals which the plant has been able to extract from the soil, during the growing process. These minerals are UNABLE TO COME FROM ANYWHERE ELSE.

If the soil happens to be deficient in PHOSPHORUS or SELENIUM, for optimum plant growth, research has shown that pastures, grown on such soils will generally be deficient in both minerals, for horse feeding purposes. In a very specific soil type in Victoria, CALCIUM is lacking for plant growth and CALCIUM deficiency has been detected in horses grazing such soils. The exact same situation exists with relation to all other minerals required for horse nutrition, if the individual mineral is not present in the soil in optimum amounts for plant growth, then that pasture will be deficient in that mineral for horse nutrition.

The only EXCEPTION to this rule is the CALCIUM and PHOSPHORUS content of grains. GRAINS always contain low levels of CALCIUM and very high levels of PHOSPHORUS. Nature designed grains this way, not because they are used for horse feeding but because PHOSPHORUS, as a plant nutrient, is responsible for efficient water use. Hence HIGH PHOSPHORUS levels in grains, in botanical terms SEEDS, allows the germinating seed to survive under more adverse soil moisture conditions than if the PHOSPHORUS level was less.

SODIUM CHLORIDE

also known as COMMON SALT or TABLE SALT, consists of sodium (Na) and Chlorine (Cl). Both these elements play an important part in maintaining the OSMOTIC PRESSURE of the body cells. This simply means maintaining the turgidity or INTERNAL CELL PRESSURE at a satisfactory level, so that transfer of food nutrients, to the individual body cells and the removal of waste products, from the individual body cells, is continuous, ensuring optimum growth and performance.

BLOOD also contains higher proportions of SODIUM and CHLORINE, than other minerals. Chlorine is also contained in some substances in the GASTRIC JUICES. These gastric juices are essential for breakdown and absorption of the food nutrients by the horse, and hence, a sub-optimal Chloride level, in the horse, could lead to food nutrients being excreted in the faeces and the urine and not being absorbed by the digestive tract.

The horse is UNABLE to store salt in its body in any reasonable amount. As salt is continually used and excreted by the horse, it is necessary for the animal to receive a continual daily intake.

Salt requirements depend on:

1. type and amount of work being undertaken
2. daily temperature
3. degree of sweating
4. humidity of the air

Horses, in work, have been known to lose up to 100 grams of salt in a 24 hour period. These particular horses were fed a diet which contained only 35 grams of salt per day, hence these horses were subject to a severe salt stress after only one days' work.

If animals receive insufficient salt, on a daily basis, the body cells cling excessively to the salt already inside the individual cells and excretion of salt in the urine is reduced. In sub-chronic conditions, where the horse is affected by lack of salt intake, but not sufficiently to be noticeable, the horse will not perform to its' ability. The owner will not notice any difference in the external appearance, only that performance is not up to expectations.

Symptoms of CHRONIC SALT DEFICIENCY in the horse are:

1. abnormal skin texture.
2. reduced speed of eating.
3. decreased water intake.
4. excessive appetite for salt

In SEVERE ACUTE SALT DEFICIENCY in horses, the symptoms include:-

5. muscle contractions.

6. peculiar chewing habits.
7. unsteady gaits and paces.

If salt was provided to animals with the above symptoms, a rapid recovery occurred.

As salt CANNOT be stored inside the horse, and intake by all animals needs to be on a daily basis, and the use of salt is similar in the horse and the cow, there is no reason why the symptoms of salt deficiency in the cow, as described above, should not also apply in the horse.

Salt is not an expensive feed nutrient and should be fed in all horse rations. The horse will excrete excess levels of salt, in the urine, so the problem is one of correcting SALT DEFICIENCY, not one of worrying about salt excess. For hand fed horses, either fully or partially hand fed, about 40 grams of salt per day in the ration is desirable for the average 450 kg horses, not performing much work. 40 grams of salt is equivalent to 2 tablespoons/ day, mixed into the ration. Horses sweating freely and performing hard work could need up to twice this level of daily salt addition to the ration.

Some nutritional references express salt intake as 0.5 to 1.0 % of the ration. If the horse is eating 10 kgs D.M/ day, 1.0% of 10 kgs is 100 grams.

Salt blocks and licks are sometimes provided for horses under partial, or complete grazing conditions, as a means of correcting salt deficiency.

Problems exist with the feeding of salt blocks in the paddock situation

1 Not all horses will eat salt given free access.
2. Some horses dominate in a mob and when given unrestricted access to salt blocks, prevent the weaker and or milder horses from getting access to the salt block.

(This is especially important in small paddocks with large numbers of horses where a domineering horse may prevent other horses from getting access to the salt block)

This system of voluntary intake of SALT, (self feeding) was examined in a recent scientific experiment. with mature unexercised horses for a period of up to 45 weeks. The amount of salt consumed on a daily basis, varied from 19 to 143 grams, the average level being about 53 grams. Horses tended to prefer access to free choice salt licks containing relatively low amounts of salt about 0.2 %.

The only sure way of ensuring that horses receive enough salt is to add salt daily to the concentrate or chaff part of the ration.

Salt deficiency in performance horses, especially race horses, has been mentioned on a number of occasions by veterinarians practicing in that field, as being a very common problem and probably a reason for poor performance, either as a straight salt deficiency or, more likely, as a part of a more involved nutritional and physiological problem.

Salt deficiency SHOULD NOT EXIST in the performance horse. The cost of the additional salt required to be added to a ration is very small, the compound when fed in excess is not detrimental to the animal, in fact it may assist CALCIUM and PHOSPHORUS absorption and retention in the body and it is known NOT TO AFFECT the utilisation of both MAGNESIUM and COPPER in the horse. Excess salt, above the horse's daily needs is excreted in the URINE.

CALCIUM AND PHOSPHORUS

These two minerals will be discussed together, because they COMPLEMENT or assist each other in the horse and must be available to the horse at the same time in specific amounts.

Calcium (Ca) and phosphorus (P) are responsible for BONE FORMATION, BONE GROWTH and MAINTENANCE. Horses fed rations or on pasture which are deficient or lacking in calcium and/or phosphorus will suffer reduced growth, reduced performance, malformed or thin bones, and other problems. This is commonly seen, in the horse, by way of stunted growth, bone problems including fractures, and allied conditions. CALCIUM is also required as an ELECTROLYTE, responsible for energy use during muscle contraction, and insufficient Calcium available to the horse for this purpose will mean that a horse cannot perform to the best of its ability.

Calcium and phosphorus make up about 75% of the mineral matter in the animal's body and about 90% of the minerals in the horse's skeleton. At 12 months of age, a normal foal will already contain 98% of the CALCIUM and 94% of the PHOSPHORUS, that the same horse will contain as a two year old, clearly indicating the need to ensure correct levels of CALCIUM and PHOSPHORUS in the diets of growing horses, especially in the first 12 months of age.

Hence the importance of adequate calcium and phosphorus being continually available, in the horse's ration, cannot be too greatly emphasised.

Calcium is also an important component of MILK and a plentiful calcium supply is absolutely essential for pregnant and lactating mares. Recent work has shown that some hoof wall problems require adequate levels of both CALCIUM and BIOTIN in the diet for increased strength in the hoof wall and correction of the problem.

In practice, CALCIUM is absorbed, by the horse, in the small intestine, the absorption process involving the active participation of VITAMIN D. PHOSPHORUS is absorbed, in the horse, primarily by the large intestine and secondarily, by the small intestine and also appears to play an important part in the absorption, by the horse, of VOLATILE FATTY ACIDS.

Subject to excessive levels of either or both minerals, the horse is able to store any calcium and phosphorus, not required for daily needs of growth and maintenance, inside the bone marrow. Dependent on the horses' diet, it is able to draw on this supply of calcium and phosphorus when the daily feed intake of either mineral is less than required, and the horse is able to replenish this store of the two minerals, when the diet again contains more calcium and phosphorus than the horse actually needs on a daily basis.

Whilst this mineral storage is excellent, we know very little of the actual amounts of calcium and phosphorus that can be stored in the bones. We are, therefore, unable to say whether the bones can supply enough calcium or phosphorus for one or one hundred days, when the ration being consumed, is low in both minerals. It is, therefore, desirable to ensure that the daily ration contains enough calcium and phosphorus for immediate needs.

Excessive levels of CALCIUM in the diet can cause INCREASED EXCRETION of PHOSPHORUS in the urine. In ponies fed at levels of 40 and 100 grams of CALCIUM/day, the higher level reduced the true digestibility of PHOSPHORUS in the ration by some 44%. Provided there is sufficient PHOSPHORUS in the ration, this is generally not a problem. High CALCIUM levels in the diet will, however, lead to increased water consumption and urine output as the kidneys act to attempt to eliminate the excess CALCIUM from the horse's body.

The actual availability of CALCIUM, to the horse, in most feeds is about 50-70% of the CALCIUM contained in those feeds, unless the feeds contain PHYTATE, as in grains or

OXALATE as in some pasture species, in which instances the CALCIUM availability will be considerably reduced below 70% of actual CALCIUM content.

Apart from its requirement, in conjunction, with CALCIUM in bone development, PHOSPHORUS is also required, within the horse, as part of the ENERGY TRANSFER system, being part of a number of compounds involved with energy use by the muscles.

PHOSPHORUS in the normal ration comes in two types, one form which is readily absorbed by the digestive tract, and a second form, known as PHYTIC PHOSPHORUS, which is much less digestible within the digestive tract. Most forms of PHYTIC PHOSPHORUS are excreted in the faeces.

The content of PHYTIC PHOSPHORUS compounds varies with feeds. Roughages, both green and dry contain very little PHYTIC PHOSPHORUS, in comparison to grains where the PHYTIC PHOSPHORUS levels can be very high, indicating additional care which needs to be taken to correct the CALCIUM and PHOSPHORUS levels in rations with a high grain content. The so called "BRAN DISEASE" caused as a direct result of feeding high levels of bran with no corrective CALCIUM supplement added, is due in part to the very high PHYTATE level in bran.

In terms of actual PHOSPHORUS availability, about 30% only of the P, in grain, is available to horses, about 45% in roughages and about 60% in any P supplement.

Excessive levels of PHOSPHORUS, in the ration, is known to depress the absorption of CALCIUM, by the small intestine, due to the formation of CALCIUM PHYTIC compounds which are virtually not absorbed in the digestive tract. This produces a condition, known as NUTRITIONAL SECONDARY HYPERPARATHYROIDISM (N.S.H.).

CALCIUM AND PHOSPHORUS DEFICIENCY OR IMBALANCE

Adequate bone growth in the horse is a function of the correct amounts of Calcium, Phosphorus and VITAMIN D being available to the animal. Lack of either or both of these two minerals, and or insufficient VITAMIN D generally produces the condition known as RICKETS, the severity of the RICKETS depending on the levels of the two minerals and VITAMIN D NOT AVAILABLE to the horse.

With RICKETS, the blood becomes deficient in one or both minerals, and the bones then do not grow normally in size or in strength. Weak bones may readily fracture with a work level that normal horses can accept without injury.

The initial visual signs of rickets are stiffness, swollen joints, bent knees and often sag in the back immediately behind the shoulders. Animals with RICKETS may be easily excited, breathing may be rapid and the animals may chew bones, wood and bark.

In young animals, growth will be restricted, although this will not be immediately noticed, if only marginal or complicated by other factors such as lack of protein as well in the diet. In most instances the occurrence of restricted growth MAY NEVER be noticed.

Practicing horse veterinarians indicate that the classical symptoms of RICKETS as described above are very rarely seen. In practice the Ca/P deficiency and/or imbalance is generally sub-chronic and often shown by some vague dysfunction and/or lameness. There may well be other complicating problems, with such a horse, as well as Ca and P problems.

RICKETS and its associated symptoms may be cured if diagnosed at a very early stage and correct early supplementation of any calcium and/or phosphorus imbalance takes place as well as correction of any possible VITAMIN D deficiency or excess.

However, any PERMANENT effects of low calcium and/or phosphorus levels in the previous rations will not be corrected. If a sway back or crooked legs exist, as a result of rickets, feeding Ca or P will only strengthen the malformed bones. Feeding will not cause the bones to straighten.

With some specific exceptions, CALCIUM deficiency does not exist in horses obtaining most or all of their feed intake from pasture. The one known exception has been in horses grazing on pasture growing on sandy acid soils in Victoria.

By far, the largest number of problems which occur due to a lack of CALCIUM, in the diet, are in horses which are fed rations which contain reasonable levels of grains or grain by-products, (bran and pollard), all these feeds are very low in levels of CALCIUM.

PHOSPHORUS DEFICIENCY as an individual problem can occur. Many soils are deficient in the levels of phosphorus needed for adequate plant growth. Animals, including horses, grazing such pasture, are therefore receiving less phosphorus in their feed than they normally require. PHOSPHORUS DEFICIENCY or inadequate phophorus intake reduces the digestibility of the many food nutrients leading to reduction in appetite, an overall reduced growth rate and a general unthrifty appearance including harsh light coloured coat. These symptoms are also common to a number of other problems in the horse e.g. worm infestation so careful diagnosis of the problem is required. Lack of phosphorus can also affect milk production in lactating mares, causing the mare to produce less milk than normal and often to prematurely dry up.

Animals suffering from a lack of phophorus are also supposed to chew bones, wood etc., in an effort to gain the deficient mineral.

Phosphorus deficiency MAY also be created within the horse, if the horse is eating pasture which contains high levels of MOLYBDENUM. Levels of MOLYBDENUM in pasture, of the order of 5-25 p.p.m. have been found to affect PHOSPHORUS utilisation in the horse. It is possible that the PHOSPHORUS level of the ration could be at a satisfactory level but RICKETS could still occur, due to a high level of MOLYBDENUM in the feed, affecting the utilisation of the PHOSPHORUS.

Considerable amounts of CALCIUM can be lost in SWEAT, as an electrolyte, and this can be especially severe in two and three year old racehorses and pacers. These horses are still growing, whilst being expected to perform at what is classified as heavy work rates.

Hence, these types of horses need extra amounts of calcium in the ration for use as an ELECTROLYTE in muscle function, over and above those levels required for BONE growth and maintenance.

Some people have suggested that feeding of excess protein may be related to development of skeletal disorders, especially enlargement at the ends of the bones and also contracted tendons. Recent studies have shown that there is no effect on calcium uptake by various levels of protein, PROVIDED THE ENERGY LEVEL of the ration is kept CONSTANT. If, however, both PROTEIN and ENERGY levels of the rations of young growing horses are increased above the expected values, there is the possibility of increased excretion occurring of both CALCIUM and PHOSPHORUS from the horse.

Calcium and phophorus intake is based on two established criteria, ABSOLUTE DAILY INTAKE and CALCIUM/ PHOSPHORUS RATIOS.

ABSOLUTE AMOUNTS OF CALCIUM AND PHOSPHORUS

A 450 kg. mature horse, at rest or in light work, requires 23g Ca and 14g P per day to maintain the normal body levels and efficient body operation and these amounts HAVE to be supplied within the expected 10Kgs daily DRY MATTER intake of the horse. Young growing horses will require a slightly higher amount of each mineral, relative to the appropriate body weight and lactating mares will have increased needs at the same body weight.

Whilst CALCIUM and PHOSPHORUS are recognised as being the most important minerals in development of the skeleton of the horse, such skeletal development can be affected by deficiencies of COPPER, ZINC and possibly SELENIUM in the ration, even if CALCIUM and PHOSPHORUS are present in the correct amounts.

If this 450 kg "reference" horse is fully grown, i.e. over four years of age, and neither a brood mare or an active performance horse, there can be an increase in the Calcium level of the ration compared to that of Phosphorus, as bone growth has been completed and only bone maintenance and muscle function needs to be considered. For these types of horses, Phosphorus intake has to remain at 14 grams/day but Calcium intake can rise to about 84 grams/day, without affecting the horse.

Mature fully grown horses are able to withstand a much higher amounts of Calcium in the ration than at any earlier age, PROVIDED the amount of PHOSPHORUS remains the same.

Young growing horses, under 4 years of age, but especially under 1 year of age have very critical CALCIUM and PHOSPHORUS needs in the feed. The amount of CALCIUM required cannot exceed 3 times the amount of PHOSPHORUS in the ration whilst the desirable amounts are in the order of CALCIUM BEING double the amount of PHOSPHORUS present.

BROOD MARES and any PERFORMANCE horse, actively competing, have a demand for the two minerals very similar to that of 23 grams Ca and 14 grams P per day, the brood mare for effective foetal growth and lactation, and the performance horse for bone strength and efficient muscle function.

The following Table explains the minimum quantity of the various feeds that the mature horse needs to eat to get the required level of the CALCIUM and PHOSPHORUS present in that feed in the least quantity.

The table also shows the level of CALCIUM and or PHOSPHORUS supplementation required in grams per day of the other mineral to bring the Ca/P ratio to the desired value of 1.3 Ca/1.0 P.

On a ration basis, only the green plants and their hays supply enough CALCIUM and PHOSPHORUS for mature horses on an expected daily feed intake basis, the EXCEPTIONS being kikuyu with the problem of oxalate content described earlier, and green growing oats. The pasture species described or their hays, can be fed, without worry, about correcting the level of Ca or P in the ration.

Skim milk is balanced for CALCIUM and PHOSPHORUS as well, and no corrective supplements need be fed if skim milk constituted the whole ration, which is most unlikely, due to cost and the inability of some horses to digest skim milk, leading to scours and other problems.

The basic feed grains and oil seed meals are however all deficient in Ca to some extent. Further it is not possible, with some grains, for the horse to physically eat enough feed to get the minimum quantity of some minerals. It is impossible to get a horse with a digestive capacity of 10 kgs per day to eat 19 kgs of maize, 33 kgs of barley or 23 kgs of oats in order to get the minimum quantity of CALCIUM.

Complicating this even further, is that these levels of grain feeding would not supply enough protein to all but mature resting horses, and are sub-standard or below daily requirements, regarding PROTEIN level, for horses performing any sort of work.

CALCIUM/PHOSPHORUS RATIO

At the physical levels of CALCIUM and PHOSPHORUS intake desirable for a growing horse, to 4 years of age, an ideal ratio exists between the two minerals of 1.3 parts Ca to 1 part P.

Commonly called the CALCIUM/PHOSPHORUS RATIO, this indicator is often used as a a means of expressing the needs of CALCIUM and PHOSPHORUS in the ration.

It has generally been accepted that the CA/P RATIOS in the ration should be:-

IDEAL RATIO FOR ALL HORSES	1.3 Ca/1.0 P
USUALLY ACCEPTED	
FOR MOST RATIONSranging from	2.0 Ca/1.0 P to 1.0 Ca/1.0 P
YOUNG HORSES LARGEST RATIO	3.0 Ca/1.0 P
MATURE HORSES over 4 years	6.0 Ca/1.0 P

It is desirable, from a horse feeding angle, that the use of Ca/P ratios in ration formulation and feed marketing be IGNORED. If the following explanation is carefully followed, it will have to be appreciated that we are only confusing ourselves, and others, by continuing to use CALCIUM/PHOSPHORUS RATIOS.

IF HORSE RATIONS ARE FORMULATED TO CONTAIN THE MINIMUM REQUIRED WEIGHT OF PHOSPHORUS ON A DAILY BASIS AND THE DAILY EXPECTED CALCIUM INTAKE IS THEN ADJUSTED TO BE AT LEAST 50% HIGHER, THE HORSE WILL BE RECEIVING ADEQUATE SUPPLIES OF BOTH MINERALS.

The correct CALCIUM/PHOSPHORUS RATIO will naturally occur, if the necessary physical amounts of each mineral are present in the horse feed.

The use of CALCIUM/PHOSPHORUS RATIOS in horse feeding is leading to the formulation, and sale, of horse rations which CONTAIN CALCIUM AND PHOSPHORUS in the correct ratio, BUT AT PHYSICAL LEVELS WHICH are less than the horse's daily needs, sometimes only half the daily physical requirements. Horses being fed such rations must, at some stage, suffer a CALCIUM AND PHOSPHORUS DEFICIENCY.

At this current time, horses obtaining most or all of their feed requirements from grazing pasture WILL NOT SUFFER a CALCIUM DEFICIENCY problem. Pastures, in general, contain adequate levels of CALCIUM, and the only known CALCIUM DEFICIENCY which has occurred in horses grazing pasture has been where the pasture has been growing on acid sandy soils, as in a small part of VICTORIA.

The greatest number of reports of CALCIUM DEFICIENCY occur in horses whose rations contain a reasonable amount of GRAINS or GRAIN BY-PRODUCTS. These feeds are dangerously LOW in CALCIUM compared to PHOSPHORUS, and a CALCIUM supplement should always be added in correct amounts to the diet. As these horses are always hand fed, and even if grazing also provides some daily feed intake, it is convenient and simple to add CALCIUM to the hand feed, ensuring constant and adequate daily intake.

CORRECTING CALCIUM AND PHOSPHORUS LEVELS

In practice, more attention is paid to the correction of calcium levels, because under stabled conditions, grain is generally fed at reasonable levels, leading to a calcium deficiency in the ration. However, there is the possibility of CALCIUM EXCESS problems occurring in brood mares and horses under 2 years of age grazing pastures, predominantly legume in content or being fed rations based principally on legume hay, particularly ALFALFA (LUCERNE), PHOSPHORUS DEFICIENCY problems occurring in brood mares and young horses being grazed on pasture of principally grass composition, including winter cereals, oats, barley and wheat, or being fed hay or chaff made from those pastures.

Various supplements are available, including finely ground limestone or calcium carbonate and calcium gluconate. The former is probably the supplement of choice, being available at most produce outlets, readily assimilated by the horse, and reasonable in price.

For correction of both calcium and phophorus deficiencies, dicalcium phosphate or bone meal can be used.

Ca AND P REQUIREMENTS FOR A 450 KG HORSE
(at rest or light work)
Expected feed intake at 10 kgs per day of dry matter.

Feed	Ca/P	Min. Feed Levels	Grams of mineral required to balance ration to a ratio between 3/1 to 1/1 Ca	P
Lucerne hay	4.2	3.88 kgs	0	18
Paspalum	1.04	6.36 kgs	0	0
Subterraneum clover	3.43	6.08 kgs	0	7
Rye grass	2.53	4.66 kgs	0	0
White clover	3.47	4.11 kgs	0	0
Kikuyu (oxalates?)	1.69	5.38 kgs	0	0
Green oats	0.47	9.20 kgs	41	0
Oaten chaff	1.00	7.48 kgs	5	0
Oaten grain	0.30	23.00 kgs	76	0
Barley grain	0.22	32.80 kgs	109	0
Maize grain	0.52	19.16 kgs	35	0
Linseed meal	0.46	5.60 kgs	42	0
Soybean meal	0.74	3.15 kgs	18	0
Skim milk powder	1.31	1.57 kgs	0	0

OXALATES AND CALCIUM DEFICIENCY

In sub-tropical and tropical regions, horses suffer from a condition called "BIG HEAD". "BIG HEAD" is the end result of an induced CALCIUM DEFICIENCY, in horses, caused by the grass component of tropical pastures containing substances called OXALATES and is the common term for the condition, technically, known as NUTRITIONAL SECONDARY HYPREPARATHRYOIDISM.

OXALATES bind CALCIUM in the digestive tract and make it unavailable for the the normal functions of BONE formation and maintenance and for use as an ELECTROLYTE in the horse. Where the grazing intake of the horse is such that the CALCIUM level, is ideal but OXALATE is present in the pasture, the OXALATE reduces the availability of the CALCIUM to the horse BEFORE THE CALCIUM IS ABSORBED in the digestive tract. If there is insufficient CALCIUM in the pasture to "satisfy the appetite" of the OXALATE, CALCIUM is then withdrawn from the bones of the horse.

OXALATE problems are now known to occur in horses when the CALCIUM/OXALATE ratio in the grass is 0.5/1.0 or less, and this generally occurs when the total OXALATE concentration, in the DRY MATTER, exceeded 0.5%. OXALATE has also been found in lucerne hay but at concentrations which in general are much below the level needed to affect CALCIUM uptake by the horse.

OXALATES are also known to depress the absorption of PHOSPHORUS from the diet but the effect on the horse is not nearly as marked as with OXALATE effect on CALCIUM absorption.

MEASUREMENT OF CALCIUM AND PHOSPHORUS

1. Analysis of hair
2. Analysis of urine
3. Ration analysis
4. Blood analysis

Problems exist with all three methods:

1. HAIR ANALYSIS can be affected by:-

age of animal, colour of hair, location of hair on the body and season of the year.
The results are too variable for practical use.

2. URINE ANALYSIS is based on the fact that about 30% of the CALCIUM absorbed by the horse is excreted in the horse's urine. However, urine concentrations of minerals depend on the horse's water balance and is essential, when using urine analysis for mineral status determination to recognise and make allowances for this problem. Drugs to increase urine flow cannot be used, as these alter the levels of calcium and phosphorus excretion and hence do not lead to correct results. Short term starvation of horses on pasture (only 2-4 hours) can reduce markedly the level of calcium excreted.

The use of this test for horses on pasture makes it necessary to sample a representative number of horses from the mob to reduce the errors caused by restricted water intake or short term starvation.

3. RATION ANALYSIS. The levels of calcium and phosphorus in virtually all feed components used for horses are generally listed in all nutritional books or can be readily obtained from laboratory analysis.

However there appears to be considerable variation in the calcium and phosphorus levels published for the same feed in the same country. The following table compares the calcium and phosphorus levels expressed as mgs/KG in some common horse feeds for one area of one country.

	No. 1			No. 2			No. 3		
	Ca	P	Ratio	Ca	P	Ratio	Ca	P	Ratio
OATS	.83	5.06	.16	1.2	2.3	.52	.6	2.5	.20
MAIZE	.19	2.75	.52	1.0	3.3	.30	.6	3.0	.20
BARLEY	.44	3.74	.11	.7	3.1	.22	.7	3.0	.23
BRAN	1.40	11.88	.11	2.0	11.9	1.6	1.2	8.0	.13
SOYBEAN MEAL	2.79	6.49	.42	7.3	9.8	.74	2.7	6.3	.42
LINSEED MEAL	3.98	8.53	.46	4.1	8.9	.46	3.8	8.1	.46
MOLASSES	7.48	.79	9.46	2.4	6.6	15.84	11.5	.7	16.42

A careful look at this Table may be confusing to some, but in fact it reveals a considerable variation in the calcium and phophorus content of each feed. The major variations are:

The P level for oats varies from 2.3 to 5.86
The Ca level for maize varies from .19 to 1.00
The Ca level for soybean meal level varies from 2.7 to 7.3
The Ca level in molasses varies from 2.4 to 11.5
The P level in molasses varies from .79 to 6.6

This variation, in levels of the same mineral in the same feed, is considerable and does not help the formulation of horse rations if using general feed analysis figures for ration formulation. The Ca and P levels of some feeds will depend on which set of tables are used. With variations of up to 78% around the average value, and up to 735% increase on the least value, as in the actual P level of molasses, it is difficult to become precise in measuring mineral supplement needs.

Variations in Ca and especially P levels in feed, are due to

1. different laboratory techniques used to determine the levels of the two minerals.
2. differing plant growing conditions, especially re soil fertility and climate in the area where the crop is grown.

In those feeding situations, where where it is critical that CALCIUM and PHOSPHORUS levels be known exactly, laboratory analysis should be carried out on all the feed samples and actual results used in ration formulation.

4. BLOOD ANALYSIS. Continuous variation exists in the levels of calcium and phosphorus detected in blood samples. Often these values are outside the normal range but do not appear to be related to any deficiency or excess of either mineral. The use of calcium and phosphorus levels in the blood as a direct assessment of the status of either mineral in the horse can be misleading and is generally not recommended.

Some veterinarians, however, may use the calcium and phophorus levels in the blood with other factors to assess possible Ca and P levels.

One particular method of assessment involves the relationship between high blood calcium levels and alkaline phosphate (AP) enzyme levels. The second method uses urinary excretion rates of calcium and phosphorus, urine specific gravity, blood phosphorus and creatinine levels to monitor the Ca/P balance in the horse.

Both methods require the experience of an animal nutritionist or veterinary surgeon to effectively appreciate the readings and to diagnose a possible result. The use of these techniques are definitely not for the untrained horse person.

LIMESTONE, SOIL pH AND HORSE NUTRITION

CALCIUM, as an important component in horse nutrition, is also a valuable mineral as far as growing plants are concerned. Calcium in the soil has the following effects on plant growth.

1 - Calcium is required by all plants for normal cell division.

2 - Calcium forms part of the material that makes up the cell walls.

3 - Calcium is one of the salt compounds inside the plant cells.

4 - Calcium forms part of the genetic coding material of the individual plant cells.

Calcium is a component of most soil minerals and particularly in LIMESTONE (calcium carbonate) and in GYPSUM (calcium sulphate). Calcium carbonate has the effect of providing calcium to the plants as a plant nutrient and, at the same time, has an effect on soil pH. Calcium sulphate, on the other hand, will also supply calcium to growing plants but has no effect on soil pH.

Soil pH is simply a measure of the acidity or alkalinity of the soil. In general chemistry, the pH of any material ranges from 0 to 14. In practical agricultural situations, the soil pH values are generally in the range of 5.0 to 7.0, but extremes do occur. Peat bogs have shown very acid readings of 3.0, whilst some arid, very dry desert soils have shown extreme soil pH values in the alkaline end of 10.5.

There are twelve generally accepted plant nutrients and it is commonly recognised that the maximum availability of all these nutrients occurs in the soil pH range of 6.0 to 7.0.

LIME, as LIMESTONE, for pasture top dressing is a natural product mined from various localities throughout the world. Due to this fact, LIME comes in all types of qualities and some limes are of little or no value on agricultural use, as the lime particles are not small enough to be absorbed into the soil in a reasonable time, and also because of the contaminants, in the form of soil, clay etc. in the lime.

To be effective, Lime needs to be cultivated into the ground to be of any value in raising soil pH, and even when this cultivation is carried out after lime spreading, there may be a period of 12 - 24 months after application, before any significant response is noticed in an increase in pH levels. Lime spread on top of the ground and not cultivated in, may take years to have any effect on soil pH in the root zone of the plants. Lime generally acts in raising soil pH for a few years, usually about 4 years, dependent on the soil type, and then a further application of LIME is generally necessary to maintain soil pH at the increased level.

In this context of optimum plant growth, the pH scale is important, PROVIDED all the 12 plant nutrients are present in the soil in optimum amounts, and that the soil pH value is, in fact, the ONLY LIMITING FACTOR to nutrient availability.

When consideration is made of the value of CALCIUM in horse nutrition, recognition must also be made of the interrelated effects of CALCIUM and PHOSPHORUS in bone formation. This has been discussed in detail earlier, but suffice to say that correcting a CALCIUM IMBALANCE in the soil, without attention being paid to the soil

PHOSPHORUS LEVEL, will only increase the IMBALANCE between the two minerals, and SKELETAL and GROWTH problems can be caused, in horses grazing pasture on such treated paddocks, not only by a lack of either or both calcium or phosphorus, but also by an imbalance between the two minerals in the pasture.

THE APPLICATION OF LIME TO A SOIL TO RAISE SOIL pH AND TO PROVIDE CALCIUM FOR GROWTH IN HORSES WILL BE TECHNICALLY INCORRECT IF THAT SOIL IS ALREADY DEFICIENT IN PHOSPHORUS FOR NORMAL PLANT

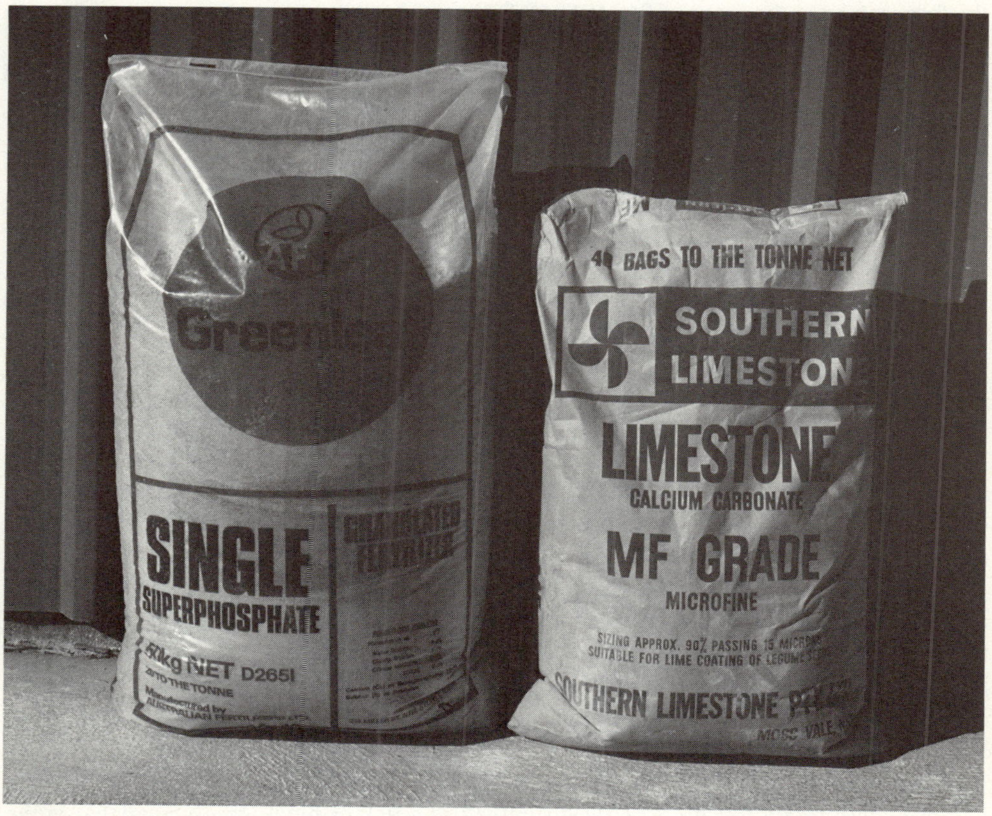

Calcium is best supplied as a feed additive from limestone, Superphosphate, applied to the pasture,is the best way to grow feed and supply Calcium and Phosphorus to the grazing horse.

GROWTH AND NO ATTEMPT IS MADE TO CORRECT THE PHOSPHORUS DEFICIENCY.

Horse people have just assumed that if CALCIUM is applied to the ground as CALCIUM CARBONATE or LIME, it will become immediately available to the horse and therefore build better bones and presumably grow better horses. There is little technical information available on this subject, largely because the supply of CALCIUM to horses, or other grazing livestock, on all types of pasture has NEVER been a problem which has been considered of sufficient concern to warrant research of any detail. There has been a CALCIUM uptake problem diagnosed in horses in VICTORIA, specifically restricted to pasture plants growing on a small and specific area of very acid sandy soils, but this is the only CALCIUM uptake problem of grazing horses reported in the technical literature

Australian prices for lime, spread on the ground, will vary from around $20 to $90 per tonne, dependent on the quality of the lime and the distance the lime has to be transported from the quarry to the farm.

At the common application rates of 2 to 4 tonnes per hectare the spread costs of lime on the farm can be in the range of $40 to $360 /hectare.

If, in this example, horses are being carried at the rate of one horse to one hectare, and that is very good carrying capacity on pasture, then the cost of providing calcium as a food nutrient by one lime application will be in the order of $40 to $360 per horse. Generally, the lime has an affect on soil pH which lasts, on average, four years, so the cost/horse /year of providing lime by this method will be from $10 to $90 /horse per year. This use of lime however, has no effect on the level of soil phosphorus.

CALCIUM AND SUPPLEMENTARY FEEDING

In the case of horses which have access to full or supplementary hand feeding, an alternative exists for the feeding of lime.

Micro-fine lime, 30 grams of which will contain 10 grams of CALCIUM, can be mixed in the feed to the level of 60 grams per horse per day. In normal horse feeding language, 60 grams is equal to 2 tablespoons.

Micro-fine lime is calcium carbonate which has been finely crushed and has had all the foreign matter and contaminants removed. It is commonly used in the lime coating process of legume seeds where it has to protect specific bacteria from destruction by heat and sunlight and is the best available form of limestone to feed to a horse.

This addition of CALCIUM to the daily feeds will ensure that the horse receives an excess of lime and should in general terms not suffer from problems. Based on current costs, this method of feeding lime to horses works out at about 0.8 cents per day, or just under $25 per horse per year, considerably cheaper than supplying CALCIUM to the horse from either the topdressing of pasture with limestone or the application of superphosphate.

CALCIUM LICKS.

Horses will rarely touch CALCIUM supplied as a lick or block, freely available in the paddock. In Queensland, a block has been formulated to supply CALCIUM in a grazing situation to horses eating pastures containing OXALATES. The block consists of CALCIUM CARBONATE, DICALCIUM PHOSPHATE, MOLASSES and SALT and consumption under free range grazing conditions are satisfactory for CALCIUM supply in this situation, provided allowances are made for the problems which occur in the feeding of horses in mobs.

NOTE -THE HORSE REQUIRES CALCIUM CARBONATE, commonly called LIMESTONE. Other lime products, including QUICKLIME and SLAKED LIME SHOULD NEVER BE FED TO A HORSE, they will damage the digestive tract. If in doubt as to which type of LIME or CALCIUM SUPPLEMENT you are feeding, place a small quantity in some water, if the mixture heats up, bubbles and lets off visible gases, that product IS NOT TO BE FED TO A HORSE.

PHOSPHORUS SUPPLEMENTATION

It is most unlikely that the ration of any hand fed horse will require the addition of PHOSPHORUS, to correct a PHOSPHORUS deficiency, simply because most grains are already high in PHOSPHORUS and most pastures and pasture hays contain sufficient of both CALCIUM and PHOSPHORUS. If however PHOSPHORUS has to be corrected in a ration, do so by adding DICALCIUM PHOSPHATE, each 30 grams of which will add 7 grams of CALCIUM and 6 grams of PHOSPHORUS to the ration. Having corrected the PHOSPHORUS problem, has probably now created a CALCIUM PROBLEM which can be corrected by the addition of MICRO-FINE LIMESTONE at the correctly calculated amount to the same feed.

DO NOT, UNDER ANY CIRCUMSTANCES, USE SUPERPHOSPHATE OR ANY FERTILISER CONTAINING PHOSPHORUS AS A SUPPLEMENT TO CORRECT PHOSPHORUS DEFICIENCY IN A HORSE RATION. THESE PHOSPHORUS SOURCES HAVE NOT HAD THE FLUORINE CONTENT REMOVED AND MAY PRODUCED PROBLEMS IN THE HORSE, DUE TO EXCESSIVE FLUORINE LEVELS.

CORRECTING SOIL PHOSPHORUS DEFICIENCY

Many soils are deficient in phosphorus, and in these soils, the limiting factor to plant growth is not the soil pH but rather the low level of natural phosphorus. Soil phosphorus levels can be increased by the application of the fertiliser called superphosphate, which provides not only phosphorus as a plant nutrient but also calcium in the form of calcium sulphate. Whilst the use of superphosphate will not increase soil pH, it will increase the level of two of the important plant nutrients, i.e. P and Ca. As well, provided improved pasture species are sown at the same time as reasonable superphosphate applications are used, is is quite likely that an increase in carrying capacity will result, up to 50% or more. In this situation the horse is able to graze pasture that contains INCREASED LEVELS of calcium and phosphorus, and it should be possible to graze more horses on the same area after pasture improvement and the continued application of superphosphate.

In Australia, the average PHOSPHORUS DEFICIENT soil would need superphosphate at the rate of 250 kgs per hectare for about four years. At a superphosphate price of around $240 per tonne on the ground, this programme would use 1 tonne in four years, or /hectare/year price of $60. However, in normal pasture improvement situations, the expected increase in stocking rate would occur so that the carrying capacity would end up being in the order of one horse to 0.66 hectares - a 50% increase.

On this basis the cost per horse per year of supplying calcium by this method would be $45.

The application of superphosphate is NOT to correct a lime or calcium problem, but to supply PHOSPHORUS which is already present in less than desirable levels in the soil. Increased SOIL PHOSPHORUS levels allows and encourages plants to grow larger and stronger and to SUPPLY PHOSPHORUS to the horse to allow the CALCIUM/PHOSPHORUS ratio in the overall feed intake to approximate the needs of both minerals, by the horse, for efficient growth.

The individual property cost of lime as opposed to superphosphate, will vary depending on the location of the property to the lime quarry, and/or the superphosphate works. Transport and spreading costs will play an important part in the choice of calcium supply. It will be an individual property decision as to the best method to use.

The important points to remember when considering the use of lime applied to pasture are:

1. CORRECT THE SOIL PHOSPHORUS LEVEL FIRST. An increase in soil pH will not increase availability of phosphorus, if the soil already is deficient in the mineral.

2. Application of lime to a pasture may extend the Ca/P ratio, due to the increase in the calcium level in the soil and no increase in the phosphorus level. This can lead to bone growth and maintenance problems, due to the horse feeding on pasture with an imbalanced Ca/P ration.

3. Lime very rarely acts instantly to raise soil pH. Lime may take up to two to three years to effectively change soil pH.

4. If it is necessary to correct a horse ration for calcium, it will generally be more economical to feed limestone supplements to the horse either directly mixed with the supplementary feed, or as a prepared block with molasses and salt, rather than top dress pasture with lime.

HIGH LIMESTONE SOILS

It is commonly accepted, in certain sections of the horse industry, that particular areas are excellent for producing horses, due to the LIMESTONE CONTENT of the soils and or the WATER.

As mentioned earlier in this section, CALCIUM is very rarely a problem as far as plant growth is concerned, whereas LOW PHOSPHORUS LEVELS can be of considerable concern in a number of soil types, both as a limiting factor in plant growth, and from this fact, a limiting factor in animal growth.

There are many documented cases where the increase in the soil PHOSPHORUS level, by the application of superphosphate or a similar fertiliser containing PHOSPHORUS, has provided a noticeable increase in animal growth, WITHOUT THE APPLICATION of additional CALCIUM in the form of LIMESTONE to the soil to the soil.

Observations over many years of numerous soil tests from many horse regions in Australia lead to a conclusion that GOOD HORSE COUNTRY is NOT HIGH in natural limestone but in fact has HIGH NATURAL PHOSPHORUS levels.

Whilst no research appears to have been carried out on this topic, it would appear logical that soils with high natural levels of PHOSPHORUS would probably have higher levels of CALCIUM and PHOSPHORUS in the soil and therefore in the plants growing on such soils, leading to the the production of better horses.

Practical observation confirms that all the good horses are produced from properties where the soils will either have high natural phosphorus levels or alternately on soils where the low natural phosphorus levels have been increased by the application of phosphorus containing fertilisers.

IRON

IRON is essential to horse nutrition as it is involved in the following body processes:

1. Blood haemoglobin, which carries oxygen throughout the body, contains iron.
2. Iron is necessary, in minute amounts for efficient functioning of all body cells, as the nuclei in each cell contains the mineral.
3. Iron is contained in some enzymes that are responsible for the use of food nutrients in the digestive tract of the horse.

Iron is present in animals in very small amounts, in fact micro-amounts. About 70% of the iron in the body is contained in the red blood cells and, in this form, is continually being re-used by the horse with only a very slow loss or wastage. All horses, from the rapidly growing foal to the mature horse, require a diet containing about 40 p.p.m., IRON on a daily basis, to satisfy their iron requirements. This daily need is only exceeded when the horse carries a heavy internal parasite burden (is wormy) or in situations where, for some reason such as injury, the horse has suffered severe blood loss.

Analysis of all the common horse feeds reveal iron levels well over 40 p.p.m. of iron. In fact some of the feeds contain up to 500 p.p.m. as in lucerne hay.

1. Feeds below 40 p.p.m. Maize grain, skim milk.
2. Feeds 40 - 100 p.p.m. Oats, sorghum.
3. Feeds above 100 p.p.m. Barley, bran, pollard, soybean meal, sunflower seed, all pasture species, and the hays or chaff made from such species.

IRON DEFICIENCY

Lack of iron, in the horse' diet, will decrease haemoglobin level as well as red blood cell count, and symptoms may include very pale mucous membranes-lips, gums, eyelids etc.-lethargy, loss of body condition and a tendency to become tired earlier than normal, the exact same symptoms of internal parasite infestations. Once the haemoglobin level and red blood cell count are increased to normal values, additional iron in the feed, or as any form of supplement, will not increase either component. Iron is often added to a horses' diet in the mistaken belief that it will increase either the number of RED BLOOD CELLS and or the amount of HAEMOGLOBIN in the horse. When the results of a BLOOD COUNT are examined, the critical factor, with RED BLOOD CELLS and HAEMOGLOBIN levels are BELOW NORMAL FIGURES, not ABOVE NORMAL FIGURES. Each horse can only carry a certain amount of blood and that blood can only carry a certain quantity of RED BLOOD CELLS and once those respective levels are reached, NO ADDITIONAL AMOUNT OF IRON IN THE DIET WILL MAKE ANY DIFFERENCE to either blood component.

Deficiency of iron in horse diets very rarely occurs. The only documented cases involve the effect of very high levels of PHOSPHORUS in the ration where iron was prevented from being held in reserve, within the lining of the digestive tract.

Iron deficiency symptoms generally occur when the horse has suffered some problems with the haemoglobin content of the blood. This can occur from loss of blood due to injury, heavy internal parasite infestations not treated by correct and continual drenching, or by some specific veterinary problems such as small cell anaemia.

These occasions are generally well recognised by some horse people, and some appropriate iron supplement fed for short periods of time, up to three weeks, until the horse gets back to normal, refer ANAEMIA in chapter titled NUTRITIONAL DISORDERS.

IRON EXCESS

IRON has been fed at levels of up to 545 mgs /horse/day, to mature horses, for a period of 42 days, some 13 times the normal daily requirement. This extremely high level of feeding IRON DID NOT affect the HAEMOGLOBIN level or the PACKED CELL VOLUME of the blood. Where the same levels of IRON were fed to the horse, in conjunction with LIVE YEAST CULTURES, again no significant increase was found in either blood component. In fact, the weekly fluctuations in HAEMOGLOBIN LEVEL and PACKED CELL VOLUME were considerable, considering that the horses were all fed and treated the same.

IRON is normally held in reserve in the lining of the digestive tract and when required for the production of new red blood cells, the IRON is bonded to specific proteins and transported to the bone marrow. The body contains a self regulating mechanism, known as HOMEOSTASIS which only allows a certain quantity of IRON to be held in the digestive tract for later use. Any IRON, fed to the horse in excess of the normal needs will be stored at and in various other tissues, within the horse, where firstly it will NOT BE accessible for use by the horse as the bonding proteins, specific to the digestive tract cannot get to it, and secondly the excess iron can cause toxicity problems.

There are indications that iron fed in excess to horses, i.e. over and above their normal daily requirements, may decrease growth rate, cause diarrhoea, drowsiness, partial shock, severely reduce the effectiveness of the liver to function correctly and, more importantly, the excess iron may interfere with phosphorus and other mineral absorption leading to poorly mineralised bone being produced. Similarly, high PHOSPHORUS levels in the ration can affect the availability of iron for use by the horse. Hence, iron fed, in excess of the horse's daily needs, can lead to bone disorders and fractures, and possible death.

Young foals are extremely susceptible to the administration of excess or additional IRON. Deaths have occurred, from severe liver damage, in young foals given IRON supplements within 8 hours of birth, in the mistaken belief that the additional iron would assist growth rate.

IRON AND ANABOLIC STEROIDS

There has been some use of iron supplements, given in conjunction with ANABOLIC STEROID treatments which are given to some horses to increase body muscling. The muscle building action of the ANABOLIC STEROIDS appears to give better results if additional iron is supplied to the horse at the same time as the ANABOLIC STEROID treatments are being applied. The practice of the administration of ANABOLIC STEROIDS to horses in some competitive horse sports is now BANNED and so the need for iron administration in these instances will no longer be required. However in some horse activities ANABOLIC STEROIDS can still be used.

This practice of the use of muscle building compounds in some horses can lead to a problem when the horse is taken off the compounds, most horses so treated will, after removal of the drugs, develop a harsh coated appearance, appear to lack muscling and be lethargic and generally NOT RESPOND to most known methods of feeding to get a horse well conditioned. These horses appear to have muscles where the energy use functions have been completely changed by the previous administration of drugs and the only way to get them back, to what appears a normal physical state, is to subject the horse to a further treatment of ANABOLIC STEROIDS and iron. If it is possible to find out from the previous owner and or trainer of the horse, exactly what was given to the animal, it will help to sort out the problem but most people are reluctant to admit that they use these types of drugs on their horses. If such compounds are to be used, they should only be used under veterinary supervision.

MAGNESIUM

MAGNESIUM is responsible for BONE formation, being involved with CALCIUM and PHOSPHORUS as part of the mineral content of body cells. MAGNESIUM is also needed, as a form of ELECTROLYTE, for the use of GLYCOGEN for energy production by the muscle cells. The absorption of MAGNESIUM, in the diet, takes place in the small intestine of the horse. Horses require about 6.5 grams daily of magnesium, and with the exception of whey, all common horse feeds contain sufficient magnesium for practical needs. HYPOMAGNESIA or MAGNESIUM TETANY (magnesium deficiency) is a problem with sheep and cattle, but horses grazing the same pasture have not been affected by any lack of MAGNESIUM in the diet. Symptoms of MAGNESIUM DEFICIENCY in horses HAVE ONLY been produced in foals fed on specially prepared diets, designed to produce such conditions. Symptoms include CALCIUM deposits within the blood vessels, hyperirritability, glazed eyes and possible collapse.

POTASSIUM

POTASSIUM is required in the horses' body as an ELECTROLYTE, in that it is responsible for maintenance of the body cells at the correct acidity, or pH level, and for ensuring, in conjunction with SODIUM CHLORIDE, that each individual body cell maintains the correct OSMOTIC PRESSURE to allow interchange of food nutrients into, and waste product out of, each body cell. Our reference horse at 450 kgs. requires about 27 grams, and again, with the exception of whey, all horse feeds contain well in excess of the horses' daily needs. This applies whether the horse is pasture fed or fully hand fed.

SULPHUR

Sulphur forms an integral part of the amino acids, methionine and cystine, contained in the PROTEIN component of the ration protein, and is also present in the VITAMINS, THIAMINE and BIOTIN, both belonging to the B group. Apart from the presence, as indicated above, the exact function of SULPHUR in the horse is not clearly defined but it is thought to be involved in the production and maintenance of the outer tissues of the horse. Similarly no data exists as to the amount of SULPHUR required by the horse at any stage of growth and or development.

SULPHUR deficiency has never been diagnosed in the horse, as the mineral is present in many different feeds. Feeding of high quality proteins, as in mixed pasture, soybean meal or lucerne hay, will prevent any likely sulphur deficiency.

ZINC

ZINC is required in the horse as part of the ENZYME systems which control many of the activities of the body, including digestion of feedstuffs. ZINC has also been found, in high concentrations, in skin and hair and in lesser levels in muscle, blood, bone and some of the internal organs. Horses appear to need about 18 grams of zinc per day for a 450 kg. animal or, fed at a rate of 41 mgs of zinc per kg. of diet. Grains are generally below this level, whilst all other main horse feeds contain up to 110 mg/kg of feed.

In practical feeding terms, a zinc problem may occur if the horse is on high grain rations, but it would be little problem in horses fed a mixed diet where the grain level of the ration was 50% or less. ZINC Toxicity has been reported in foals fed large quantities of zinc - about 90 grams per day. These foals developed bone and joint problems including stiffness, lameness, enlarged ends on the long bones and increased tissue levels of zinc. Care should therefore be exercised in feeding zinc supplements to horses, especially to horses with a low grain intake in the diet. ZINC toxicity has also been involved in causing secondary COPPER deficiency in young horses, of a type which does not respond to additions of copper to the ration of the affected horses. The symptoms of ZINC deficiency are very similar to those produced in the foals fed excess levels of COPPER so care should be taken when considering ZINC as a component of the horse's ration.

COPPER

COPPER is required for the production of bone, cartilage, elastin (the re-inforcement of major blood vessels), effective utilisation of iron, in the horse, and formation of the hair colour pigments. Liver Copper levels appear to be high at an early age, decreasing as the horse gets older. Studies have revealed Liver COPPER levels as follows:-

FOETUS (unborn foal)	319 p.p.m.
YOUNG FOAL to 4 months	406 p.p.m.
OLDER FOALS	172 p.p.m.
ADULT HORSES	31 p.p.m.

Adult horses only need about 10 mgs of copper per day, and this is adequately provided in all feeds. However the Copper requirements of young growing horses may well be in excess of this level. On land known to be deficient in COPPER for cattle grazing, adult horses showed no visible signs of Copper deficiency yet foals reared on such land showed enlarged joints and changed pastern and fetlock angles and structure. In another specific trial on growing horses, to determine the effect of COPPER on bone growth and skeletal development, the foals which DID NOT receive COPPER in the creep feed, did not show any external signs of lameness and nothing unusual showed up on X-ray of the legs, before slaughter. At slaughter, however, all the foals on the diet not supplemented with COPPER had 350% more bone lesions than the foals which received the copper supplementation. Most of these bone lesions, seen at slaughter were too small to be detected on X-ray but it was suggested that these bone lesions could develop further as the horse gets older, causing leg and lameness problems. In cases of severe COPPER deficiency in foals, CONTRACTED TENDONS, were an obvious symptom and responded to added dietary COPPER within one week of treatment. OSTEOCHRONDOSIS, or inflammation of bone and adjacent cartilage is another condition where lack of COPPER in the ration has been incriminated as a cause. There is the possibility that additional levels of COPPER,in excess of normal values may have to be fed to young growing horses, who are on high protein rations.

Toxicity, to the horse, from COPPER was not produced at feeding levels of about 800 p.p.m. Copper in the diet. Copper can be stored in the liver for considerable periods of time, dependent on dietary intake.

The actual amount of COPPER available to the horse, depends on the source of the copper and interaction of COPPER with ZINC, IRON, MOLYBDENUM and SULPHUR. High levels of MOLYBDENUM, in the diet, increases the rate of copper excretion from the body, and excessive levels of ZINC can prevent a specific type of copper deficiency which does not respond to any copper therapy.

MOLYBDENUM

As far as can be determined, MOLYBDENUM has no positive part to play in horse nutrition. It can, however, play a very negative part in that horses fed pasture, containing between 5 and 25 p.p.m. of MOLYBDENUM had considerable reductions occur in levels of both PHOSPHORUS and COPPER, leading to the production of RICKETS.

Later research work indicated that MOLYBDENUM was unlikely to interfere with COPPER METABOLISM in horses, but the experiment only went for 20 days and it is quite possible that intake, by horses, of MOLYBDENUM from pastures, over a longer period of time can still cause reduction in COPPER levels in horses.

Molybdenum is a very important micro-nutrient in plant nutrition, being essential for the efficient growth of the RHIZOBIAL bacteria which grow on the roots of legumes. If MOLYBDENUM is not present in the soil or applied by fertiliser, then the RHIZOBIAL bacteria is unable to survive and so legumes cannot be grown. Horses grazing such pasture for any length of time are likely to pick up high levels of MOLYBDENUM.

MANGANESE

This mineral is involved, in very small quantities, in the metabolism of the ENERGY from CARBOHYDRATES AND FATS and formation of BONE and CARTILAGE tissue but the actual MANGANESE requirements of the horse have not been established.

A deficiency of MANGANESE in the ration, in animal species other than the horse, can lead to the development of enlarged joints, contracted tendons and reduced or shortened length of bone.

COBALT

COBALT forms part of VITAMIN B12, also known as CYANOCOBALAMIN, which is involved with the production of RED BLOOD CELLS. the amount of COBALT required, by the horse, each day is minute and there has never been a COBALT deficiency diagnosed in horses, even in horses grazing pastures which were deficient in COBALT for ruminant growth and reproduction.

SELENIUM

SELENIUM is required by the horse in very small amounts. Selenium acts, in combination, with Vitamin E in the maintenance of muscle tissue and in the development of antibody production in the horse which protects the horse from various infections, including tetanus and influenza and selenium, combined with some of the amino acids, plays an important part in soft tissue structure.

Considerable difference of opinion exists as to the SELENIUM requirements of horses. Levels of from 0.1 to 2.5 mg SELENIUM/day for a 450 kg horse have been mentioned in the scientific literature. In terms of P.P.M., one source has suggested a SELENIUM daily requirement of 0.1 to 0.5 P.P.M. SELENIUM/DAY, or converted to metric measurement a SELENIUM intake of 2.4 uG/kg body weight/day. A daily SELENIUM intake of 45-50 mg for the same 450 kg horse would be considered toxic.

Fortunately most of the feeds analysed for selenium, contained in excess of the horses' daily needs, and research work has also shown that horses can tolerate up to ten times the acceptable selenium level in their food, without showing toxic effects. U.K. information provide SELENIUM levels in oats and hay at 0.03 mg/kg D.M. which means that a 450kg horse eating about 9 kg of DRY MATTER/ day would have a SELENIUM intake of 0.45mg/day.

SELENIUM DEFICIENCY

Mild SELENIUM deficiency will cause diarrhoea, often not responding to the normal treatments for this condition.

Severe SELENIUM deficiency has been diagnosed in WHITE MUSCLE DISEASE or W.M.D., also known as NUTRITIONAL MYODEGENERATION, in horses under 12 months of age, and lately deficiency of selenium has been implicated in the "TYING UP syndrome" which can affect some more mature horses.

Selenium deficiency associated with white muscle disease in foals has been diagnosed in parts of the U.S.A, Victoria, Western Australia and New Zealand. The disease appeared in specific conditions, where the mares were grazing in areas where certain soils were known to be selenium deficient, containing less than about 0.5 uG (micrograms SELENIUM)/GRAM of soil. WHITE MUSCLE DISEASE, which can ocur in foals up to about 8 months of age, nearly always had a seasonal incidence, generally occurring in Spring when it was felt the accelerated growth of the pasture, may have reduced the total selenium intake of the horses. The season of the year probably was not important, what was important was that SELENIUM DEFICIENCY, as WHITE MUSCLE DISEASE, was most obvious in newly born foals which were born in the Spring. The pastures concerned did not contain lucerne, which is recognised as containing adequate levels of selenium for horse needs. WHITE MUSCLE DISEASE, in foals, can be corrected if early diagnosis is made when the horses are bred on soils known to have a SELENIUM deficiency problem. WHITE MUSCLE DISEASE is very difficult, if not impossible to cure, if NOT DETECTED IN THE VERY EARLY STAGES. In stabled horses, on mixed rations, there appears to be no relationship between selenium nutrition and white muscle disease.

Selenium is often administered to racehorses in conjunction with Vitamin E as a treatment for "TYING UP". In some cases, this treatment has had a beneficial effect but should only be carried out under veterinary supervision.

SELENIUM TOXICITY

SELENIUM EXCESS in the diet, produces a condition known as SELENINOSIS, ALKALI DISEASE, BOBTAIL DISEASE or BLIND STAGGERS and can be caused by the horses eating plants which accumulate large amounts of SELENIUM. In the U.S.A., where any plant which contains over 5 p.p.m. of SELENIUM is considered potentially toxic, a number of plants have the ability to accumulate SELENIUM, in levels which are dangerous to horses. These plants include members of the ASTRAGALUS family, including milk vetch, woody aster (XYLORHIZA) and goldenweed (OONOPSIS), all of which grow in the low rainfall areas of the western U.S.A. Fortunately most of these plants are most unpalatable and will not be eaten by the horse, unless there is nothing else available. There is also a strong correlation between alkaline soils and plants which are SELENIUM accumulators.

SELENIUM TOXICITY can also be caused by the administration to the horse of SELENIUM overdoses, either by injection or in the feed. SELENIUM TOXICITY is a problem which is occurring far too frequently in horses as owners and trainers incorrectly administer the mineral, without being fully aware of the consequences.

SELENIUM can accumulate in the body and its excretion rate is extremely slow, excess accumulation producing symptoms which include loss of appetite, loss of weight, loss of hair, with the mane and tail falling out first, disintegration of the hoof wall, elevated temperature, respiratory failure, blindness, paralysis and possibly death.

SELENIUM should only be administered to a horse under strict supervision of a professional who is fully aware of the possible consequences of the mineral, ONCE TOO MUCH SELENIUM HAS BEEN ADMINISTERED TO THE HORSE, IT IS TOO LATE TO STOP SELENINOSIS FROM OCCURRING.

IODINE

IODINE is essential for the production of the hormone THYROXIN which is produced in the thyroid gland. This hormone influences practically every organ in the body, and in turn affects metabolic rate, oxygen consumption, uptake and neutralisation of glucose by the muscle cells, and increases protein synthesis.

IODINE DEFICIENCY is normally seen as GOITRE in adult animals, while foals, from mares which have suffered IODINE deficiency may be born dead or very weak. Weak foals are often unable to suckle and die from lack of milk whilst foals born dead are sometimes hairless. These IODINE DEFICIENT FOALS have come from mares which do not show any symptoms of IODINE DEFICIENCY themselves. Permanent Iodine deficiency may also occur. Lack of sufficient IODINE in a 5 month old foal has been diagnosed as being responsible for obvious skeletal problems, could not be corrected by adding IODINE to the ration and was blamed on inherited genetic problems.

In adult horses, thyroid hormones are not necessary for survival, but they are essential for development and survival of the foetus, and for the satisfactory growth of young foals after birth. If the foal survives birth and is still deficient in IODINE supply, symptoms can include reduced body function, poor growth and lowered disease resistance.

Iodine is normally required in the diet at a rate of 0.1 mg. per kg. of diet. Fortunately there are very few areas where iodine deficiency exist, those areas are commonly known and normally IODISED SALT, with very low levels of iodine is fed to overcome the deficiency problem.

Iodine is not a mineral to be fed at random to the horse. Iodine when, fed in excessive quantities in the horses' diet, has been proven to cause CONTRACTED FLEXOR TENDONS in foals and problems of this type have been diagnosed in horses fed supplements based on seaweed meal which is high in iodine. In these types of cases, ceasing to feed this seaweed based supplement removed the problem and the animals generally recovered.

GOITRE or similar symptoms can be produced in the horse by

1 - iodine deficiency,

2 - iodine excess,

3 - goitrogens in the feed (in unheated soybean or linseed)

4 - by some drugs sometimes fed to horses, including sulphonamides and phenlybutazone commonly known as "bute".

Iodine is best deleted from all mineral supplements fed to the horses and any diagnosis should be left to a veterinarian.

FLUORINE

Fluorine in minute quantities plays a part in the development of sound teeth and bones. Fluorine, in excess of normal requirements, has been known to cause bone lesions, lameness and general unthriftness. For practical purposes it appears that sufficient exists in normal feeds and that there is no need for fluorine supplements to be fed to horses.

CHELATED MINERALS

CHELATION, or also called ORGANICALLY COMPLEXED, refers to the situation where a mineral, instead of being in its normal inorganic chemical form, as CALCIUM in CALCIUM CARBONATE, has been bound to a small piece of organic substance, such as PROTEIN or CARBOHYDRATE.

A CHELATED MINERAL has an advantage of being absorbed more readily, by the horse's digestive tract, IF THE ORGANIC COMPONENT, to which the mineral is attached, IS MORE READILY ABSORBED THAN THE MINERAL ITSELF, in the inorganic form.

If however the CHELATED MINERAL is attached to some ORGANIC COMPOUND which is LESS READILY ABSORBED by the digestive tract than the MINERAL IN THE INORGANIC FORM, then that chelated mineral will not be of any additional value to the horse.

Unless ALL THE NECESSARY TECHNICAL information is available about the type of CHELATION which has occurred with each mineral, the feeding of CHELATED MINERALS to a horse may not be advisable.

8. VITAMINS

VITAMINS are complex chemical compounds which are essential, in conjunction with the other feed components, in the operation and function of many body processes.

VITAMINS are commonly divided into two basic groups FAT SOLUBLE and WATER SOLUBLE.

FAT SOLUBLE VITAMINS include VITAMIN A, VITAMIN D, VITAMIN E and VITAMIN K. These particular vitamins, if given in excessive doses where some or all is not immediately used by the horse, will dissolve in the fat in the inside of the horse and can be retained in that fatty tissue for some period of time. The main deposits of such vitamins are generally found in the fatty tissue associated with the liver, which is not surprising as the liver is the first part of the horses' waste product disposal system. Any chemical compound, circulating in the blood, and in excess of the horse's actual needs at the time, is first screened out by the liver. The ability of the body fat to absorb and retain any of these EXCESS FAT SOLUBLE VITAMINS can lead to HYPERVITAMINOSIS. This especially applies to VITAMIN A, VITAMIN D and VITAMIN K where problems, sometimes very severe, can occur as a result of excess levels of A and or D being present. At this time, there is no known problem of excessive levels of VITAMIN E, probably because it is involved with muscle function and is possibly "worked out" of the horses' system, with exercise.

WATER SOLUBLE VITAMINS include VITAMIN C and all the VITAMINS of the B COMPLEX. Storage of unused quantities of these vitamins in the horse is not nearly as extensive as it is of the FAT SOLUBLE VITAMINS. Any WATER SOLUBLE VITAMINS, in excess of the horses' requirements, are generally excreted, from the horse, in the urine, within 24-48 hours so the horse rarely ever suffers from a problem of excess levels of any of the B VITAMINS or VITAMIN C.

VITAMIN A

VITAMIN A, also known as RETINOL, is required in the animal for normal body cell function and in the production of new tissue, especially in the outer body cells such as skin, hair, eyes etc. Vitamin A is also essential, in reasonable levels, to assist disease resistance, prevent nerve degeneration and to ensure that reproduction and lactation progress satisfactorily. No animal is able to survive with all its normal body functions, unless adequate supplies of Vitamin A are available.

VITAMIN A DEFICIENCY

VITAMIN A deficiency can occur when the ration availability to the horse approximates about 50% of normal requirements and can cause many symptoms, some of which may also be due to other possible causes.

These conditions include Night or moon blindness. This is a classic condition of Vitamin A deficiency. Horses find it very difficult to see in dim light. Simply, the lack of Vitamin A affects the horse's ability to see properly. The condition was originally called "moon blindness" when seen in army horses in India. It was originally thought to occur with the cycles of the moon, but was subsequently found to be due to a Vitamin A deficiency.

Lack of Vitamin A will also cause a possible partial degeneration of the nervous system, leading to horses with wobbly gaits, lameness and similar conditions, decreased growth, decreased RED BLOOD CELL count and decreased blood plasma levels of IRON, ALBUMIN and CHOLESTEROL.

Respiratory conditions can worsen, if a Vitamin A deficiency exists in the horse. The tissues of the respiratory tract are weakened allowing attack from organisms that cause respiratory problems such as pneumonia. Other conditions that can occur are poor growth, (often associated with other causes), scaling and flaking of hoof tissue and skin. In severely affected animals, the hair may even fall out. Lack of sufficient VITAMIN A, in the diet, has also been involved in horses which have suffered TENDON injuries.

VITAMIN A EXCESS

The symptoms of VITAMIN A EXCESS are similar to those of VITAMIN A DEFICIENCY.

Levels of Vitamin A, fed in excess of certain quantities, can prove dangerous to the horse. Total combined daily intake, from pasture, grains and supplements should not EXCEED the equivalent of 540 mg RETINOL for an average 450KG horse. Excess VITAMIN A, in the diet of the horse, can cause depressed growth, reductions of the levels of iron, albumin and cholesterol in the blood and eventually death.

In practical terms, VITAMIN A should not be fed to the horse at levels more than 1.5 to 5 times the N.R.C. specifications. otherwise there is the possibility of sub clinical VITAMIN A problems occurring. i.e. the horse is being affected but in such a manner that the effect cannot be detected and or diagnosed from other possible causes by visual means. It is possible, for the problems of VITAMIN A EXCESS to occur in horses if the horse is being fed a ration already containing CAROTENE PLUS A FEED SUPPLEMENT which has HIGH LEVELS OF VITAMIN A. The problem of VITAMIN A EXCESS is compounded by the fact that horses are able to self regulate the amount of VITAMIN A which they make from the BETA CAROTENE content of green plants, they make sufficient for their needs and excrete the rest. However with artificial sources of VITAMIN A, as in feed supplements etc, all or nearly all of the VITAMIN A is available to the horse and the horse DOES NOT possess any self regulating mechanism to protect against an overdose. Each ration situation needs to be individually calculated to determine any potential problem.

VITAMIN A AND CAROTENE

Vitamin A does not occur as such in plant tissue. All plants contain a number of yellow coloured compounds which are collectively called Carotene. Inside the animal, Carotene, principally in the form of BETA CAROTENE, is converted to Vitamin A in the small intestine and the liver. Carotene is present in all green plant tissue and other closely related compounds, which can also be changed to Vitamin A inside the animal, are found in maize (corn) and in carrots.

In terms of relative BETA CAROTENE contents and the variations which can occur in growing conditions of plants the VITAMIN A activity of green pasture and carrots is about the same on a DRY MATTER basis, with the VITAMIN A activity of yellow maize (corn), only about 10% of that of CARROTS and green grass, again on a DRY MATTER basis.

The horse is able to self regulate the conversion of BETA CAROTENE into VITAMIN A and rarely is there ever a problem of VITAMIN A EXCESS in horses which obtain their VITAMIN A requirements from green feed intake. The liver acts as a store for Vitamin A in the body. Hence it is not necessary that Vitamin A be supplied on a daily basis.

Cattle have been known to exist for up to 60 days on a Vitamin A deficient diet before developing the usual early symptoms of "moon blindness". Horses after adequate green feed intake are able to store Vitamin A in the liver for up to nine months for use in future periods of restricted Vitamin A intake.

DESTRUCTION OF VITAMIN A AND CAROTENE

Both Carotene and Vitamin A are stable in green, actively growing feed. Artificial Vitamin A is also stable if kept in sealed containers. However, both Carotene and Vitamin A will break down and lose potency under most practical storage conditions. When green crops are made into hays, some Carotene is lost due to oxidation.

Further losses of Carotene may occur in storage. With fresh hay, the green colour,so prized by horse feeders as an method of determining the value of the hay, is an indication of the Carotene level of the hay. During storage however, loss of Carotene from hay is generally more rapid than loss of green colour, and hence the green colour, in stored hay, is generally not a good indication of the Carotene level. Rain damaged, weathered or bleached hay will always be lower in Carotene than green material, and hay which heats or moulds in storage, generally looses all the Carotene content.

Whilst conditions of hay making and storage vary considerably, a rough rule of thumb is that hay can lose around 66% of its Carotene level in the first six months of storage. Thereafter the loss of Carotene is very small.

Loss of Carotene level also occurs in prepared feeds such as dehydrated lucerne and pellets. Not only is Carotene destroyed in the artificial heating process, but decomposition still occurs in the periods after manufacture, as for hay.

The Vitamin A precursor in maize is more stable than in hay. Over a one year period, maize stored correctly only loses about 25% of the potential Vitamin A level as compared to hay.

Artificial Vitamin A as a feed supplement, may also be subject to breakdown. Loss of Vitamin A content in prepared feeds or feed supplements may occur, due to oxidation. This will take place when the feed or supplement in not sealed after each use. Failure to re-seal feed supplement containers, especially the inner plastic bag, can lead to losses of Vitamin A from the supplement. Vitamin A loss can also occur due to the effect of other Vitamin and/or mineral components in the feed mix. Any feed supplement which is based on limestone, with added Vitamin A, will have the Vitamin A destroyed by the limestone upon mixing.

Vitamin A requirements increase in the horse, in times of stress or medium to heavy work loads, during pregnancy, and lactation in mares. Cod Liver Oil, which is an excellent source of Vitamin A for dogs, cats and poultry, SHOULD NOT be fed to herbivores or grass eating animals, including horses, for long periods. A number of reports indicate that continued feeding of Cod Liver Oil, to horses, can cause muscle degeneration and lowered milk fat levels. Muscle degeneration is the last thing any reasonable horse owner wants to occur in their animals.

VITAMIN A CONTENT OF FEED AND HORSE REQUIREMENTS

One estimate of VITAMIN A storage and requirement has suggested that if a horse has had access to good fresh green pasture for 4-5 weeks, where the BETA CAROTENE level can be expected to be about three times the horse's daily needs, there will be enough VITAMIN A stored in the liver to last the normal horse from three to six months.

N.R.C. Standards indicate Vitamin A needs, of the horse in the region of 11,000 to 34,000 I.U. (International Units) per day, but later research work indicates that needs in practical terms are more likely to be about three times the N.R.C. levels. These increased levels appear to be necessary, to prevent sub-clinical Vitamin A deficiencies. These are problems caused by Vitamin A which are not noticeable to the horse owner, do not produce visual symptoms, but can affect the well being and performance of the horse.

Mature horses, at rest, therefore need about 33,000 I.U. per day whilst horses in hard work, young actively growing horses, and pregnant or lactating mares can require up to 102,000 I.U. per day. These levels of Vitamin A can be provided by daily consumption of 0.75 kg. to 2.00 kg. of green feed or good quality hay.

As a mature horse at 450 kgs. requires a daily roughage intake of at least 2.25 kg. (0.5% of body weight) to maintain gut fill and gut mobility, any such horse being fed that quantity of green feed and/or hay will not require Vitamin A supplementation.

This comment does not apply to the feeding of oaten/wheaten hay of chaff. Both these feeds are extremely low in the natural Vitamin A precursor as they usually contain very little green tissue at the time of harvest.

VITAMIN A DEFICIENCY will only exists in horses which:-

1 have not had access to green feed for about 4 or 5 months.

2 are stabled and NOT FED about 2.5 kgs/sun cured hay or 12 kgs green feed/day.

3 are fed a diet which does NOT CONTAIN which does not contain any green feed, sun cured hay, carrots and or yellow maize.

VITAMIN B COMPLEX

The original Vitamin B now consists of many compounds, and the group is now known as the B Complex. The whole group of Vitamins is able to be synthesised, or produced, by the intestinal flora in the horses' digestive tract. Average horses, fed good quality feed, should not require any additional sources of Vitamin B Complex. The horse is able to make its own requirements, within its digestive tract. However, it appears that performance horses may NOT BE ABLE to make the vitamins of the B COMPLEX at the same rate at which they are being used. Supplementation of the rations of performance horses with certain B Complex Vitamins has become a common practice in some areas of horse competition. The main problem, however, is to know which B vitamin to feed, there are some 9 separate compounds, some of which are of value and some of which are not. It is NOT simply a matter of giving the horse a B COMPLEX, the horse must be given the correct VITAMINS of the B COMPLEX to get any result and this will be dependent on the rations being fed and the type of work the horse is being asked to perform.

B COMPLEX VITAMINS are present as co-enzymes in nearly all the metabolic processes that take place in the horse. They are involved in the utilisation of all main food nutrients, protein, fats and carbohydrates. Whilst B vitamins are produced in the gut of the horse, about 25% of those vitamins produced in the horse are absorbed by the animal. The balance appears to be passed out in the faeces. One of the practical problems in looking at the B Complex in horse nutrition is to ascertain whether the horse is receiving insufficient, sufficient or excess B Complex from production in its own digestive tract, plus any supplements which are being fed to the horse. Racehorses in particular, are often known to go "track sour"and overfeeding of B Complex is generally involved in this problem. "Track sour" horses generally follow a pattern of playing with their food, losing performance and then losing weight. These horses when removed from the stable situation with hand feeding and placed on pasture, inevitably improve.

VITAMIN B1

Also called THIAMINE - appears to be one of the vitamins lacking in horse rations. Horses, especially racehorses, stabled and hard fed, for any length of time and also horses being fed on poor quality hay have developed Thiamine deficiency (detected by blood analysis). In obvious Thiamine deficiency the symptoms are poor appetite which is often very noticeable, impaired fertility and unco-ordinated gait.

Daily needs of the Thiamine are not definitely established, but it would appear that the average large horse needs about 20 mg. of Thiamine per day for normal work. Grains and grain by-products appear to be low in Thiamine, whilst green pasture and good quality hays are normally a good source of the vitamin. 1 tablespoon of DRIED BREWER'S YEAST/day should satisfy any THIAMINE needs of stabled horses and, if THIAMINE is the problem, a reasonably quick response will be obtained. THIAMINE is often given to performance horses and brood mares even if the ration appears to contain sufficient levels. There appears to be no known problems with feeding this vitamin in levels above normal daily needs.

VITAMIN B2

Also called RIBOFLAVIN - important in absorption of energy by the intestine. RIBOFLAVIN deficiency in the diet, of the horse, has never been diagnosed. Good quality hay or pasture contains more than adequate amounts of Riboflavin and supplementation on this type of feed with RIBOFLAVIN does not appear necessary.

VITAMIN B6

Also called PYRIDOXINE - involved in protein metabolism. Vitamin B6 deficiency has not been reported in horses and both grasses, hays and grains are good sources of the vitamin. Use of B6 supplements are usually not required.

VITAMIN B12

Vitamin B12, also known as CYANOCOBALAMIN, is required, in extremely small amounts, for normal production of red blood cells. Larger amounts of VITAMIN B12 are also required by the horse in training for metabolism of one of the fatty acids which is produced at increasing levels when the carbohydrate energy level of the ration increases, as in racehorse training.

The vitamin is not present in any plant material, but is manufactured in the lower part of the horse's intestine. Cobalt, contained in VITAMIN B12, only needs to be present, in the normal feeds, in micro amounts to allow production of adequate quantities of Vitamin B12. The animals' need for the Vitamin B12 appears to be very small, except when doing hard physical exercise. Horses fed diets containing virtually no Cobalt or Vitamin B12 for a period of two years showed no reduction in the levels of Vitamin B12 in the blood at the end of the two year period.

These horses were also prevented from practicing COPROPHAGY, i.e. from eating small portions of their own faeces.

Significantly lower blood concentrations of VITAMIN B12 have been found in Thoroughbreds in training as compared to similar horses grazing in pasture. It could well be that the use of "HARD FEED" in racing stables has some effect on the ability of the large intestine to produce VITAMIN B12, probably due to a reduction in either or both fibre amount and or cellulose type.

Under normal conditions of little exercise, COPROPHAGY then fibre digestion in the large intestine of horses, supplies, some if not all, the Vitamin B12 requirements of the horse with low levels of activity. VITAMIN B12 supplementation of the ration could well be required for horses whose levels of work require a reasonable degree of physical activity.

Vitamin B12 injections have often been given to horses, but experimental evidence shows that most of the injected Vitamin B12 is EXCRETED in the urine and is not, in fact, used by the horse.

It appears that the Vitamin B12 requirements of horses are much less than those of cattle. Horses have remained in good health whilst grazing pastures so low in Cobalt, that cattle grazing that same pastures have died.

FOLIC ACID

FOLIC ACID, also know as FOLACIN, has many functions in the animal including playing an important part in the formation of red blood cells. A deficiency of FOLIC ACID in the diet may cause a reduction in the red blood cell number (anaemia), although the red blood cells remaining appear to be larger than usual. Folic acid requirements of the horse are not known, but average to good quality pasture is an excellent source. Poor quality hay or pasture has a reduced level of FOLIC ACID, indicating a possible FOLIC ACID loss from plants as they mature and set seed. There may be a case for the feeding of folic acid to performance horses, on a high grain diet, or on a diet which contains low quality roughage. Exercise and increasing work load stimulates the formation of red blood cells, hence increasing the need for folic acid. Grains are generally low in folic acid, hence a supplement may be of advantage in these situations. Studies have found that the amount of FOLATES in the blood of grazing horses is considerably greater than in the blood of stabled horses. FOLIC ACID supplementation of stabled horses have been in the order of 100 to 1000 mg/day of FOLIC ACID, given on a repetitive daily basis mixed with the rations, as injectible forms of FOLIC ACID were not present in the blood 24 hours after administration.

NIACIN

NIACIN, also known as NICOTINIC ACID and NICOTINAMIDE, is a component of the two enzymes which are important for normal body function. NIACIN can be made inside the horse from the amino acid TRYPTOPHAN, and hence any horse fed reasonable protein levels in the feed, especially lucerne hay and/or soybean meal, will not suffer a niacin problem. One study of niacin balance in the horse showed that the amount excreted in the urine can be greater than the amount of niacin eaten by the horse. This extra niacin produced, comes from the conversion of tryptophan to niacin, in the intestinal tract. NIACIN DEFICIENCY has never been diagnosed in the horse and a deficiency is not expected in normal horse feeding situations.

PANTOTHENIC ACID

Sometimes called PANTOTHENATE, Pantothenic acid is required in compounds which are an essential part in the absorption of fat, carbohydrates, and certain amino acids in the horse. The actual daily needs of pantothenic acid, by the horse, are not properly established, and a PANTOTHENIC ACID DEFICIENCY has never been reported in the horse. Good quality hay and pasture contain more than adequate levels of pantothenic acid, whilst grains generally contain about half the quantity found in hay and pasture. Pantothenic acid deficiency has not been diagnosed in horses, and hence there is no apparent need to provide the compound as supplements in the ration.

BIOTIN

Formerly known as VITAMIN H, BIOTIN is an essential co-enzyme involved in the use of energy and protein by the horse. It is also of importance in the correct development of hoof keratinization or hoof wall strength. The horse is only able to synthesise relatively small amounts of BIOTIN in the digestive tract, in comparison to its needs, as a performance horse, for efficient energy use.

Recent scientific work has shown considerable benefit from daily feeding of low levels of Biotin to horses with badly cracked hooves, e.g. sand cracks and quarter cracks. At initial feeding rates of 10-15 mg BIOTIN / day,over a four to six month period, dramatic improvement will occur in HOOF WALL strength and cracks, thin walls etc. will become a thing of the past. Once the HOOF WALL texture and strength has returned to "normal", the daily dose rate for such horses can be reduced to 1-2 mg BIOTIN/horse/day and desirable hoof wall texture will be maintained. This same level of BIOTIN supplementation 1-2 mg/day is also adequate for efficient energy use in performance horses. It has also been proven that adequate levels of CALCIUM in the ration are desirable for BIOTIN to be effective in correcting some types of hoof wall problems.

CHOLINE

Choline is important in metabolism and digestion of fat, within the digestive tract, and for maintaining cell structure. Deficiencies of choline have been reported in rats and chickens, but have never been reported in horses. Choline is either present in adequate levels in the feed, or else is synthesised in the horse's digestive tract. There appears no known current reason why CHOLINE should be added to the ration of any horse.

VITAMIN C

Vitamin C, more commonly known as ASCORBIC ACID, is an essential vitamin for humans, but not for the horse. Horses are able to synthesise or manufacture VITAMIN C in their digestive tract from glucose. Hence a horse adequately fed on energy will not suffer a Vitamin C deficiency. VITAMIN C function, in the horse, is in the formation of connective tissue and is reputed to be involved in the ability of the horse to withstand stress of both a physiological and pathological type, e.g. as in a training programme, or with a sudden decrease in daily temperature.

Some Vitamin C supplements - pure ascorbic acid- have been used with success in the treatment of bleeders in the racing industry. Ascorbic acid added to the drinking water on a daily basis has been able to control some forms of bleeding. The administration of ASCORBIC ACID, by mouth in one large dose, of 20 grams did not affect the level of VITAMIN C in the blood, as most to the VITAMIN C was excreted from the body. If however daily doses were given, so that the body learnt to recognise the additional VITAMIN C there were significant increases in the VITAMIN C level of the blood. No adverse effects were noted in the horses continually fed 20 grams ASCORBIC ACID/day.

Vitamin C supplements have also been claimed to improve reproductive performance and to decrease the effect of some respiratory problems.

There is, at this stage, no scientific evidence to verify these claims, so the value of Vitamin C as being responsible for the above claims, may be well due to a change in some other factor in the horses diet, and/or management, which occurred at the same time as supplementation with Vitamin C commenced.

VITAMIN D

VITAMIN D, sometimes called CALCIFEROL, is required, in conjunction with the correct amounts and proportions of CALCIUM and PHOSPHORUS in the horses' daily diet, for optimum bone and skeletal development.

Vitamin D is required in relatively large amounts in actively growing horses, as well as for pregnant and lactating mares, when compared to mature fully grown horses.

Sunlight is the most common source of the pre-cursors of Vitamin D. Sunlight acts on substances in the horses' skin, converting these substances to Vitamin D. It is not necessary for the animal to get full sunlight as it is the ultra violet rays in the sunlight which is the important factor. Likewise any feeds such as hay which are sun-cured, also contain reasonable quantities of Vitamin D pre-cursors. It is known that horses are able to store Vitamin D in the liver but the relative storage level of Vitamin D is not nearly as great as that of Vitamin A.

The VITAMIN D requirements of the horse have been estimated at about 300 I.U. (mg)/50kg live weight, a 450 kg horse requiring about 2700-3000 I.U. (mg)/day. Vitamin D requirements, in humans, can be supplied, by access to 20 minutes of sunlight/day. No comparable figures exist for the horse, but it may be reasonable to assume that about 2 to 4 hours sunlight per day should provide the horse with sufficient Vitamin D for all requirements.

VITAMIN D DEFICIENCY

Very rarely, if ever, does one see the problem of a straight VITAMIN D deficiency. A deficiency of VITAMIN D in the ration will be complicated by the ration levels of CALCIUM and PHOSPHORUS as the three feed components work to-gether in bone formation and maintenance. Deficiency(ies) of one one or more of these TWO MINERALS and ONE VITAMIN can cause the condition commonly called RICKETS. The classical symptoms of RICKETS include stiffness, swollen joints, bent knees, sag in the back behind the shoulders.

Affected animals may also have rapid breathing, become easily excited and may chew bones, wood and bark from trees.

In practice, there has to be a considerable problem with any one of the levels of CALCIUM, PHOSPHORUS and or VITAMIN D in the diet to produce such obvious symptoms. Often a deficiency of VITAMIN D is observed, in a sub clinical situation, as some vague lameness and or body dysfunction and can only be clarified by an assessment of the previous management programme of the horse. VITAMIN D deficiencies are likely to occur in any horse which does not have reasonable access to sunlight, i.e. horses which are stabled and or fully rugged and hooded all the time, in stabled horses which do not have access to sun cured hay, or to horses in far northern latitudes where sunlight can be very limiting in the winter months.

Since vitamin D is provided free by nature from sunlight, any likely Vitamin D deficiency can be overcome by removing the horse rugs, where applicable, and letting the animal graze or be exercised, without any rugs for a few hours each day. There may be a reason to add Vitamin D supplements to horse rations in areas of the far northern and far southern latitudes, especially in winter, but any such additions should be very carefully calculated so as to not produce an excessive level of VITAMIN D in the horse.

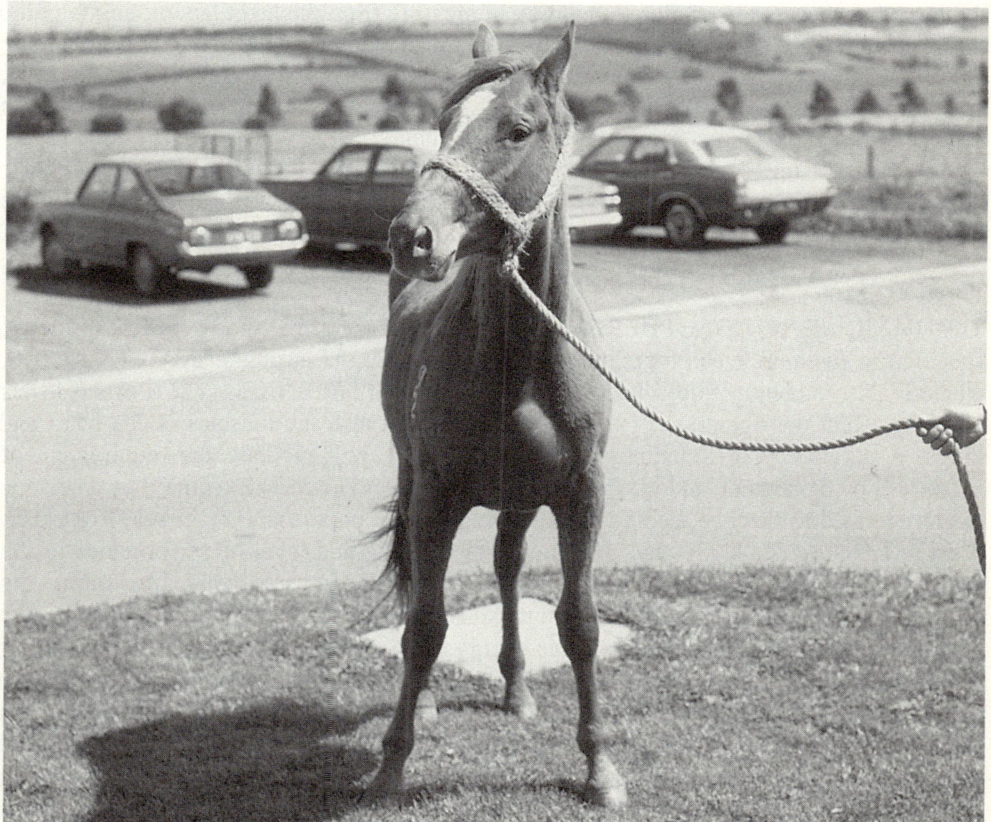

Two year old thoroughbred, provided with excess vitamin D – the owner's treatment for lameness. Refer colour plates.

VITAMIN D EXCESS

Vitamin D, when fed in excess of the horses' continuing daily needs, can have some dramatic effects on the health of the horse. The excessive Vitamin D can cause calcium to be deposited in soft tissues such as blood vessels, heart, lungs and kidneys in horses of any age, and can cause irregular bone development which will be permanent in growing horses. Excess vitamin D is also responsible for a general weakness in the condition of the horse, accompanied by a loss in body weight. The toxic level of VITAMIN D has not been established in the horse, but in other animal species, it is 10 times normal requirements.

There are several reported cases of these sorts of problems occurring, in practical situations, from the USE and or OVERUSE of mineral vitamin supplements containing what appear to be reasonably high levels of VITAMIN D, fed to the horse at the same time as the horse has access to reasonable amounts of sunlight.

Research studies have also shown that mares fed about ten times the accepted level of Vitamin D during pregnancy, have produced foals which have died shortly after birth, due to deposition of calcium in the blood vessels. Rupture of the large blood vessels coming from the heart has then occurred, due to build up in pressure from the heart, attempting to pump the same amount of blood through a much smaller diameter artery, the diameter restricted by the CALCIUM deposition inside. Growing horses, when fed excess levels of Vitamin D, develop ossification of the bone joints - simply too much calcium is laid down, the joints become stiff and the animal becomes permanently lame.

Any changes in the horse, such as CALCIUM deposit in the blood vessels, irregular bone development etc. are PERMANENT and IRREVERSIBLE, so extreme care should be taken when feeding VITAMIN D supplements to a horse.

VITAMIN E

VITAMIN E or TOCOPHEROL is necessary for normal body cell respiration, specifically, the muscle cell function involved with the use of unsaturated FATTY ACIDS, where E acts, in conjunction, with very small amounts of SELENIUM. VITAMIN E levels not only affect the operation of the body muscles but also the muscles of the heart and lungs. A deficiency of Selenium, in the horse's diet, will increase the requirement of Vitamin E by the animal, and vice versa. The amount of VITAMIN E required by a horse is directly related to level of feeding and or storage of the polyunsaturated FATTY ACIDS, previously fed to the horse, and the amount of exercise and level of performance of the horse. VITAMIN E acts as an anti-oxidant within the muscle cells, preventing the destruction by oxygen of some of the breakdown products of FAT metabolism. In this regard, VITAMIN E allows more muscle energy to be obtained from the fat component of the ration, and it therefore controls the use by the muscles of some of the energy breakdown products of FATTY ACIDS. The higher the level of feeding of FATS in the ration, the greater will be the need, of the horse, for adequate and increasing amounts of VITAMIN E to allow effective use of the energy source of those fats.

In a Swedish experiment, with performance horses, where VITAMIN E depletion studies were carried out on the same horses over an 8 month period, the highest VITAMIN E levels were found in the fat tissues, VITAMIN E being one of the fat soluble vitamins, followed next by liver deposits and then muscle deposits. VITAMIN E was most effective when given daily by mouth at levels of around 1500-1800 mg/horse/day.

VITAMIN E is also important in the ability of the horse to resist infectious diseases. E is involved in the efficient operation of the horse's immune defence mechanism. Absorption of VITAMIN A from the intestines is also dependent on the availability of VITAMIN E in the ration. The horse is unable to make VITAMIN E within the digestive tract so the complete requirements of VITAMIN E must come from feed intake.

The VITAMIN E levels of various feeds is extremely variable with Lucerne and Lucerne hay being excellent sources of Vitamin E. The average horse's normal requirements appear to vary from around 300 I.U. (or mg) VITAMIN E /animal/day. As good quality lucerne hay contains an average of 140 I.U.(mg)/ kg, the average horse has to eat only 2.2kg of lucerne per day to receive its Vitamin E needs. Fresh green pasture contains slightly less Vitamin E than lucerne hay but the levels of VITAMIN E in other horse feeds may vary considerably. OATS has been known to have levels as low as 6 I.U. (mg)/KG.

Vitamin E is the most unstable of the fat soluble vitamins, and ground or cracked feeds will allow oxygen to enter and destroy the Vitamin E. In manufactured horse feed supplements, Vitamin E is used to prevent oxidation or decomposition of Vitamin A in compounded feeds.

VITAMIN E DEFICIENCY

Deficiency or insufficient VITAMIN E in the daily diet causes a number of problems. VITAMIN E deficiency, in the initial stages, causes breakdown of the structure of cell wall, resulting in the most common visual problems of ANAEMIA and WHITE MUSCLE DISEASE.

VITAMIN E DEFICIENCY has also been associated with STRESS in horses, as in travelling, performance etc.

Vitamin E, in previous times, was called the "anti-sterility" vitamin and was supposed to play a vital part in reproduction. Stallions in particular were supposed to produce more potent semen when fed Vitamin E in the diet. There is no evidence to prove this theory. Vitamin E and Selenium act together in the prevention of WHITE MUSCLE DISEASE (refer Selenium in the section on minerals).

VITAMIN E EXCESS

VITAMIN E does not appear to be toxic in large doses, and in fact levels up to 4500 I.U. per day, or 15 times average daily requirements, are sometimes fed to eventing horses and racehorses. Here the Vitamin E is supposed to assist and improve muscle activity and athletic performance.

VITAMIN K

VITAMIN K, also known as PHYLLOQUINONE, is responsible for the formation of the blood clotting factor. Vitamin K is produced, in more than adequate quantities, in the digestive tract of the horse, and practical problems with Vitamin K deficiency in the horse are very rare. Any deficiency of Vitamin K, in the horse will always be manifested as internal bleeding which is often very difficult to control.

There is no practical need to supplement any horse ration with Vitamin K. Vitamin K has been used, in some cases, to cure "bleeders" of the problem of blood appearing at the nostrils after physical exercise Blood appearing at the nostrils of a horse, after exercise, is a result of thin walls of the blood vessels of the lungs and Vitamin K has no effect on increasing the thickness of such blood vessels. All performance horses "bleed", within the lungs, after hard exercise, some unfortunately "bleed" to a greater extent than others, causing blood to be seen coming from the nostrils.

Injectible Vitamin K or menadione (synthetic Vitamin K), given after the horse has bled, appears to cure bleeding, but in fact the bleeding would naturally cease anyway as the animal is normally not under stress when the injection is supposed to be working.

Horses, treated with VITAMIN K injections, often develop COLIC within 48 hours of the injection. Symptoms noted include arching of the back; if stabled, repeated backing into a corner, mild but persistent abdominal pain and frequent lying down. Laminitis has also been known to develop in horses treated with VITAMIN K injections to control bleeding. The most damaging part of VITAMIN K injections is damage to the RENAL system (excretion of urine) which is generally irreversible.

OTHER POSSIBLE VITAMINS

People are always looking for the magical cure or the super compound which will solve all the present feeding problems or, alternatively, produce something extra that nothing else has produced before. The following substances currently fit into this category. As more is learnt about each substance, and they are better understood, they MAY become accepted feed components in their own right.

VITAMIN B15

Also known as PANGAMIC ACID. Originally isolated from apricot pips or seeds. It has been promoted to specially increase stamina and performance. No evidence exists to support this theory, and recent studies have shown that Vitamin B15 is probably a mixture of compounds and not a separate compound in its own right. Some reports for the U.S.A. suggest that in fact pangamic acid or Vitamin B15 may be harmful when fed to horses.

VITAMIN B17

Also called LAETRILE. Little knowledge is available and certainly has no known value for horses.

VITAMIN P

Obtained from citrus fruits. Belongs to the bioflavonoid group of compounds. The, name Vitamin P, was applied to substances claimed to increase the resistance of the blood capillaries and hence reduce the permeability to Red Blood Cells. This theory has since been abandoned as it was found that all substances with 'Vitamin P' activity are bioflavonoids.

Substances in this group include Rutin, troxerutin and hesperidin and have been used, on some occasions, in the treatment of "bleeders".

9. ELECTROLYTES

ELECTROLYTES are basically body salts, essential for the efficient operation of NERVES, KIDNEYS and MUSCLES. These salts, which are a combination of MINERALS and other chemical elements, are present in most feeds and water which the horse consumes.

ELECTROLYTES are generally present in the feed as components within the individual plant cell walls and are released, for absorption by the large intestine, by the cellulose breakdown process which occurs in that part of the digestive tract to produce VOLATILE FATTY ACIDS. Other body fluids, as well as blood, also transport these salts around the horse's body.

The kidney acts as the electrolyte store and maintains, in reserve, any salts not required by the body.

Electrolytes move throughout the body in the following manner:

1. Ingested by the horse.
2. Absorbed into the blood stream and carried throughout the body.
3. Used by the specific body cells in normal body function.
4. Excess electrolyte not used by the horse is stored in the kidney and can be used by the animal at a later time.
5. Used electrolytes are returned to and excreted via the kidneys in the horse's urine.

This ELECTROLYTE FLOW structure only applies when the required amounts of MINERALS, as distinct from electrolytes, are present in the ration. EXCESSIVE MINERAL LEVELS, greater than the horse needs, is able to upset ELECTROLYTE balance and usage.

ESSENTIAL ELECTROLYTES

Salts of SODIUM (Na) and POTASSIUM (K) are important for the transmission of nerve and muscle commands throughout the body. They are both responsible for maintaining the OSMOTIC PRESSURE or fluid balance of the individual body cells which affects the whole operation and function of the horse. SODIUM (Na) is principally concerned with fliud balance, outside the body cells and POTASSIUM (K) inside the body cells.

MAGNESIUM (Mg) salts are needed to assist the correct use of energy by the individual body cells. Signs of deficiency of MAGNESIUM in the diet include excessive sweating without apparent reason, increased irritability of the horse, glazed eyes, abnormal general behaviour and possible eventual collapse. Such problems can occur at and after stress, such as strange surroundings, travelling, auction sales etc.

CALCIUM salts (Ca) maintain the normal function of body cell walls or membranes, especially in relation to the passage back and forth of SODIUM and also assist in converting the energy in the muscle for muscle contractions. Insufficient CALCIUM in the diet, for electrolyte use, in MUSCLE function will mean that the horse is unable to contract its muscles as efficiently as if sufficient Calcium was present and this must affect performance.

BI-CARBONATE (HCO_3) acts on and neutralises the acid products from energy use by the muscles, specifically LACTIC ACID. The use of BICARBONATE, as an electrolyte is a very contentious and debated subject.

SODIUM (Na) and CHLORINE (C1) maintain body cell OSMOTIC PRESSURE, essential for overall body function and also assist in the control of kidney function and urine flow.

PHOSPHORUS (P) is also termed an ELECTROLYTE by some nutritionists but the levels of PHOSPHATE, in the blood serum show considerable variation which cannot be traced to any one physiological event, and feeding trials have shown no response, to date, to the recognition of PHOSPHORUS as an ELECTROLYTE.

Electrolytes are lost from the body in many ways, e.g. as sweat, saliva, bile, in urine and in various gastric secretions. The rate of loss depends on a number of interrelated factors.

A horse at rest, with adequate feed intake, is able, in most circumstances, to maintain some form of balance between availability of the ELECTROLYTES in the ration, absorption of the electrolytes from the gut, effective use by the body and then excretion of the used products from the animals.

When horses are asked to increase their work rate, increase in electrolyte needs occur, and losses are also increased. Increased sweat and urine output are the main reasons for the greater need for electrolytes, but the demand can also be affected by periods of hard work, hot weather, travelling stress and other similar factors.

EXCESSIVE LOSS of electrolytes may also occur in horses with diarrhoea and sometimes after the over use of drugs, especially kidney tonics.

ELECTROLYTES AND SWEAT OUTPUT

All working horses generally sweat at some stage in their preparation. The cooling effect, produced by the evaporation of sweat from the body surfaces, is necessary for the horse to regulate and maintain its body temperature within safe limits. Horses working hard, especially for reasonable periods of time, produce a lot of excess body heat as a result of the breakdown of energy in the muscles, and that body heat is dissipated or lost from the horse by the sweating mechanism.

When the body temperature increases, the horse will initially compensate for the increase by increasing heart work rate, which in turn increases the amount of blood circulating within the horse and increases blood flow to the skin, to allow more effective heat loss. As work continues and heat is built up inside the horse, the amount of blood directed to the skin, to assist cooling, is increased at the expense of a reduction in the blood flow to the working muscles.

Body temperatures of a horse, during hard physical exercise, may be increased by up to 5% above average. An increase in body temperature, of this degree, in a horse at rest a would normally mean a sick horse which requires immediate veterinary attention. In a horse working hard, the increase in body temperature is controlled by the amount of sweat that the horse produces. Sweat losses can vary from up to 10 litres for aracehorse on race days or days of fast work, and up to 30 litres for endurance horses during and after long endurance rides.

ELECTROLYTES

Research work, on endurance horses in particular, gives some idea of the quantity of salts that can be lost in sweat. A horse losing 10 litres of sweat per day can lose up to 57 grams of SODIUM salt, 30 grams of POTASSIUM salt and 106 grams of CHLORIDE salt. Some adjustment of these salts does occur within the body, by water and salt redistribution, but over a period of time the levels of the salts required CANNOT be met by the normal components of the horse's daily rations.

Supplementation, especially of POTASSIUM and CHLORIDE in particular, is desirable in these types of competition conditions to maintain the correct salt levels in the body.

Other theoretical figures, on the expected SWEAT production/hour of activity, for thoroughbreds, are as follows:-

WALKING	3 LITRES
TROTTING	15 LITRES
CANTERING	20 LITRES
GALLOPING	50 LITRES

NOTE, these are THEORETICAL calculations, very few horses are capable of cantering, yet alone galloping, for one hour without a change to a slower gait.

Based on, these theorectical calculations of sweat output, 20 litres of sweat would contain something in the order of 200 grams SODIUM CHLORIDE (NaCl) and 75 grams POTASSIUM CHLORIDE (KCl). On average rations and maximum daily DRY MATTER intake, it would take the average horse from 7 to 9 days to obtain that quantity of those two salts from the feed, whereas the energy used during that level of salt loss could be obtained from two days average feed.

Expressed in another way ELECTROLYTE LOSS via sweat can amount to approximately the following quantities:-

AVERAGE ENDURANCE RACE	about 20 teaspoons salt
CROSS COUNTRY PHASE of 3 DAY EVENT	about 5 teaspoons salt
THOROUGHBRED RACING	about 2 teaspoons salt.

Very rarely is there a problem which can be due to one ELECTROLYTE. All electrolyte problems involve the interaction of two or more of the salts.

The body salts excreted in SWEAT generally are SODIUM (Na), POTASSIUM (K), CHLORINE (Cl), as the main electrolytes and then MAGNESIUM (Mg), whilst horses which sweat very heavily also excrete CALCIUM (Ca). In fact, the composition of salts excreted in the sweat changes as the work rate of the horse increases.

POTASSIUM (K) losses are considerable, not only from sweat but also by excretion in the urine. Green feed contains consistently high levels of POTASSIUM and the horses' excretory system has been developed to excrete POTASSIUM. Levels of up to 150 grams (6 ozs.) of POTASSIUM can be excreted each day, even in a horse which has not sweated to any extent and the efficiency of POTASSIUM excretion is such that the kidneys will still remove POTASSIUM from the body even if there is a deficiency of POTASSIUM in the daily feed. Since most other horse feeds, grains, hays etc. contain much lower levels of POTASSIUM than green feed, any horse, working reasonably hard, on a ration which does not contain green feed and does not have a POTASSIUM SUPPLEMENT, will have a deficiency of POTASSIUM in the body.

Horses which suffer heavy losses of POTASSIUM (K), SODIUM (Na) and CHLORIDE (Cl) could well be too fatigued and weak to even want to drink despite the biological need to do so. These horses are virtually on the edge of EXHAUSTION and should be treated accordingly.

Horses with heavy work demands, producing large quantities of sweat, can suffer an increased build up of BI-CARBONATE (HCO3) or alkaline salts in the blood. This can cause an additional complication called "ALKALOSIS". Alkalosis develops slowly and it is a result of long periods of sweat output and can in itself cause the horse to perform at less than optimum levels, due to the following:-

1. BICARBONATE will decrease level of HAEMOGLOBIN in the blood and therefore reduce amount of oxygen available to the tissues.
2. BICARBONATE will decrease total blood flow.
3. BICARBONATE will decrease respiratory drive, lowered breathing rate and therefore lowered oxygen intake.

All this adds up to a decreased supply of OXYGEN to the muscle tissues, in particular, this in turn affects LACTIC ACID removal AND MAKES THE LACTIC ACID PROBLEM WORSE, than before BICARBONATE was administered.

ELECTROLYTES AND THE WEATHER

Racehorses in tropical countries have been known to have similar sweat loss and electrolyte problems to the endurance horses in the more temperate areas of the world. With the vast range of climatic zones throughout the world, and with horse competitions of various kinds, occurring in different seasons throughout the year, it is natural that a horse performing at its peak in the middle of a hot summer will sweat more and use more electrolytes than the same horse performing at the same work rate in the middle of winter.

ELECTROLYTES AND TYPE OF WORK

Type of work refers to speed or rate of work and the length of time that work takes place.

The type of work that a horse performs has a marked influence on the need for electrolytes and on the loss of such compounds from the animal during work.

The muscle fuel - GLYCOGEN - is converted to energy inside the horse by one of two methods.

The first method of GLYCOGEN conversion to muscle fuel, is known as the "ANAEROBIC" pathway and this involves the conversion of glycogen to energy only in the ABSENCE of oxygen within muscle. The conversion method used depends on the rate of activity of the horse, the speed of that activity, and the conditioning or training of the horse.

The second method is known as the "AEROBIC" pathway and involves glycogen and associated compounds, such as fat and lactic acid, being converted to energy in the PRESENCE of oxygen within the muscle.

The "ANAEROBIC" energy pathway generally occurs when the speed or pace of the horse exceeds 320 metres per minute (18 km/hour). This is applicable at a fast canter and gallop and hence, in practice, applies to racehorses, eventers on a cross country course, and polo and polo crosse horses in a hard game.

ELECTROLYTES

Up to 50% of the energy produced in the initial 3 minutes of extreme and rapid muscular activity, as occurs in a horse race or a show jump, is produced by the "ANAEROBIC" method.

Electrolyte Flow Chart

ELECTROLYTES
LOST FROM BODY BY
SWEAT, SALIVA, BILE, URINE

↓

AFFECTED BY

INCREASED WORK RATE
INCREASED SWEATING
HOT WEATHER
TRAVELLING STRESS

DIARRHOEA
DRUG OVERUSE
KIDNEY TONICS
BAD TEMPERED HORSE
HANDLERS

↓

LOSSES OF

CHLORIDE — SODIUM — POTASSIUM — MAGNESIUM — CALCIUM — BI-CARBONATE

AFFECTS

- CHLORIDE, SODIUM → KIDNEY FUNCTION AND URINE CONTROL
- SODIUM, POTASSIUM → NERVE & MUSCLE COMMANDS
- MAGNESIUM → ENERGY USE OF BODY CELLS
- CALCIUM → ENERGY FOR MUSCLE CONTRACTION
- BI-CARBONATE → METABOLISM OF ACID PRODUCTS FROM ENERGY USE IN MUSCLE

↓

REPLACE BY

↓

ALKALINE SALTS IF HORSE IS IN HARD WORK – LARGELY AT PACES ABOVE A CANTER

ACID AND ALKALINE SALT MIX IF HORSE WITH LOW OR MEDIUM WORK LOADS – PACES GENERALLY LESS THAN A CANTER.

This "ANAEROBIC" method of conversion of glycogen to muscle energy, however, causes the production and accumulation of lactic acid in the muscles and the blood. This increase of acid in the blood is known as "ACIDOSIS" and the lactic acid build up in the blood is at times considerable. In well conditioned and properly trained horses, LACTIC ACID levels in the muscle tissue will reduce to normal resting levels within 2 hours of the completion of physical exercise. However, in unfit and or poorly trained horses, LACTIC ACID may be detected in the urine for periods of up to 24 hours after the period of "anaerobic" conversion or intense and fast muscular activity.

Excess lactic acid may reduce overall performance, cause unexpected fatigue, muscle stiffness and soreness, and interfere with waste product excretion from the urine.

"AEROBIC" pathway converts glycogen, fat, and also lactic acid into energy, using oxygen in a way which produces up to 18 times MORE ENERGY per unit of glycogen than the "ANAEROBIC" system.

The "AEROBIC" system of glycogen conversion to muscle energy is therefore a much more efficient system, up to 18 times better, than the "ANAEROBIC" system and also because oxygen is present and allows the conversion of fat and the unwanted lactic acid to muscle energy as well. "AEROBIC" energy conversion takes place at speeds below 320 metres per minute (18 km/hour) corresponding to a fast trot, medium canter or slower paces. An endurance horse would be a horse which has continuing "AEROBIC" function of glycogen use by the muscles

Performance horses, in most phases of early training, will therefore, produce most, if not all, of their muscle energy needs by the "AEROBIC" pathway, and this system is greatly improved by conditioning the horse slowly with steadily increasing work demands as the horse gets fitter. Steadily increasing work loads will lead to an increase of oxygen carrying capacity, increased haemoglobin cell numbers, heart size, blood vessel size, etc.

The use of BICARBONATE ($HCO3$) as an electrolyte, normally given in the form of SODIUM BICARBONATE, commonly called BAKING SODA, is certainly not clear. The theory is to provide BICARBONATE so as to neutralise any LACTIC ACID build up in the muscles. In practice, the information currently available appears to disagree with this use of BICARBONATE.

Horses which do long periods of exercise, in hot conditions, suffer considerable losses of CHLORIDE (Cl) from the body and associated with this loss of CHLORIDE, is a retention of BICARBONATE, within the body, by the kidneys. In horses which do short sharp bursts of work, as in racing thoroughbreds, the build up in LACTIC ACID in the muscle is over such a short period of time that maybe BICARBONATE has not enough time to work to control the lactic acid build up. Such horses are known to have lactic acid levels return to normal after about 2 hours of rest, no matter how strenuous the exercise. On the other hand, some practical trainers are claiming good results in standardbred horses, fed reasonably high levels of BICARBONATE, about 150 grams, about 2-3 hours before a race. High levels of BICARBONATE are DEFINITELY not advisable. One racehorse suffered declining performance and became unmanageable and uncontrollable after a period on daily supplementation of 240 grams (0.5lbs) SODIUM BICARBONATE. The horse returned to normal after the BICARBONATE feeding ceased.

The apparently excessive emphasis on the use of SODIUM BICARBONATE in performance horses must have something to do with the fact that the compound can be purchased at any food shop, as BAKING SODA, is relatively cheap and does not need professional advice re administration. The above examples are probably a good indication of what can, very quickly, go wrong in horse feeding, IF CONSIDERATION IS NOT TAKEN OF ALL THE FACTORS INVOLVED WHEN USING ANY FOOD NUTRIENT.

ELECTROLYTES AND DIARRHOEA

DIARRHOEA, of any type can lead to the excretion, from the body of considerable amounts of fluid, and ELECTROLYTES. POTASSIUM is the main electrolyte lost, in an attack of DIARRHOEA and and treatment of any case of DIARRHOEA, should always include electrolyte replacement as part of the medication.

ELECTROLYTE SUPPLEMENTATION

The need for electrolyte supplementation of the horse is influenced by the speed and type of work, and, from this, the method by which muscle energy is produced by the horse.

For most pleasure horses, which do little active work and really do not raise a sweat, there is in general no need for any ELECTROLYTE supplementation of the ration, the horse can, as it has done for years, obtain all its electrolyte needs form the basic feedstuffs.

Individual horses may well have specific ELECTROLYTE needs which are not covered by the above examples. Success from the use of electrolytes has not been confined to performance horses. Some horses, with what would be termed very low work loads, have shown response to specific electrolyte treatments, clearly indicating the importance of ACCURATE assessment of a horse's problem.

To simplify the matter of ELECTROLYTE USE:-

HORSES in cool conditions on high quality feed HAY need ELECTROLYTES, which should contain high levels of POTASSIUM and reasonable levels of SODIUM and CHLORIDE, plus smaller levels of MAGNESIUM. The greater the percentage of grain, hay and chaff, "hard feeds" in the ration and the less the percentage of fresh green feed, the more the need for electrolyte supplementation will be.

For horses which SWEAT considerably, are nervous and/or undergo periods of long slow work, the electrolyte will need to contain high levels of CHLORIDE and POTASSIUM. A common mix which will suit this type of horse is simply one of 2 parts (66% of total weight) POTASSIUM CHLORIDE and 1 part (33% of total weight) SODIUM CHLORIDE, fed at 25-50 grams (1-2 ozs)/day increasing to 100grams (4ozs)/day with increasing work.

CALCIUM levels in the ration should always be monitored. Calcium is a very important electrolyte, but, according to some well respected veterinary equine practitioners, many people cannot get the CALCIUM level right in the rations, as noted from the number of bone problems they see. If this is the situation with the need for large amounts of CALCIUM, there is probably a considerable number of performance horses who are not competing at optimum levels due to insufficient CALCIUM being in the ration for use as an electrolyte.

POSSIBLE RESPONSE TO ELECTROLYTES

Accurate details of the horse's history, especially in the current training programme are of immense value. Details of feed types and consumption, training times, behavioural changes etc. are all of the value of assessing the possible need for electrolyte supplementation.

Dehydration, sunken eye, loss in condition, lethargy and decreased sweating ability are all important signs in diagnosing a possible electrolyte deficiency.

A common problem is where rations which contain only common salt, SODIUM CHLORIDE (Na Cl) often lead to a mild POTASSIUM deficiency, as a result of heavy stress and sweating.

BLOOD TESTS

Blood tests are the most accurate method of diagnosing electrolyte deficiencies. Refer to the section on blood tests.

SOURCES OF ELECTROLYTES

The salts that make up the electrolytes are present in varying concentrations in all common horse pasture, hay and grains.

The two different methods of energy use by the muscles, AEROBIC and ANAEROBIC make it desirable that two different types of electrolyte mixtures be available for the horse, dependent on the level of work and the condition of the horse.

An ALKALINE mixture of salts is designed to correct and prevent ACIDOSIS in horses working at fast paces, e.g. medium canter and above. An ACID mixture contains no alkaline salt and includes high levels of POTASSIUM and CHLORIDE designed to counteract the development of ALKALOSIS that occurs in free sweating horses during long periods of exercise and in hot weather.

Trotters and pacers due to their long periods of training are probably best supplemented in training with the heavy sweat acid formula. A choice of using the acid or alkaline formula in thoroughbred racing depends on the weather conditions, the training programme and the type of horse, sprinter or stayer.

If the weather is hot and/or the horse is a free sweater, racing supplementation could consist of the acid salt whereas, if the weather is cooler and the horse does not sweat as freely then the alkaline salt may be more appropriate.

The thoroughbred in training is more likely to need continual supplementation of the acid salt in the early stages of a preparation, and the change to alkaline salt when actual racing starts. The feeding of the alkaline salt usually continues during the thoroughbreds actual racing campaign as the horse is performing the greater majority of its training and racing at fast paces.

Choice and actual use of the different mixtures depends on individual horse variations and climatic conditions.

IT IS VITALLY IMPORTANT THAT THE HORSE RECEIVE THE CORRECT ELECTROLYTE, considering all the factors involved. GIVING THE HORSE THE INCORRECT ELECTROLYTE MAY GIVE A WORSE RESULT THAN GIVING THE HORSE NO ELECTROLYTE AT ALL.

METHODS OF ELECTROLYTE SUPPLEMENTATION

CAUTION - NEVER PROVIDE ELECTROLYTE SUPPLEMENTATION, OF ANY TYPE TO A HORSE, UNLESS THAT HORSE HAS UNRESTRICTED ACCESS TO WATER.

ELECTROLYTES WILL ENCOURAGE HORSES TO DRINK AND LACK OF WATER AT AND AFTER THE ELECTROLYTE SUPPLEMEMTATION COULD WELL MAKE THE HORSE WORSE RATHER THAN BETTER.

1. SALINE DRIPS INTO THE JUGULAR VEIN

Often given prior to the race or on the day after a race. This is not a favoured practice, due to the possibility of injury to the horse, and also because the amount of solution given to the horse is so small when compared to total body fluids as to be ineffective.

The practice of intravenous injection requires extreme care so as not to introduce infection into the blood, causing more severe and longer term problems than a short term electrolyte deficiency. Secondly, the continual use of intravenous injections of any kind on a horse can make a horse difficult to handle, requiring the use of extreme restraints to allow injections to be given into the vein. With some horses, it is sometimes impossible to find a section of the jugular vein which is not calloused, due to the continual administration of intravenous injections.

Generally a saline drip consists of 1-2 litres of fluid is given into about 60 litres of blood or 300 litres of total body fluid.

The amount of saline administered as a drip or drench in comparison to total body fluid is INSIGNIFICANT - at the most 0.66% of total body fluid, and secondly the extra fluid is generally filtered out of the blood, by the kidneys, when given prior to a race, going to the bladder to be EXCRETED in the urine. At least 6-8 litres of electrolyte solution needs to be given to the animal in the vein to have any worthwhile effect on the level of body salts. To administer this quantity would be an extremely slow process but this volume is needed to ensure that some electrolyte is left in the blood for use by the horse after excretion of most of the administered solution, by the kidney to the bladder has taken place. "Darrow's" solution is in effect an electrolyte type mix and the comments above apply to "Darrow's" solution as well.

2. SALINE DRENCHES

A popular method of administration, usually some hours before a race or performance or on the morning after. The method is beneficial provided the drench is given from 36 to 48 hours prior to racing. Saline drenches require administration by stomach tube, with the attendant problems of abrasion of the internal tissues by the tube, with possible occurrence of internal bleeding and also the possibility of administering the drench into the lungs, instead of the stomach. SALINE DRENCHES have the same problem as the administration of SALINE SOLUTION into the vein, the administration of large quantities of electrolyte, which the kidney does not recognise as being of value to the horse, will lead to filtering out of those electrolytes from the blood and eventual excretion from the horse, via the urine.

3. ELECTROLYTES in the FEED.

The easiest method for humans to administer and horses to receive electrolytes Divide the daily dose between the morning and afternoon feed. Start at low levels and increase the dosage over a period of days, dependent on the type of work, until the recommended dose is reached. In this method, the electrolytes are held in reserve, within the horse, as the overall salt level has been slowly increased and the salts are therefore available, in a ready reserve, for instant use by the horse when needed. Horses in peak condition and performance may be given increased doses of electrolytes, up to double dose, in the two days prior to the actual race or performance.

4. ELECTROLYTES in the WATER.

Horses which consume the average bucket of water 8-12 litres twice/day, do not get enough water for this method be successful. Heavily sweating horses can lose up to 20-30 litres/day in sweat alone and generally can drink up to 50 litres/day. The recommended normal dose in this method is to dissolve the daily dose in 25 litres of water. Dehydrated horses will drink normally and are able to consume at least 25 litres of water per day and will respond to electrolyte administration in this manner. After the horse has consumed the 25 litres of water containing the electrolyte mix, the horse can then be given additional water, without electrolyte added. There could be a palatability problem with this method of administration, the horse refusing to drink the treated water.

ONE of the main problems with performance horses suffering from partial dehydration or insufficient water intake is an electrolyte problem. Fix that problem and partial dehydration will be a thing of the past.

ELECTROLYTES SHOULD BE GIVEN TO A HORSE ON A CONTINUAL BASIS, IN EVERY FEED OR ON EVERY DAY OF A TRAINING AND COMPETITION PROGRAMME. IF ADMINISTRATION IS COMMENCED AT LOW RATES AND DOSAGE INCREASED, AS DESIRED, THE KIDNEYS LEARN TO RECOGNISE THE INCREASING LEVELS OF THESE COMPOUNDS WHICH WE CALL ELECTROLYTES AND WILL TOLERATE INCREASING LEVELS, WELL ABOVE NORMAL WITHIN THE BODY.

PRACTICAL PROBLEMS WITH ELECTROLYTES

1. Select the correct electrolyte mix for the horse's individual circumstances. You need to determine whether your horse is converting glycogen into muscle energy AEROBICALLY or ANAEROBICALLY.
2. Some electrolytes are separate acid and alkaline solutions and are not to be mixed together until immediately before administration. Likewise, do not add other ingredients to a specific electrolyte mix as the compounds could react with each other canceling any potential benefit and the mix solution could be of nil value to the horse and would be similar to giving the horse a drink of water.
3. Start on half normal dose divided over two feeds and increase electrolyte intake, subject to level of work and any individual horse palatability problems.

potential benefit and the mix solution could be of nil value to the horse and would be similar to giving the horse a drink of water.

3. Start on half normal dose divided over two feeds and increase electrolyte intake, subject to level of work and any individual horse palatability problems.
4. Measure the dose accurately. Measures are normally provided, use them. Do not rely on "handfuls" or similar measures.
5. When electrolytes are added to water, add the full dose to at least 8 litres of water. The correct amount of electrolyte added to lesser quantities or water may be unpalatable, and not consumed by the horse.
6. Change the water supply before adding more electrolyte. This is to avoid the build up in salt concentration, with consequent refusal of the horse to drink the water with electrolyte added, due to palatability problems.
7. Some horses may refuse to take electrolytes in water, an individual palatibility problem.
8. When giving electrolytes in the feed, some palatability problems may occur. Overcome this by the addition of small amounts of molasses to the feed. Always ensure that the horse has adequate water supply when electrolytes are added in the feed.
9. Do not add extra salts of any type when using electrolytes. Too many problems can occur which can produce more severe salt imbalances in the horse than existed before the electrolyte treatment commenced.
10. Be careful in the use of kidney balls and other diuretic compounds as the effect of these on the kidneys can alter the internal ELECTROLYTE BALANCE, i.e. the way in which the horse uses and and excretes ELECTROLYTES.
11. Electrolyte supplementation in feed is much preferred to supplementation in the drinking water. If the concentration of the electrolyte in the drinking water is incorrect and the horse is not drinking reasonable quantities of that water, the amount of electrolyte that the horse will receive will be insufficient to be of any value. Electrolyte given in the feed however is much more controllable by the feeder and the horse is able to drink as much water as needed for the individual circumstances.
12. ALWAYS ENSURE THAT ADEQUATE SUPPLIES OF WATER ARE AVAILABLE TO ANY HORSE, AT AND AFTER ELECTROLYTE ADMINISTRATION.

10. BLOOD COUNTS AND BLOOD TESTS

Blood specifically performs the following functions:

1. To carry oxygen to the tissues.
2. To transport hormones of growth, reproduction and action inside the horse.
3. To carry the food nutrients from the digestive tract to all parts of the body, after the food particles have been broken down in the digestive tract, by micro-organisms and enzymes.
4. The removal of waste products from the operating tissues, e.g. the muscles, the heart, the lungs etc. to the organs that excrete those waste products out of the horse, e.g. the liver, kidneys etc.
5. Assists is the control of body pH or commonly known as ACIDITY and or ALKALINITY.
6. Assists in the control of temperature and water balance within the animal.
7. Aids in assisting the bodies' defence mechanism against infection from bacteria and virus.

Because the function of BLOOD, within the horse, involves so many different purposes, the amount of the various components in the BLOOD is in a continual state of flux, involving constant change.

In addition, as the BLOOD comes into constant contact with virtually every cell in the horse's body, the components of the BLOOD sample will represent the chemical and physiological activities occurring within that horse.

EACH HORSE HAS A SEPARATE AND INDIVIDUAL BLOOD COUNT AND BLOOD TEST DETAILS and any such information should only be used for that one horse and is only of value when the details of a number of tests are available.

Details provided from analysis of blood samples are frequently used by horse owners, as a means of determining the fitness or otherwise of a horse. Information contained in such records, BLOOD TESTS especially, are of value in monitoring and changing feeds and or feeding methods of the horse.

It is very obvious, from experience, that the average horse owner really has no idea of what a BLOOD TEST or BLOOD COUNT is all about. I have seen numerous horse owners place unquestionable faith in a piece of paper, with a lot of figures on it, which they do not understand. This chapter is not meant to be a full veterinary explanation as to the content or appreciation of blood test results. That is the duty of the veterinary surgeon in conjunction with the client as results, from blood tests or blood counts can mean many things and will vary with each individual horse.

This section is, however, designed to explain just what BLOOD COUNTS and BLOOD TESTS are all about and how the practical horse feeder may use the results, so obtained, to assess the health of his horse and take corrective action, either by himself or in conjunction with his veterinary surgeon.

BLOOD COUNTS AND BLOOD TESTS

BLOOD TESTS and BLOOD COUNTS DO NOT INDICATE HOW FIT A HORSE IS. They measure the concentration or amounts of certain components in the blood and in turn determine any abnormal levels of these blood components. The correct analysis and or appreciation of these results works on the principle that if there are no differences in the results, from the levels expected in a normal healthy horse, then the horse has NO PROBLEMS as far as the blood components are concerned. There may well be many other factors affecting a horse's performance which cannot be detected by a blood test, e.g. insufficient protein in the diet and hence reduced muscle function. Litres of top quality blood flowing to undernourished muscle will not produce a horse performing at his best.

Results from blood tests or blood counts are only of value if a SERIES of blood samples, from the one horse, are analysed over a period of time. These series of samples will provide an INDIVIDUAL HORSE PROFILE of the components, in the blood, being analysed and will allow assessment of any variation in normal expected levels. The use, for diagnostic purposes, of one blood test from one horse, is of little value as there are no average values available for the same horse for the same records to use for comparison.

The RESULTS obtained from blood tests and blood counts can also vary, dependent on the conditions and the temperament of the horse, at the time of sampling. Sampling errors can be quite dramatic in blood tests or blood counts and it therefore important to understand why.

The results of BLOOD TESTS and BLOOD COUNTS can be affected by:-

1. Time of day of sampling. If you are consistently monitoring the health of a horse by results of analysis of blood, try and get the blood samples taken about the same time each day. preferably before work or of an evening when the horses' physiological function will be similar, at each sampling.
2. Condition of horse. The same horse in differing physical condition will produce differing results for the same blood components.
3. If the sample is taken for BLOOD COUNTS, they should be taken when the horse is at rest, and completely calm, and certainly some period of time after the horse has done physical exercise, a suggested minimum of at least 3 hours.
4 If the sample is to be used for BLOOD TESTS, to determine any one of the biochemical and electrolyte levels in the blood, as an aid to trying to sort out the reason for a horse TYING UP, a series of base samples taken as above with the horse at rest completely calm and at least 3 hours after exercises should be taken. Additional samples are then taken at various times after exercise, dependant on what results are being sought. Samples can be taken immediately after exercise and about 2 , 6 and 24 hours, after exercise, if a full evaluation of the biochemical components are required.
5.If the results are to assess RED BLOOD CELL details, it is absolutely essential that the horse be calm at the time of sampling.

The horse has the ability to store considerable quantities of red blood cells, about 40% or more of total red blood cells, in the spleen, during periods of rest or low levels of activity and to release these red blood cells very quickly into the blood stream. Conditions conducive to this massive release of red blood cells into the blood stream include exercise and excitement. Even the horses' reaction to hand feeding MAY be sufficient to cause an increase, due to excitement, in red blood cell output from the spleen. Any blood sampling under any of these conditions, of excitement and or exercise, will produce incorrect results for red blood cells, often an error of 40% may occur.

Blood has such an important function in the horses' body that a lot of people place complete faith in a blood test, without realising that there are other equally important parts of body function and nutrition that all combine to produce a top horse.

BLOOD COUNTS

These are the most common routine tests available to horse owners. BLOOD COUNTS are exactly what the name says, a count of some of the components of the blood, namely the BLOOD CELLS. BLOOD COUNTS determine the RED and WHITE BLOOD CELL levels and associated details in the blood. Technically, these results relating to the red and white blood cells only, are known as HAEMATOLOGICAL READINGS. Biochemical tests are generally not carried out in the performance of Blood Counts.

Haematological readings consist of details on the red and white blood cells. RED BLOOD CELLS contain haemoglobin, the iron containing pigment, which is responsible for the movement of oxygen around the horses' body. The red blood cells are produced in the bone marrow, in a continuous process which can take about 6 days or slightly longer to produce one red blood cell. The red cells live in the horse for about 150 days and the average horse contains about 18 kgs. of red cells in its' body. Efficient RED BLOOD CELL production requires not only IRON, but also COPPER, COBALT and FOLIC ACID.

ANAEMIA or reduced red blood cell numbers is a secondary abnormality in that it is always associated with some other problem which has caused the ANAEMIA. These primary abnormalities are generally associated with a chronic infection which can affect any of the following:-

a) Inadequate nutrition or incorrectly balanced rations.
b) Bone marrow problems, not producing enough RED BLOOD CELLS.
c) Excessive removal of red blood cells by worms, lice, acidosis, blood loss from injury etc.

RED BLOOD CELLS are analysed by the following criteria.

RED BLOOD CELL COUNT or R.B.C.

Measures the number of red blood cells in the sample at the time of sampling. The normally accepted range for red blood cell count is in the order of 7- 11 x 10 to the power of 12/litre.

HAEMATOCRIT, PACKED CELL VOLUME or P.C.V.

This is a second method of measuring red blood cell numbers. The proportion of red blood cells in the total sample is measured by centrifuging a small quantity of blood and reading the volume of the red blood cells in the bottom of the centrifuge tube, in relation to the total volume in that tube. Normal values are in the range of 0.30 - 0.50 L/L or sometimes expressed as 30 - 50%.

HAEMOGLOBIN CONCENTRATION

This chemical is responsible for the red colour of the blood cells and carries oxygen from the lungs to the various body tissues. The change in colour of the blood is measured on a machine and the results are used on the basis that dark red blood is able to carry more oxygen to the tissues than is blood of a lighter colour. Normal haemoglobin values in the horse are in the range of 110-170 gms/litre.

There is generally higher levels of R.B.C., P.C.V. and HAEMOGLOBIN CONCENTRATION in male horses than in female horses and there are often breed differences. R.B.C. of two and three year old thoroughbreds is often in the range of 9 whilst the same reading for COLD BLOOD breeds will be of the order of 7.

The above three tests are the basis for assessing the red blood cell content.

There are also three other readings, termed DERIVED INFORMATION, as the details can only come from the above three tests, that may be obtained from testing for red blood cells, but, in the opinion of a number of veterinary surgeons, they only repeat the information provided by the initial three criteria.

These readings are:

MEAN CORPUSCULAR VOLUME or M.C.V.

Assessment of red blood cells size. Small sized red blood cells are generally associated with iron (Fe) deficiency, but in practice this condition is apparently very rare, and if present is generally related to a problem called SICKLE CELL or SMALL CELL ANAEMIA which is genetically related and cannot be corrected by nutritional changes.

MEAN CORPUSCULAR HAEMOGLOBIN CONCENTRATION or M.C.H.C.

An estimate of the haemoglobin contained in the individual blood cells.

MEAN CONCENTRATION HAEMOGLOBIN or M.C.H.

An estimate of the haemoglobin contained in the individual red blood cells.

To emphasise the need for blood samples to be taken from the horse at rest, when attempting to assess the RED BLOOD CELL LEVELS, the following R.B.C. details of blood samples taken from a number of horses indicates the release of red blood cells, from the spleen, as a result of physical activity and the affect this can have on R.B.C. levels in a blood test.

Horses at rest	40% of total R.B.C.
Endurance horses	45%
Trotting or pacing horses	55%
Three day event horses	60%
Gallopers	65%

Horses are generally considered anaemic if the R.B.C. is below 30%. Any horse which proves to be anaemic, on a blood test, should then be examined further to determine whether the problem is GENETIC and therefore unable to be corrected. If the problem is NOT GENETIC, or inherited, in origin, immediately, have the protein content of the ration increased, PROTEIN builds and maintains tissues, including blood, and the horse should be thoroughly wormed, at least three times at three week intervals with larger than normal doses of the new and safe drugs available for these purposes. Under no circumstances, should iron tonics or supplements be fed to anaemic horses until the above two courses of action have taken place. IRON, by itself, will not increase red blood cell content, as the iron is only a very small part of the individual red blood cell. If the body of the red blood cell is not there, obtained from protein in the diet, and if the worms are sucking the blood out of the horse as quickly as it is made, then no IRON, no matter what quantity, will fix the problem.

Also remember, from earlier in this book, that IRON when fed for 6 weeks, at levels some 13 times above the normal horses' needs, had NO EFFECT on the amount of either HAEMOGLOBIN or on the PACKED CELL VOLUME in the horse and in addition EXCESS levels of IRON in the ration can affect the growth of young horses and may have the ability to fix phosphorus in the horses' body, thereby upsetting the amounts of calcium and phosphorus, leading to the possibility of RICKETS and similar problems.

WHITE BLOOD CELLS

also known as LEUKOCYTES, WHITE BLOOD CELLS are the first line of defence, in the horse's body, against DISEASE. White blood cells are a mixed population of five main cell types which individually attack the various bacteria and viruses that cause common infections in the horse. The assessment of white blood cell counts determines the levels of the five main cell types and relates these levels to the expected normal range. Deviations from the norm are then used as an indication of possible problems in the horse. White blood cells numbers, the total number of the five types, are generally present in the horse in the range of 6.0-12.0 x 10X9/ litre or sometimes expressed as 6000-12000/mmX3. Any deviation outside this range is an indication that the horse may be suffering some form of infection or sub-clinical illness. A sub-clinical disease in one which affects the horse's performance but is usually not noticed by the horse owner.

Total white blood cell counts of up to 20000/mmX3 have been detected in some horses indicating rather large bacterial and or viral infections and therefore disease and illness in that particular horse.

White blood cells are produced not only in the bone marrow but can also be manufactured in other body tissues. Lymphocytes, in particular, can be produced in the spleen, lymph nodes and liver, where they are stored for rapid use against disease.

WHITE CELL TYPES

NEUTROPHILS

The most common of the white blood cells and can make up to 55-60% of the total white blood cell count. These cells act as the first line of defence, in the body, against any infection. Neutrophils possess the ability to pass through the walls of the blood vessels and digest unwanted bacteria. Any increase in neutrophil count is a sign of some form of infection and, in practice, neutrophil count has been known up to 90% of the total white blood cell count. Neutrophils are capable of causing damage to the lungs and the condition, commonly called HEAVES, has sometimes resulted from lung tissue damage, due to the number of NEUTROPHILS, attempting to control some type of low level long term infection within the body.

LYMPHOCYTES

Present in the horse in two forms - "large" and "small". "Large" lymphocytes, found in the lymph nodes and the spleen, until an infection develops when they move into the bloodstream, and act as defence against unwanted bacteria entering the body. "Small" lymphocytes continuously move in the blood and have the ability to remember previously introduced bacteria that have been attacked by monocytes. The small lymphocytes are able to initiate the production of anti-bodies in the animal. Lymphocytes, in a fit horse make up to 30-35% of the total white cell count.

The lymphocyte count reduces during the early stages of infection when they are active in fighting against the invading bacteria. If the total number of white blood cells are considered normal, but there is a reduced number of lymphocytes present, indications of the horse being under stress may well be the diagnosis. An acceptable ratio also exists between the lymphocytes and neutrophils and careful assessment of that ratio in conjunction with other details can be of value to the veterinary surgeon in diagnosing problems in the horse.

MONOCYTES

In fit horses, Monocytes are present in the blood in low concentrations - around 5-8% of total white cell numbers. Monocytes act on infections in two ways. Firstly, they can engulf and destroy invading bacteria in a manner similar to the action of the neutrophils. Secondly, the monocytes are able to assist in the production of anti-bodies against the infection. Increase in monocyte count generally occurs when a chronic or long term infection is present. Increased monocyte levels may also be associated with fungal infections such as ringworm, fistulous withers and poll evil - Brucella infection - and possibly tuberculosis.

BASOPHILS

Normal levels are about 0-2% of the total white blood cell count. These cells probably play a part in starting the the bodys' reaction to injury, infection, and tissue damage. Basophils contain a chemical which can dilate the blood vessels and allow extra blood to flow to an injured area, and may also contain an anti-coagulant which has the effect of decreasing clot formation at the site of the injury. This allows blood to flow freely to the injured area. Any increase in the basophil count is normally associated with an increase, at the same time, in the eosinophil count in the white blood cells.

EOSINOPHILS

Normal levels are about 0-5% of the total white cell number. These cells act to control the extent of the inflammation and/or tissue reaction at the site of injury or infection. Increase in eosinophils levels are common in bad internal parasite infections, in some cases of external parasite infections, especially Queensland Itch, and may also rise when an animal is being fed on dusty feeds. Adverse reactions to drugs may also cause an increase in the levels of the eosinophil component of the white blood cells. Horses in hard work may have a negligible or zero content of eosinophils in the blood, and administration of cortisone may also reduce the levels of this type of blood cell to zero, possibly masking diagnosis any infection or disease which the horse may have.

BLOOD TESTS

This generally consists of an assessment of the red and white blood cells, as carried out on the BLOOD COUNT analysis described above, PLUS details of one or more of the many BIOCHEMICAL tests which can be performed on the blood sample. These many BIOCHEMICAL TESTS are carried out on, either, the SERUM, which is the liquid remaining after blood has been allowed to clot or on the PLASMA, which is the liquid remaining after unclotted blood has been centrifuged.

BIOCHEMICAL TESTS are able to determine in the PLASMA protein levels, hormone levels, sugars, the various electrolyte contents, enzymes and mineral content, specific cardiac enzymes, liver function enzymes as well as other more detailed and specific analysis.

BIOCHEMICAL READINGS FROM BLOOD TESTS

A number of biochemical tests can be performed on blood and the results can be useful, in conjunction with other information, including details of previous feeding history in assessing a whole range of problems in the horse.

A.S.T. TEST

Formerly called The G.O.T. Test, this determines the ASPARTATE AMINO TRANSFERASE enzyme in the blood. This enzyme is an important part of muscle function and assessment will allow determination of whether muscle damage is present or not. Muscle damage can be caused by stresses, sprains, overuse of drugs and/or tonics and many other reasons. Horses may have damaged muscles, i.e. muscles not functioning properly, but not show any external symptoms.

Normal values for fit horses are in the order of 300 units per litre or less. Care is required in the interpretation of this reading as values for A.S.T. may remain high for up to 2-3 weeks following muscle damage.

C.K. or C.P.K. TEST

This involves another enzyme, CREATINE KINASE, that also increases in level following muscle damage. This test has an advantage in that the elevated levels only occur for 12-24 hours after the muscle damage has occurred.

A.P. TEST

Determines the enzyme, ALKALINE PHOSPHATASE which splits and mobilises phosphate within the body. The level of this enzyme increases when there is bone or liver damage.

L.D.H. TEST

Measures the level of the enzyme LACTIC DEHYDROGENASE, which can exist in the blood in 5 slightly different forms, known as ISOENZYMES, because each originates in a different part of the body. Increased levels of L.D.H. indicate some form of soft tissue damage, the origin of which can be more accurately determined, by detailed tests to measure the levels of each of the ISOENZYMES.

T.P. or T.P.P. TEST

Measures TOTAL PROTEIN, also called TOTAL PLASMA PROTEIN in the blood. This is NOT a guide to the nutritional status of the horse, but rather an indication of the extent of dehydration of the horse, if any. Horses which are dehydrated, i.e. have insufficient body water content, will show increased levels of Total Protein compared to normal values. Normal levels for T.P. are about 6- 7 grams/decilitre.

A:G RATIO

A stands for ALBUMIN and G for GLOBULIN, two proteins which circulate in the blood. ALBUMIN is the binding protein in the blood which holds the water and electrolytes in solution. GLOBULIN is the protein component in the blood which carries the ANTI-BODIES which form the basis of body's IMMUNE system. In healthy horses, the ALBUMIN content of the blood should always exceed the GLOBULIN content. The ALBUMIN:GLOBULIN RATIO provides figures which can be used as an indicator of the presence of infectious diseases in the horse, whilst a fall below the expected level of ALBUMIN alone will be an indicator of possible LIVER damage.

Values obtained from the TOTAL PROTEIN test and the ALBUMIN:GLOBULIN ratio are often used in conjunction, with each other, to monitor the progress of diarrhoea, colic and other similar intestinal problems.

FIBRINOGEN

FIBRINOGEN is that part of the blood protein, responsible for the clotting of blood, reduced levels indicating a genetic or nutritional reason for poor blood clotting powers. FIBRINOGEN has an inflammatory action, rising in level during the acute or most severe phase of the disease. A change in the FIBRINOGEN level in the blood will affect the SEDIMENTATION RATE or settling out rate of the RED BLOOD CELLS, due to its effect on blood viscosity.

BLOOD GLUCOSE LEVELS

The level of GLUCOSE, in the horses' blood, is subject to short term fluctuations, dependent on the level of exercise, stress, diet and infection.

BLOOD GLUCOSE levels can be used to predict the outcome of numerous equine problems including colic, reduced tolerance to exercise, weakness in foals, excessive urination and thirst and liver dysfunction.

In the case of colic, when blood glucose levels exceeded 30 mgs/decilitre,the hope of recovery was poor and when the blood glucose levels exceeded 600mg/decilitre, there was the possibility that damage to the central nervous system had occurred.

BILIRUBIN

BILIRUBIN is the BILE pigment formed from the destruction of RED BLOOD CELLS in the liver. Determination of the BILIRUBIN level in the blood sample allows a determination of liver function and also any excessive destruction of red blood cells.

LACTATE

This test involves the determination of the level of LACTIC ACID, produced in the muscle as a result of ANAEROBIC MUSCLE activity, increased levels of which can reduce muscle performance, induce fatigue, produce muscle stiffness and soreness, interfere with waste product excretion and cause TYING UP.

PLASMA MINERALS

It is possible to test for the mineral levels in blood plasma, particularly the TRACE MINERALS. Research on the levels of COPPER, ZINC and MANGANESE, in blood plasma, show that the levels of these three minerals are far TOO VARIABLE in blood plasma to be used as a SOLE MEANS of diagnosing deficiencies in the horse.

ELECTROLYTES

These have been discussed in detail earlier in this book. Biochemical determination on blood samples, taken on a horse AT REST will allow some indication of the total body content of individual electrolytes of the particular horse before exercise.

These RESTING RESULTS can then be compared with results for the exact same electrolytes, in blood samples. taken from horses immediately after hard work and in the following 24 hour period to possibly determine the specific electrolyte needs of that horse.

The salts normally measured are:

SODIUM (Na) - this is the principle electrolyte outside the walls of the individual body cells. It has a very active role in fluid balance - refer to Chapter 14 - and it is imperative that performance horses, in particular, have adequate sodium levels.

POTASSIUM (K) - this is the main electrolyte inside the body cells. Diarrhoea and sweating will cause considerable loss of potassium and horses with these conditions should be supplemented with potassium where necessary. Increased or decreased levels of potassium may also indicate heart malfunction. If any change from normal values is detected in the POTASSIUM level in the serum, normally a kidney excretion and or urine clearance test is carried out to determine if there is any kidney damage present.

THE ABILITY TO DETECT LARGE LOSSES OF BOTH SODIUM AND POTASSIUM IS OFTEN DIFFICULT USING BLOOD TEST RESULTS. RESULTS FOR THESE TWO ELECTROLYTES CAN BE SO VARIABLE AS NOT TO BE OF ANY PRACTICAL VALUE.

CHLORIDE (Cl) this is the major electrolyte lost in body sweat. Fortunately common salt is sodium chloride so the feeding of salt to all horses, especially performance horses, should overcome the deficiency problems associated with either sodium or chloride deficiency.

BI-CARBONATE (HCO3) the level of this salt will indicate whether in fact the horse is suffering from ACIDOSIS or ALKALOSIS. Acidosis occurs in the case of colic and diarrhoea whilst alkalosis can occur in the case of endurance horses and animals trained for peak performance activities. Excess levels of bi- carbonate have also been incriminated in affecting temperament and in fact horses which are difficult to manage have often been found to have high bi-carbonate levels in the blood.

MAGNESIUM (Mg) important in controlling the use of energy by the muscle cells. Some performance horses have very specific Magnesium requirements, often considerably higher than than the normal expected levels of supplementation. Either their body cells require more Magnesium than the average, to work effectively, or alternately they are unable to get sufficient Magnesium from the digestive tract. This could be due to, either the feeding of a ration low in Magnesium or else due to, the inability of that particular horse to absorb and utilise the Magnesium in the diet. Some horses are known as "bad travellers", they will sweat uncontrollably in a float during transport and will arrive at their destination covered in sweat and often with pronounced muscle movement and tremors, symptoms very similar to mild forms of TYING UP. These types of horses appear to be using higher than normal levels of Magnesium during this period and Magnesium supplementation has been very effective in controlling the problem.

CALCIUM (Ca) not only is Calcium of importance in the horse in the formation and maintenance of bone but it is also important as an electrolyte in the use of energy for muscle contraction. As all horse movement depends on muscle contraction, any deficiency of Calcium in the diet will affect the ability of the horse to perform adequately and to the limit of its genetic ability.

The use of blood tests to diagnose electrolyte problems requires expert knowledge of the principles of horse feeding and physiology and interpretation of such blood tests is definitely the premise of the animal nutritionist or veterinary surgeon who are trained for such activities.

The inclusion of ELECTROLYTES in this section is to inform the horse feeder that the tests are available.

11. THE HIDDEN HANDICAPPER

The feeding of horses has taken some large steps forward, over the past few years, compared to the practices of the 1970's and before.

In that period, the horse could have been fed anything dependent on tradition, old wives tales, secret recipes, hearsay information or any other reason to try something new.

The "solution" to all the problems of the horse, or if the horse did not have any problems, to make the horse perform better always lay in the unexplainable but mystical qualities of some new feed or feed additive.

Unfortunately the exact same "folklore" of feeding horses still exists to-day but fortunately the general attitude to horse feeding is changing as horse people become aware of the availability of technical information on feeding and how that information can be used to help their horses, either to perform better, or for the cost conscious, to perform at the same level but at a reduced financial cost.

FEEDING A HORSE CORRECTLY is similar to MAKING A SUCCESSFUL CAKE.

To make a cake, there is a recipe or series of nominated steps:-

1 - a list of ingredients is required.

2 - the exact amounts of each ingredient is nominated.

3 - the order and length of time of mixing is stated.

4 - the correct oven temperature is provided.

5 - adjust oven temperature and cooking time. using experience as a guide to produce the best cake.

Provided all these details are followed to the letter, a successful cake will result from the exercise.

With feeding horses we can go through the same steps.

1 - require a knowledge of each of the food nutrients the particular horse needs.

2 - need to know the exact amounts of each food nutrients a horse needs for a particular task.

3 - require a knowledge of the order in which the various feed components are given to the horse.

4 - have some idea of the training programme for the horse, as this affects the level and time of feeding some food components to get the best results.

5 - need to monitor the training programme and adjust the feeding and training programme, as required, and guided by experience to produce the best from the horse.

It is at this stage that the comparison of a cake and a horse go their separate ways.

The details of a "successful" cake making exercise have probably been worked out over time, with a number of failures occurring before the desired "recipe" which produced the required end product was finalised. The cake also probably went from the basic ingredients to a finished product in a matter of hours and the changes from a number of separate ingredients to the finished product could be readily seen.

The average horse person likes to see things happen and usually reasonably quickly. Responses to changes in horse management need to be visual and obvious. The action of some chiropractors, with the tennis ball and the baseball bat, pounding the horse for some undefined complaint, the use of a particular piece of gear which is so severe the horse has to behave or it will be injured in some way, and other similar examples of "instant action" all provide, to some people, a visual action which provides some a sense of achievement. Firstly the owners can see things happening, whether these actions help the horse or not is another matter, and secondly the time frame for a "result" is short, often a matter of minutes.

WITH HORSE FEEDING, ANY SIGNIFICANT CHANGES ARE OFTEN SLOW TO HAPPEN AND CERTAINLY ARE NOT HIGHLY VISIBLE.

Sufficient technical knowledge now exists to allow determination of the needs of each individual horse for all the food components which go to make up horse rations.

Similarly, data exists which gives the amounts of each of these 40 or so individual feed components in all common horse feeds. If the data does not exist, laboratory analysis can readily and rapidly determine what is in each feed, including any new or, as yet, undiscovered "super compound".

Knowledge is available of the reactions and interactions of each of the feed components with each other. Those components which affect the use of other components, either favourably or unfavourably, are well known, those which have to be fed first before any other to get the best result are all documented.

The varying demands of the different types of horses, for specific feed components at various stages of a training programme, are now able to be expressed in terms which can be related to the feed components required.

THE PROBLEMS WITH FEEDING HORSES ARE:-

1. Unlike the separate and individual ingredients which go into making a cake, it is not possible to distinctly and individually see the PROTEIN or the IRON or any other of the 38 other feed components in the ration. These components are nevertheless contained in all the basic horse feeds and have been present in those feeds for hundreds of years.

The horse has been able to survive, perform and reproduce satisfactorily for generations, existing all the time on vegetation and the seeds (grain) of such vegetation. In fact, racing times of thoroughbreds showed a slow but continual improvement until about the 1920's when man started to become scientific and commenced feeding the horse all sorts of supplements. Since that date, racing times have shown virtually no improvement, despite modern technology and its benefits. Man has appeared to have forgotten all about what natural vegetative feeds contain, and has resorted to the feeding of all types of artificial feeds and supplements, most of which contained feed components, already in the natural feeds. At the same time little attention has been paid to the fact that the components of some feed supplements destroy others, or when combined, with the levels of the same feed components, in the natural feed, may be prove damaging to the horse.

2. Any response to a change in feeding practices is generally slow to happen, occurring over weeks and sometimes months and NOT HOURS, as with the cake, or minutes as with the chiropractor. Further, most horse people are too impatient to wait for the change or do not know how to recognise and or evaluate the change.

As a result, many people continue to feed as usual, rations based on tradition, adding a new feed as soon as it becomes known, all in the hope of improving performance.

The MAIN PROBLEMS of horse feeding:-

INSUFFICIENT LEVELS of any of the 40 feed components in the ration.
EXCESSIVE LEVELS of some 14 feed components in the ration.
DESTRUCTION of some feed components by additives.
INCORRECT ORDER of administration.
NOT CO-ORDINATING FEEDING AND TRAINING.
are either not understood, not wanted to be understood, or completely ignored.

NUTRIENT DEFICIENCY

If the horse suffers from a deficiency or imbalance of any one of the 40 or so known feed components which constitute properly balanced horse feed, a sequence of events will commence in the horse as follows:

NUTRIENT DEFICIENCY

↓

BIOCHEMICAL DEFECT

↓

FUNCTIONAL DEFECT

↓

MICROSCOPIC ANATOMICAL DEFECT

↓

MACROSCOPIC (VISIBLE) DEFECT

↓

DEATH

A deficiency of VITAMIN B1 or THIAMINE in the horse will provide a practical example of this procedure.

NUTRIENT DEFICIENCY	THIAMINE or VITAMIN B1
BIOCHEMICAL DEFECT	prevents breakdown of PYRUVIC qACID, a by-product of energy use, leading to increased levels in the tissues.
FUNCTIONAL DEFECT	poor appetite and reduced growth, NOT HIGHLY VISIBLE or easily recognised, the same effects could be cause by numerous other problems in the horse.
MICROSCOPIC ANATOMICAL DEFECT	microscopic lesions develop in nervous tissue.
MACROSCOPIC (VISIBLE) DEFECT	goes off feed, loses weight, muscle tremors.
DEATH	the final and end result if the condition is NOT CORRECTED.

In any situation, involving a deficiency or an excess of any feed component in the horses' ration, there will be considerable undesirable changes, SUB CLINICAL, which will have occurred inside the horse, BEFORE ANY VISIBLE SYMPTOMS are noticed, diagnosed and treated.

The response to any treatment will depend on:-

1. reason for the problem.
2. length of time the problem has existed.
3. age of horse.
4. any other complicating factors in the ration and or training programme, including drug administration.

THE BIOCHEMICAL, FUNCTIONAL and STRUCTURAL DEFECTS in horses, associated with nutrient deficiencies are SPECIFIC to each NUTRIENT or FEED COMPONENT and only careful and thorough evaluation is able to correct the problem.

It is much more desirable, simpler and certainly less expensive in the long run, to ensure that each horse is receiving the correct ration, fully balanced for all its needs so that possible nutritional problems DO NOT OCCUR.

The phrase HIDDEN HANDICAPPER describes most feeding techniques used by horse people. When the rations and the training programmes of some horse people are assessed, there is, in many cases, a feeding problem, small but very significant,which is restricting the performance of the horse.

Explanation of, and correction of, these problems more often than not removes the HIDDEN HANDICAPPER from restricting the horse's performance.

The following chapters of this book should help the reader to eliminate the HIDDEN HANDICAPPER from affecting the performance of your horse.

12. INTERNAL PARASITES - WORMS

All horses have worms.

All horses get re-infected with worms.

The first step in any nutritional evaluation is to ensure that the horse is as free from worms as possible.

If you are feeding worms, inside the horse, as well as the horse itself, it is impossible to expect the horse to perform to the best of its ability.

Horses, unlike other grass eating animals, or ruminants, DO NOT develop any acquired immunity or resistance to the majority of internal parasites. For this reason ALL HORSES have to be constantly protected from massive worm build-ups, within the digestive tract, by continual and repeated drenchings, once termed an ANTHELMINTIC UMBRELLA.

Whilst this book is not intended to be a study of internal parasites of horses, it is important to mention some practical aspects of worm control which are often neglected by horse owners, and are vitally important to ensure correct horse health and efficient feed utilisation.

Worms in horses are present in three forms:

1. Mature Adult Worms - present in the digestive tract and sometimes observed in the faeces after drenching. These adult worms cause little damage inside the horse, with the exception of the large ROUNDWORM which can block the intestines of foals, but are essential to lay eggs and produce the next generation.
2. Immature Worms - are present in the digestive tract and sometimes other organs - generally not seen by the naked eye, but often passed out in the faeces after worming, provided sufficient quantities of drench are used.
3. Migratory Worms, in some worm species, a specific stage of the migratory cycle - these are microscopic worms invisible to the naked eye and are generally in the blood stream, blood vessels, and other organs such as the heart, liver, lungs, kidneys etc. Drenching with normal dose rates does not affect these worms.

Each species of worm or INTERNAL PARASITE in the horse is generally present in the three stages outlined above.

External visible symptoms of worm infestation, in horses, generally include, poor condition, pale coloured mucous membranes, lips eyelids etc., lethargic appearance, lack of energy, harsh or "steely" coat-dull in appearance, possibly a liquid, foul smelling faeces or alternately a very hard dry faeces. These symptoms are SIMILAR to many other problems which can affect a horse, lack of protein in the ration, electrolyte imbalance, etc. VITAMIN B deficiency, slight SELENIUM poisoning and so the list goes on.

An infestation of RED WORM (STRONGYLUS species) DOES NOT produce the above visible symptoms. A horse, severely infected with RED WORM, can appear well muscled, shiny coat, perform as expected and show no visible signs of worm infestation.

RED WORM is probably the most dangerous worm to have inside a horse and it is also the most difficult to control.

Any INTERNAL PARASITE control programme for a horse should be based on effective control of all stages of the RED WORM, (adults, immatures and migratory stages). Anthelmintics are now available which can control the RED WORM effectively, in all stages, and if the red worm is controlled, all other worm species will also be controlled at the same time.

The LIFE CYCLE of the worm in simple terms is:

Adults living in the digestive tract lay eggs which pass out with the faeces.

Dependent on the worm species, the worm eggs live for various periods of time within the faeces, on the pasture, and generally after rain, hatch, and swim in a droplet of water onto grass leaves. The horse eats the grass and ingests the active small larval worm.

The larval stages of the worst worms penetrate the tongue and other mucosal or similar tissue and enter the blood stream.

This migratory stage of the worm may then be carried around the body, in the blood stream, stopping along the way in the many body organs, and slowly destroying the various tissues. Migratory worms, of some species, can move in the blood stream and through the various organs for periods of up to 8 months damaging body tissues all the time.

Eventually the migratory worm matures and finds its way to the digestive tract. The migratory worm then becomes an immature worm and lives for further period within the gut itself. Finally the immature worm matures to become an adult, lays eggs and the whole cycle repeats itself.

Most damage to the horse is done by the microscopic migratory stages of the worms as they burrow in and move through the various body tissues.

The damage done by the adult stages, whilst of concern, is generally not as great as the damage done by the migratory stages.

In practical terms, the smaller the worm, the more damage that species will do to the horse, and following from this, the smallest stage of the worm, the migratory stage, does more harm than the older and larger stages in the same species life cycle.

WORM EGG COUNTS

It is possible, by examining faeces collected from a horse, under a microscope, to be able to get some idea of the internal parasite infestation, both in terms of numbers and species of worm present.

Whilst the results from one egg count MAY be of interest, they are really not of any value as the egg production from the adult worms is extremely variable within a 24 hour period. It could be that the faecal sample was taken at the time when the egg output was very low and a false result would be obtained. Similarly, the faecal sample could be taken at a time when the egg output was very high, again giving a false result. To get a correct result, from FAECAL WORM EGG COUNTS, a sample of each faeces, voided by the horse over a twenty four hour period should be bulked to-gether and examined. In general, if the WORM EGG COUNT is ABOVE 100 eggs/gram, the horse either needs drenching or else the anthelmintic being used is not effective against the worms present in the horse and a change to a drug of a different chemical family is recommended.

In practical terms, by far the greater percentage of FAECAL EGG counts, from horses, will contain large numbers of worm eggs, indicating the need to drench the horse. It may well be better, in terms of overall cost to spend the money, normally used to pay for egg counts, to pay for extra drench and to get onto a regular and continual drenching programme, of every 2 or 3 months.

ANTHELMINTICS or DRENCHES are the drugs used to control worms.

The two important factors in the use of anthelmintics are:

1. Dose rate
2. Toxicity of the drug to the horse.

Some modern anthelmintics (or worm drenches), in current use, for horses are now being sold with varying dose rate instructions.

The lowest rate is capable of controlling the adult worms only but has no affect on the immature or larval stages.

The intermediate rate will control not only the adult worms but also the immature stages, but not the migratory stages.

The heavy or largest dose rate will control all three stages of the worms.

The main feature of these modern drenches are their safety. Some of these drenches can be used in the horse up to 50 times normal strength, without affecting the animal.

Secondary features are: palatability to virtually all horses at normal dose rates. This means that the anthelmintic can be mixed with feed at these rates. The drenches can also be easily administered by modern small drenching guns with little waste.

These new types of anthelmintics are a big advance on products previously used. The older type worm drenches were, in the main, not nearly as safe to use on horses. The amount of anthelmintic required to kill the adult worms was often close to the level of the drug which could affect the horse in some way. It was, therefore, necessary to be VERY CAREFUL not to overdose for fear of harming the animal. Since most of the instructions for administration were based on body weight estimates and as many horse people are unable to estimate body weight, within a reasonable margin, the possibility of overdose and possible adverse effects on the horse was always present.

As these products generally only removed adult worms, the immature and migratory stages of the parasites remained in the horse. This fact then allowed these migratory stages to slowly become exposed to low levels of the drug which was in the horse, and then to develop resistance to the drug.

The safety margin of most of the new drugs allows the use of dose rates which will clear all stages of the parasite from the horse. In this situation, very few immature or migratory stages are left in the animal, provided the correct dose rate of drench is given. With this situation there is no chance of the migratory stages in particular becoming continually exposed to low dose rates of the drug, with the possibility of resistance developing.

The palatability of the newer drugs also makes administration much easier.

Information on these drugs is available in the manufacturers promotional material, and on the labels. Your local veterinary surgeon should be able to help.

INTERNAL PARASITES AND WORMS

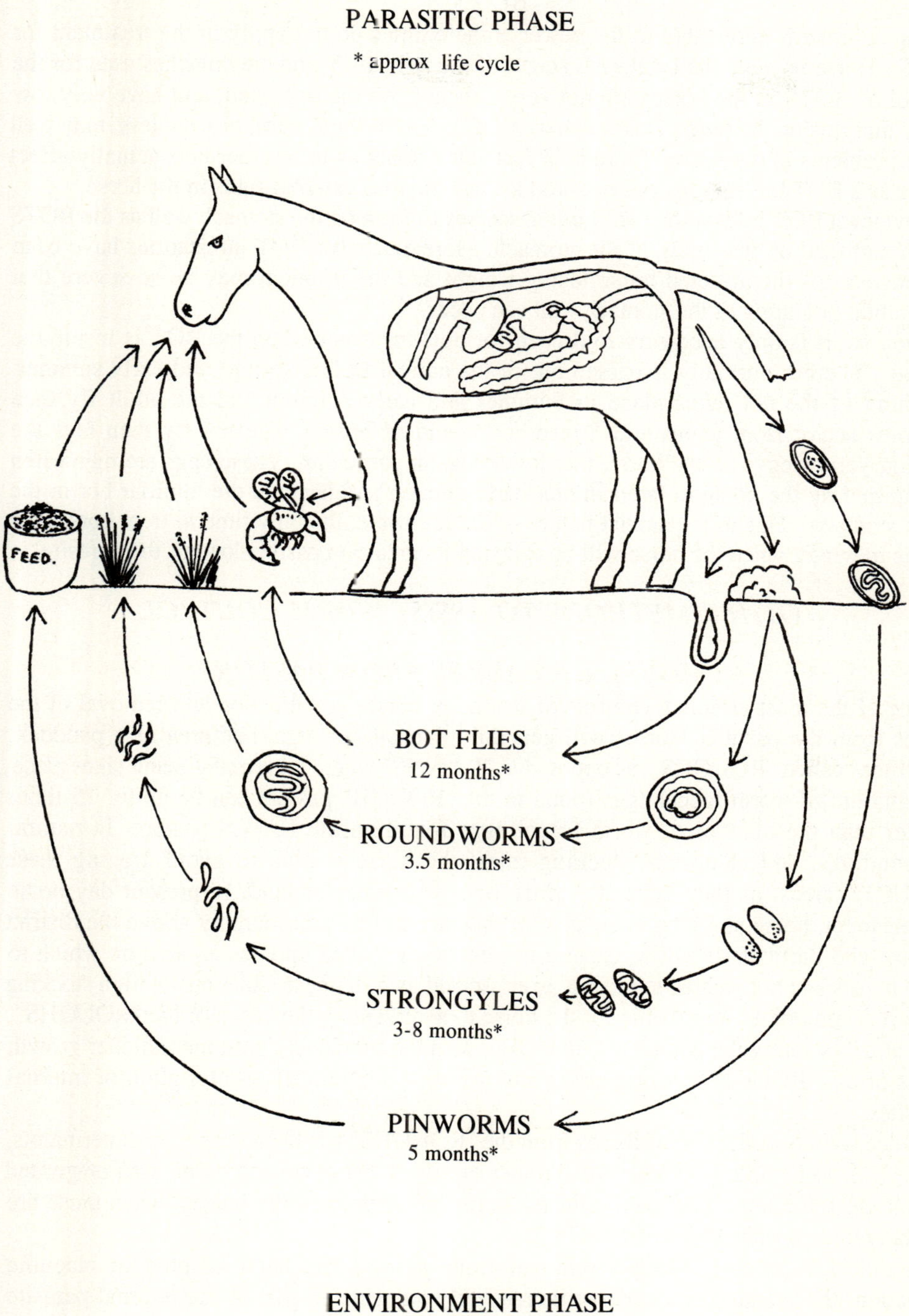

INTERNAL PARASITES

BOTS

The comments applicable to the newer anthelmintics do not apply in the treatment for BOTS. Horse bots are the LARVAL stages of the BOT FLY and the drenches used for the control of BOTS in the horses are not very palatable on the one hand, and have very low safety margins on the other. Doses in excess of 25% of normal rates, or even less, may well cause problems in the horse. There is in fact some doubt as to whether bots actually affect horses as a BOT infestation does not produce any obvious external signs in the horse.

Low level BOT infestation can cause abscesses to form on the stomach wall as the BOTS attach and feed on the lining of the stomach. More extensive BOT infestations have been responsible for the affected horse losing weight and the problem may be so severe that perforation or tearing of the stomach wall can occur.

Even so, it is only necessary to drench for bots in winter when the BOT is inside the animal. The bot normally is passed out of the animal in late spring and early summer. Hatching of the bot takes place in Summer and early Autumn and the adult fly then becomes active from about mid December to end of March. The bot fly then lays the familiar yellow eggs on the horse, the lower legs in particular. These eggs are then eaten or ingested by the horse in late summer-early autumn and become the familiar bot in the horse stomach. Due to the annual nature of the life cycle, the only time to treat horses for bots is in winter when the horse will be carrying its greatest possible load of the parasite.

OTHER METHODS TO ASSIST WORM CONTROL

REMOVAL OF FAECES FROM PASTURE

One of the most effective controls of worms in horses is collection and removal of the faeces from the pasture. Horses will generally deposit faeces in one area of a paddock, sometimes called "ROUGHS", as opposed to "LAWNS" where preferred grazing takes place. The amount of worm faecal eggs found in the "ROUGH" pasture can be up to 15 times greater than the number of worm faecal eggs found on the LAWN pasture. In natural surroundings, and at normal stocking rates, the horse is able to avoid grazing these "ROUGH" areas, as they generally graze over vast areas of land. In present day horse management, horse stocking rates/ acre or /hectare can be considerably above the district average and particularly where pasture is sometimes looked upon as an area on which to stand horses and not an area to provide exercise and feed. In these situations of high stocking rates, it is sometimes impossible for the horse to avoid eating the edges of the "ROUGHS", even at times eating the complete "ROUGH", with the previously prominent higher growth levels of the "ROUGHS" disappearing and meaning a continual re-infestation of internal parasites.

Twice weekly collection of faeces from the "ROUGHS" has been shown, in experiments, in the U.S. to be able to double the number of horses being carried on an area of ground and, at the same time, markedly reduced worm infestations in the horses, when these are regularly treated with ANTHELMINTICS.

In the U.S. where FAECES removal from pasture has been adapted to machine collection, the practice is becoming increasingly valuable as part of the internal parasite control programme.

PASTURE HARROWING

Pastures grazed by horses should be regularly harrowed, by some method, in order to break up and spread the faeces. This can be done with pasture harrows which are specifically designed for the purpose and can be pulled behind a tractor, four wheel drive vehicle or similar. However, cheaper and effective substitutes can be readily made from old car tyres wired together or weld mesh, or any similar article weighted, down with old fence posts.

The benefits of pasture harrowing are two fold:

1. To open up and spread the faeces so that the worm eggs and worm larvae are not protected from sunlight. Sunlight has a very good effect on destroying worm eggs and hence the chance of infection of horses has to be reduced where pastures are regularly harrowed.

2. Pasture harrowing will spread the faeces around the paddock and eliminate the problem of excessive plant growth around the dung patches where the horse generally will not eat. By spreading the dung around, a more even distribution of the fertiliser nutrients in the faeces over the area isachieved, and therefore better overall pasture growth.

PADDOCK SPELLING

Removal of horses from the paddock for a period of time is a follow up from the practice of pasture spelling as used in the cattle and sheep industries. Paddock spelling is however decreasing in importance as an aspect of worm control in horses, because the eggs of some worms that affect horses can live for up to 4 years on pasture. It is just not practical on most horse properties to spell a paddock completely for 4 years.

This fact, therefore, means that once pastures are contaminated with equine worms eggs, any horse grazing such pasture, unless it has been spelled for at least four years, will be getting re-infected with internal parasites.

IT IS IMPORTANT THAT ALL HORSES SHOULD BE ADEQUATELY DRENCHED AT REGULAR INTERVALS FOR EFFECTIVE WORM CONTROL ON PASTURE.

Section Two

Practical Aspects

13. FACTORS AFFECTING FEED CONSUMPTION.

Horses are like humans, they will have individual likes and dislikes as to feed preferences and eating habits. These feed preferences and eating habits will be determined, some by NATURAL or INHERITED FACTORS which affect all horses and some by ENVIRONMENTAL or ACQUIRED FACTORS, something which has happened to the horse at or after birth and the horse has learnt either from watching other horses or because of a repetitive act involved with feeding.

The horse is an animal which has adapted in the natural surroundings, to eating moderate amounts of feed, at frequent intervals, as shown by the small size of the horse's stomach, in relation to the total volume of the digestive tract and by the fact that horses, when grazing can spend up to 16 to 20 hour/day grazing. Grazing horses, are not confronted with sudden changes of feed availability, as can occur in some present twice a day hand fed situations.

NATURAL or INHERITED FACTORS

PALATABILITY

PALATABILITY is the overall acceptance by the horse of a particular feed, indicated by a ready and obvious desire to consume that feed.

PALATABILITY is the end result of a number of different factors, all which combine to-gether to affect the horses' like or dislike of a particular feed. These factors include appearance, smell or odour, taste, texture, temperature and possibly any sound the feed may make when disturbed.

These six factors are, in turn, affected by the physical and chemical nature of the feed, which may or may not be modified by individual physiological (biochemical) and psychological (personal preference) differences.

APPETITE

APPETITE normally refers to the horses' internal factors, both physiological and psychological that either stimulate or inhibit hunger in the horse. The factors, which control appetite are very difficult to define individually and even more difficult to measure.

HUNGER

HUNGER is the physiological or biochemical state which results from the absence of a food or foods of a general or specific type

and which is satisfied, cancelled, abolished or erased by the provision of that food or foods to the horse.

TASTE

TASTE is the result of complex mixtures of organic and inorganic compounds, contained in the feed, some of which are yet to be fully defined.

Taste buds, in the tongue and also in the palate and other parts of the oral cavity or mouth, allow the taste assessment of compounds which are able to dissolve, either completely or partially in the saliva.

Taste can also be markedly affected by odours or smells, and in pigs where the only research work has been done, milk consumption of suckling piglets has been increased by the addition to the ration of the sow, of a flavouring which appeared in the milk.

Horses are known to prefer certain flavours, molasses. licorice, aniseed, strawberry, banana and apple are all natural or artificial flavourings which are added to horse feeds to ensure consumption. In some instances, it has to be the flavouring which is of value to the horse because, in some flavoured feeds and feeds supplements, there is little else of value. As to flavours which horses tend to dislike, the smell and taste of fat, in particular, is generally found offensive.

ODOURS

ODOURS are produced by volatile compounds, compounds which are able to slowly decompose under certain conditions and emit or give off a smell of some description. ODOURS are so complex and consist of so many volatile substances which are sometimes very difficult to analyse, due to the instability of the compounds, that there is no general agreed basis for any type of classification of odours in feeds.

It is, however, generally accepted that animals have a much keener and sharper sense of smell than humans.

SIGHT

The importance of SIGHT as it affects the intake of food, by animals, is not fully understood. It is also of little relevance to the food intake of a horse as the horse is unable to see the feed which it is eating. The location of the horses' eyes in the skull are such that the horse, with head down, in a grazing position, has a BLIND SPOT in front of the mouth extending about 1 metre in front of the nose.

TOUCH

TOUCH can play an important part in the horse's ability to select feed to eat. The TACTILE HAIRS, those short hairs which grow on the lips of the horse have a very important function in allowing the horse to differentiate, when grazing, between plants to eat and plants not to eat. When the horse is grazing, the position of its eyes DO NOT ALLOW the horse to see exactly what it is biting in each mouthful, the nose gets in the way. The grazing horse is eating BLIND.

TACTILE HAIRS provide the horse with a sense of touch, partially overcoming the lack of ability to see want is being eaten, allowing ingestion of plants of preference and rejection of plants which the combined senses of the horse advise are undesirable.

In show ring circles, there is a continuing habit of completely removing the TACTILE HAIRS from the horses' nose, presumably to make the horse look better. Such a practice, whilst cosmetically accepted, can prove dangerous to a horse which is allowed access to grazing whilst the TACTILE HAIRS are clipped. Such a horse will not have a valuable feed selection aid, designed by nature for a purpose and MAY ingest some type of plant which could have adverse consequences, possibly of a serious and permanent nature to the horse.

PHYSICAL FEATURES AND TEXTURE.

TEXTURE and PARTICLE SIZE of feed will affect consumption. Most horses will readily take to the consumption of PELLETED FEEDS, even if the horses are completely unfamiliar with them.

Horses also take more readily to cracked or rolled grain rather than whole grain and feed preparation or mixing methods which can reduce dust content also will increase the intake of such feeds. The horse has a digestive tract specifically designed to handle the digestion of feeds which contain relatively large amounts of cellulose.

There are a number of feed treatment processes which modify or change the nature or the make-up of the feed. Most of these processes are used on the basis of getting the horse to be able to utilise the feed nutrients better but, at the same time as allowing this to happen, such treated feed can be eaten much more rapidly than normal and also pass through the digestive tract faster than normal. Most of these processes which can affect feed consumption are detailed below.

CHAFFING or CHOPPED HAY.

This is a simple mechanical process which involves cutting hay into small lengths. Chaffing does not alter the chemical composition of the hay in any way and does not impart any magical qualities to the feed. Chaffing only reduces the length of the feed and increases the number of sites of entry of the saliva and digestive juices which attack cellulose.

Chaff is always more readily eaten by the horse but the amount fed should only be enough to be satisfactorily mixed with the grain and concentrate to allow consumption by the horse.

Feeding of excessive levels of chaff can lead to teeth problems as the amount of chewing required to prepare the chaff for digestion is much less than if hay and or grass is part of the diet.

GRAIN PROCESSING

Chapter 4 provides full details of the various methods to processes grain, all of which will increase rate of feed consumption over whole grain by changing and or reducing the cellulose or fibre content to a form more readily attacked by the enzymes in the saliva and the digestive tract.

PELLETS

These are commercially available and are favoured by the "one horse" owner, as only one bag of feed needs to be kept in the feed shed. Pelleted feeds are manufactured by initially mixing all the components, generally after grinding, in a suitable mill. Molasses is then added to produce a mixture of desired consistency, basically a mix that will flow, and cooking is then undertaken by steam. Before cooking, an anti-oxidising agent is generally added to prevent too rapid a deterioration of the feed components in the cooking process. After heating, the mixture is then forced through the dies on the pelleting machine. As the mix comes from the dies in long threads, it is cut to the desired length.

PELLETS can be produced of varying thicknesses, length, and texture hardness, dependent on requirements.

PUFFED PELLETS are produced by subjecting the pellets to steam under pressure. This expands the pellet to about twice the volume, by incorporating air, into the mixture. The practice of PUFFING has been used for some time in the human and dog food industries and is an expensive process and its use in horse feeding is only favoured for those horses which are fast compulsive eaters. PUFFED PELLETS reduce the rate of feed intake per mouthful, slow down the rate of eating and help to overcome digestive problems, including colic, which can arise from rapid ingestion of feed, refer chapter on FACTORS AFFECTING FEED CONSUMPTION.

Pelleting allows uniform mixing of the many compounds in the final feed.

DISADVANTAGES of pelleted feeds are:-

1. Horses tend to eat pelleted feeds more quickly than normal feeds. Care needs to be taken in feeding pellets to horses which are fast eaters, as digestive problems may occur.
2. Pellets may not satisfy the horse's inherent need to chew as with grass or hay and the horse may resort to satisfying this need by TAIL and MANE CHEWING, WOOD CHEWING, BARK EATING etc.
3. Fast eating horses can be more prone to get COLIC, the feed enters and passes through the digestive tract faster than normal.
4. Pellets, because they are concentrated in size, may expand in the stomach and cause possible problems. This will be especially so if a number of horses are fed from the one feed trough with pellets. The fast eaters may well be susceptible to digestive upsets.
5. The heating process may well destroy some of the vitamins added to the original mix. It may be that the vitamins, detailed on the label of a bag of pellets, are not present in the final feed.
6. Pelleted feeds are often more expensive than most other horse feeds. If all the technical components of the different feeds are equal, the horse feeder has to determine if the extra cost of the pellet feeds are worthwhile.
7. Care needs to be taken when introducing horses to pellets. Colic, and other problems, may occur if too many pellets are fed too quickly. Horses should be slowly introduced to pellets, by gradually increasing the weight of pellets and reducing the weight of hay in the ration, until the desired weight of pellet feeding is reached, preferably over at least a three week period.

ADVANTAGES of pelleted feeds are:-

1. Generally highly digestible but this is usually dependent on the quality of the feeds which form the original mix. There is no way it is possible to tell, from looking at a pellet, whether top quality or second grade materials were used to make the feed. The reputation of the manufacturer is the only criteria that may be used to assess this matter.
2. All feed components are well mixed, but this same comment can be made with a number of other prepared feeds. Pelleting ensures that all the ingredients are mixed to-gether, in a physical manner, which DOES NOT allow any sorting out of the feed components with specific palatability problems. The disadvantage of this is unpalatable feeds can be incorporated into pellets as the taste will be disguised by the more palatable components.

3. Palatability, due to the addition of molasses to improve the consistency of the final mix just before pelleting and generally leads to reduced overall wastage of feed.
4. Of value to horses which are subject to HEAVES and other respiratory conditions, generally due to dust in the feed. Pellets are virtually dust free and do have a place in the feeding of this type of horse.
5. Reduced storage space.

EXTRUDED FEED

This is a dry feed preparation and is used extensively in dry dog and cat foods, the reason any type of extruding process would be used in the horse feeds would be to allow addition of much higher levels of fat to be incorporated than can be mixed in other types of prepared foods where FAT breakdown and rancidity occurs.

MINERAL IMBALANCE

Detailed studies have shown that APPETITE for COMMON SALT is the only specific mineral hunger documented in horses. Selection is preferred for rations which contain 0.5% to 1.0% salt over rations which are deficient in the mineral or rations which have very high levels, of the order of 15-20%.

The horse has a NON SPECIFIC appetite for the consumption of any other mineral, it really does not care what it eats and can not distinguish between various minerals free fed and what it needs to correct any mineral deficiency that may be present. When horses, suffering from a phosphorus deficiency were given free access to various mineral salts, they preferred and consumed more calcium than phosphorus salts, increasing the problem of phosphorus deficiency.

FEED CHANGES

Changes of feed, which can affect the variety or the novelty of the ration, will often stimulate horses to consume increase amounts. Ponies fed on mixed horse pellets which were offered, after voluntary cessation of feeding, a choice of oats, sweet feed, alfalfa pellets and the original horse pellets some 10 minutes after finishing the original feed, all commenced eating all the feeds EXCEPT the mixed horse pellets. Normally these ponies would not be expected to eat for at least another two to three hours after voluntary cessation. Horses will also show a decoded preference for fresh feed, e.g. pasture as opposed to dry hard feeds.

INDIVIDUAL HORSE EFFECTS ON FEED INTAKE

FEED INTAKE of any horse is affected by one or more of the following:-

BODY WEIGHT

Feed consumption is directly related to volume of the digestive tract, a fact which most horse owners are unable to determine. As volume of the digestive tract is related in a reasonable manner to BODY WEIGHT and this can be measured, BODY WEIGHT is the common criteria used to assess feed consumption. Big horses will eat more feed than small horses, but as a considerable amount of the additional feed eaten in relation to size, is in fact in the ENERGY fraction of the ration, any increase in feed consumption, due to size will not be LINEAR, i.e. increasing in equal amounts/50kg live weight but will be in smaller and ever decreasing amounts per 50kg live weight.

INDIVIDUAL HORSE PREFERENCE

Each horse will have its likes and dislikes in feed, some due to natural or inherited factors which cannot be changed and some due to environmental or acquired factors, learnt by the horse, since birth, from either the surroundings, the feed provided or specific habits of the people doing the feeding. These INDIVIDUAL HORSE PREFERENCES are sometimes quite annoying and it is usually preferable to be able to sort them out and live with them rather than try and change the horse.

ACTIVITY OF THE INDIVIDUAL HORSE

When a horse increases its level of physical activity, it will increase the amount of feed, on a DRY MATTER basis which it consumes each day, sometimes doubling the amount or weight of feed eaten from rest of say 8 kg to full physical activity of say 16 kg. In turn, horses are able to self regulate their energy consumption, if allowed AD LIB or unrestricted feeding. The speed at which a horse will alter its individual feed intake to compensate for either weight gain or weight loss is very much an individual matter.

Each horse has an INBUILT IDEAL BODYWEIGHT, controlled by various organs and hormones in the individual, exactly the same as in humans. Some people can never get thin and other people can never get fat, due to individual hormonal differences.

Problems arise when the "IDEAL BODY WEIGHT" of the horse, as determined by the human, may not be attainable in that particular horse. Horses also have the ability to change body weight with feed intake, probably a result of environmental adaptation over time when the grazing horse had to store fat in the good times – Spring and Summer – to satisfy body demands in the times when pasture production was not as good – Autumn and Winter.

Horses, in a controlled feeding situation, have not learnt to adopt to the constant availability of feed, of consistent quality.

The amount of work, exercise and or performance expected of dry horses can increase or reduce their feed intake. Horses, being asked to do an increased amount of exercise, will if allowed free access(AD LIB) to feed always increase feed intake to attempt to satisfy the additional energy needs of the extra work. A 500kg (1100 lb) horse, at rest, requires about 16 megacalories of energy/day. The same horse, if in strenuous or hard work would need up to 36 megacalories/day, an increase in energy need of about 125%.

If the additional feed eaten DOES NOT provide the extra energy required, the horse is able to mobilize, for muscle activity, extra energy from the fat reserves within the body, leading to a loss in body weight. A similar situation of loss of body weight will also occur if the horse is asked to do more work without any increase in the weight of physical feed intake.

FACTORS AFFECTING FEED CONSUMPTION

The average thoroughbred AT REST requires about 17 MEGACALORIES of ENERGY/DAY.

When that same horse commences to work at various paces, the energy level for work will rise dramatically.

At the TROT ENERGY needs increase	X 5.0
CANTER	X 12.5
GALLOP	X 24.0
ABSOLUTE PEAK DEMAND	X 39.0

EXTRA ENERGY DEMANDS FOR WORK are related to weight of horse, or horse and rider, times the distance travelled.

EXTRA ENERGY DEMANDS ARE NOT RELATED TO THE SPEED USED TO COVER ANY DISTANCE.

Some racehorses have been known to expend up to 25 MEGACALORIES of energy in one 2400 metre race.

It is important to note that, dependent on the horse and the training programme, only about 25-30% of the daily energy intake of the horse is actually used for muscle activity and hence performance. Some ENERGY will be stored for future use and the greater proportion, often up to the remaining 75%, will go in HEAT production, firstly, as part of the digestion of fibre and cellulose in the large intestine, and secondly, as a by-product of all the many body processes which go on inside an active horse.

EXERCISE RELATED FEED DEMANDS can be classified as follows.

FEED NUTRIENTS whose ration levels DO NOT INCREASE as EXERCISE increases are:-

CRUDE PROTEIN, CALCIUM/PHOSPHORUS LEVELS and RATIO, and amounts of VITAMIN A and D and the minerals IRON, COPPER, ZINC. MAGNESIUM and SELENIUM.

FEED NUTRIENTS whose ration levels SHOULD INCREASE as EXERCISE increases are :-

ENERGY, ELECTROLYTES, WATER and VITAMINS B, C and E.

RATE OF DIGESTA PASSAGE

DIGESTA, sometimes termed INGESTA refers to the food material being utilised by the horse within the digestive tract. The average rate of digesta passage in the average horse can be divided into two parts. From the mouth to the large intestine generally takes about 3 hours. In this very short period of time, the digestive tract has to breakdown the plant material, modify and absorb, within the stomach and small intestine, ALL THE PROTEIN, CARBOHYDRATE TYPE ENERGY and FAT TYPE ENERGY, MINERALS and VITAMINS before the digesta passes onto the large intestine, and its associated organ, the caecum, where the micro-organisms attack the CELLULOSE fraction of the feed. Studies on digesta retention of maize (corn) in the large intestine show that about 10% is passed as faeces after 24 hours, 50% has passed after 36 hours and 95% has passed after 65 hours.

Other research work indicates that digesta can remain in the large intestine for up to 10 days, after consumption.

This relatively slow digesta passage in the large intestine is due to the slow breakdown of cellulose, providing VOLATILE FATTY ACIDS, (V.F.A.) which is an energy source for horses at rest.

DIGESTA PASSAGE TIME is influenced by the physical form and density (weight per unit volume) of the feed. Pellets will have a faster rate of digesta passage than fresh pasture which in turn will move faster than hay. HAY of poor quality (pasture species over mature when made), generally very coarse with fibrous stems and little leaf, will remain, being digested, longer in the large intestine than normal and depress dry matter intake. This will be of advantage for horses which are overfat, compulsive or fast eaters but will be of no advantage to the normal horse, especially if it is required to work or perform in some way.

ENERGY DENSITY OF THE FEED

This refers to the weight of the feed in relation to the volume. HIGH ENERGY DENSITY FEEDS, such as maize (corn), sorghum, and barley, where the amount of energy in the feed in relation to volume weight is high, will pass through the digestive tract FASTER than will LOW ENERGY DENSITY FEEDS, such as hay where there is a low weight for a given volume and at the same time a low energy level in the hay.

ELECTROLYTE IMBALANCE

Feed and also water intake of performance horses can be dramatically affected by lack of ELECTROLYTES in previous rations. Endurance horses as well as racehorses, pacers and eventers have been known to completely refuse to either eat or drink for some considerable time after physical exercise, due to ELECTROLYTE deficiency problems.

ATMOSPHERIC TEMPERATURES

Air temperatures can have an effect on the amount of feed consumed. High temperatures, particularly if associated with high humidity will have a depressing effect on feed intake. At the other extreme cold temperatures will stimulate appetite and feed consumption.

GENERAL HEALTH

Horses, like humans will reduce feed intake to some extent when not feeling well or affected by any condition or disease which can reduce body function. Such situations can occur as a result of worm infestation, invisible muscle damage, detectable only with blood enzyme analysis, excess levels of some feed components, especially some of the vitamins and minerals.

MUSCLE FATIGUE

MUSCLE FATIGUE or the inability of the muscles of the horse to function normally can have quite a dramatic effect on the feed intake of the affected animal.

FACTORS AFFECTING FEED CONSUMPTION

Three types of FATIGUE have been defined

1. CHRONIC FATIGUE due to mental stress, boredom and or anxiety.
2. NERVOUS OR CENTRAL FATIGUE appears to be due to a change in the nerve endings, reduction in levels of CALCIUM and or POTASSIUM in the blood, and or nervous signals, coming from fatigued muscles. This is the type of FATIGUE which appears to be overcome by the use of WHIPS, SPURS and certain stimulating drugs etc. on a horse where the onset of fatigue is extended past the normal point.
3. MUSCULAR or PERIPHERAL FATIGUE where the muscle fibre will no longer respond to any form of nervous stimulation.

The onset of MUSCLE FATIGUE in any individual horse is a function of one or more of the following problems:-

1. amount of training.
2. length and speed of work producing the fatigue.
3. protein level in the ration.
4. energy level in the ration.
5. energy sources in the ration.
6. electrolyte levels in the ration.
7. water intake of the horse.
8. whether muscle energy use takes place AEROBICALLY or ANAEROBICALLY.

Whilst MUSCLE FATIGUE is partially determined by what the horse eats before muscle fatigue sets in, what the horse eats after muscle fatigue occurs is very much dependent on what happens to the horse in the fatigued state.

Physical exertion affects a number of physiological or biochemical processes within the horse. With long term AEROBIC exercise, there were decreases in the levels, within the blood plasma, of GLUCOSE and increases in TOTAL PROTEIN, LACTATE, FREE FATTY ACIDS and HAEMATOCRIT. There were also variable movements, affected by speed of work and the environmental temperature, in the plasma levels of POTASSIUM, CALCIUM, SODIUM and MAGNESIUM.

When the horse uses muscle energy in an AEROBIC manner, it seems that the level of GLYCOGEN stored within the muscle fibres becomes limiting, generally always associated with a rise in the LACTATE level which may be responsible for muscle fatigue responsible for muscle fatigue. It is now thought that other factors are responsible for muscle fatigue, LACTIC ACID is just an end product of energy use.

When ANAEROBIC muscle activity is present, the limiting factor appears to be the amount of food components in the blood which are available to the muscle cells, associated with the ability of the muscle cell to function effectively at the low pH level, leading to an increase in LACTATE levels both within the muscle cells and within the blood. The increase in LACTATE lead to the reduction in cell pH, which in turn affected the operation of two enzymes which are responsible for muscle control.

SODIUM BICARBONATE IS often given to horses shortly before undergoing intense exercise where energy use is by ANAEROBIC methods. This results in the muscle cells developing a slight alkaline condition which, in theory, should assist the control of the accumulation of LACTATE, as LACTIC ACID.

Whilst SODIUM BICARBONATE has been shown to extend the time it takes to get a particular horse fatigued, it does not appear to have any affect on the the level of LACTIC ACID which accumulate in the muscles and, in fact, the administration of SODIUM BICARBONATE to performance horses may be dangerous.

ABSENCE OF OTHER HORSES

The horse is a herd animal, associating and moving naturally with other horses in a mob situation. Some horses have been known to not eat simply because they miss the presence of other horses. This problem, once diagnosed, is solved by one of the following methods.

1. allow the stabled horse to be able to see, at all times, any other horses which may be in the stables by removing the top half of any internal stable wall which prevents horses seeing along a row of stables and replacing with open wire mesh, which will still allow restraint of physical contact between horses but will allow visual contact.
2. if that does not increase appetite, or the horse has no stable companions to see, feed the horse outside the stable, it may be able to see the neighbour's horses and not feel so lonely.
3. buy your horse a companion, say a small SHETLAND, which will eat a lot less feed but may cure the problem.
4. if all that does not work, your horse unfortunately is strictly a social animal and has to have the company of other horses, maybe you get another horse.

14. HORSE AND FEED MEASUREMENT

For accurate horse feeding it is necessary to be able to relate what the horse needs and gets with the feed available.

Measurement of the physical details of horses are available in two forms
HEIGHT in hands, inches or metres.
WEIGHT in kilograms (KG) or pounds (LB)

It is very difficult to relate HEIGHT of horse to amount of feed consumed as there is no common relationship between a measurement for height and any measurement for feed.

It is, however, very possible to get a relationship between WEIGHT of horse and WEIGHT of feed. Both details can be expressed in the exact same units, generally KILOGRAMS in the metric system and POUNDS in the imperial system of measurement.

THE BEST WAY TO MEASURE A HORSE IS BY BODY WEIGHT.
THE BEST WAY TO MEASURE FEED IS ALSO BY WEIGHT

MEASURING HORSES

Horses are known to have a total daily food intake, in proportion to each individuals' body weight, and this is generally referred to as a daily feed intake as DRY MATTER of between 2% and 3% of the horses' body weight, although it is not uncommon for performance horses, in training, to have larger daily DRY MATTER intakes.

CALCULATION OF HORSE'S BODY WEIGHT

WEIGHING THE HORSE

Often when travelling the horse somewhere, you will pass a public weighbridge used to weigh trucks and various other materials. Unload the horse from the float and simply walk the horse onto the weighbridge. You will get an exact weight of the horse. Some performance horse trainers even have their own set of horse weighing scales installed at the stables, using body weight variations as an important part of racehorse training and it might be possible to get a horse weight from use of such a set of scales.

Horses should be weighed just before a feed and a drink of water so as to obtain a reasonably accurate weight of the horse and not the horse plus GUT FILL. A 450kg (1000 lb) horse can have a gut fill of up to 100 KGS (220 lbs) or more and if weighed immediately after a feed and a drink, the weight obtained could be up to 20%, or so, too heavy.

WEIGHT TAPES

These tapes which pass around the horses' chest, immediately behind the wither are suitable if nothing else is available but do have an error of up to 20% on the reading, dependent on the make of tape and the conformation of the horse. This error can occur when comparing readings, from the one tape, from different horses but is not present when the same tape is used on the one horse. Weight tapes are of value in assessing the weight GAIN or LOSS of any animal as any error which is in the original reading will be constant on the one horse. The use of weight tapes, is however, better than no weight at all.

ESTIMATION or "EYEBALL"

Commonly know as the "EYEBALL" method, some people have an excellent ability to be able to accurately estimate the weight of animals. If you know such a person, particularly if they buy livestock for slaughter, their weight estimate on a horse should be fairly accurate. "The problem with the use of the EYEBALL method is everyone can be right, if there are no scales around to check on the weight."

The following are some weight ranges for ADULT HORSES, to be used as a guide only.

THOROUGHBREDS	410-520 kgs
STANDARDBREDS	410-545 kgs
ARABS	410-480 kgs
QUARTER HORSES	420-540 kgs
STOCK HORSES	450-520 kgs

BODY CONDITION SCORING

BODY CONDITION SCORING is a very valuable tool to allow any horse person, no matter what level of experience to be able to evaluate the condition and weight of any particular horse.

BODY CONDITION SCORING was originally reported in the scientific journals in 1983 and described work carried out by a group of researchers in the U.S.A. headed by Don Henneke. In 1988, another study, based on slightly different principles but with a similar final objective, was undertaken in Australia by Carroll and Huntington.

THE U.S. METHOD

The U.S. work involved the formulation of a 9-step system which describes the amount of fat and muscle which can be present on specific and defined areas of the horse, areas which are readily identified with a little training for the newcomer to horses.

The specific areas and reasons for their use are as follows.

1. OVER THE LOIN

In this area, a very thin horse will have a NEGATIVE CREASE or ridge, where the upward projections on the individual vertebrae in the back are most noticeable. These bone projections are able to be readily felt with the fingers and and in a very thin horse, there will be a noticeable absence of soft tissue or FAT, which will slide readily over the bone.

This is the first visible region of the horse where an increase in muscle and fat, will occur once the level of feeding increase.

Prior to an increase in bulk in this area, the horse has already replenished the internal fat depots but that is not visible to the naked eye.

As the horse gets fatter, the muscle bulk over the loins increases in size and eventually can get to the stage where the muscle mass rises above the level of the top of the bones and a prominent depression actually exists in the middle of the loin. Some horses will have relatively flat rumps and the increase in muscle mass may spread across the loin. With these types of horses, no central depression will be seen until the horse is virtually obese.

2. RIB COVER

An extremely thin horse will have prominent ribs, easily noted and often giving the impression of nearly projecting out of the skin. As the horse increases in muscle mass, the "padding" around the ribs will increase and about level 5 on the U.S. scale, the ribs will no longer be able to be seen individually but will still be able to be manipulated with the fingers. As the horse increases in muscle mass, the area between the ribs fills with additional tissue, fat and muscle and eventually at the top of the scale, patches of fat will be able to be felt actually on the outside of the ribs, there being no space left between the ribs to fill in.

3. TAIL HEAD

This is the region of the horse which is sometimes called the DOCK, that part of the horse where the tail separates from the body. A prominent tail head will be obvious at and up to level 3. At level 1 or emaciation, it will be possible to see each individual tail bone. From level 4 on the prominence of the TAIL HEAD and the increasing muscle mass will be dependent somewhat on the shape of the croup. Horses with flat croups, as in the ARAB breed, will be more difficult to detect increase in muscle mass in this area than will the case be with horses with natural steep sloping croups. At level 4, some fat will be present around the TAIL HEAD.

4. WITHERS

A very thin horse will allow a visual outline to be seen of the top of the shoulder blade, often with a pronounced hollow or depression between the two shoulder blades. At about score 5, this visual outline will have disappeared and the shoulder will have a rounded appearance. From score 6 on, fat will be felt on the outside of muscle mass and under the skin. In the obese (very overfat) horse, lumps of fat will be obvious on the top of and between the shoulder blades, the area actually bulging with fat.

5. NECK AND SHOULDERS

Used in combination, the increase in muscle mass on the neck, immediately below the base of the mane and behind the shoulder in the vicinity of the lower ribs are a further indicator of increasing body condition. In a very thin horse, it may be possible to even see bone in these regions. At about level 5, both areas will blend smoothly into the body and then as the horse increase in muscle mass, fat deposition will increase rapidly in these two areas. At level 8, the neck will adopt a rounded appearance with fat very evident at the crest and also probably under the throatlatch and the area behind the shoulder has filled in and there is no longer any apparent depression in this region.

6. BUTTOCKS

The development in this region of the horse is the final area of interest. This is the last area to be affected by fat deposition, the horse having to score 8 before any noticeable change occurs and at level 9, the buttocks are of such increased size that they rub to-gether as the horse moves.

In summary, the following details each individual CONDITION SCORE and is taken directly from an article by HENNEKE, the leader of the development team.

SCORE 1 - POOR

The horse is emaciated with prominent spinous processes, tailhead, pelvic bones and ribs. The bone structure under the withers, shoulders and neck can be seen and no fat can be felt anywhere.

SCORE 2 - VERY THIN

The spinous processes are still prominent but fat can be felt at their bases, and the transverse processes of the lumbar vertebrae feel rounded. The ribs, tailhead and pelvic bones stand out and the bone structures under the withers, neck, and shoulders are still able to be seen.

SCORE 3 - THIN

The spinous processes stand out, but fat covers them to about midpoint, (half way up), so that the transverse processes cannot be felt. The ribs and tailhead also have a light coat of fat, ribs can be seen but vertebrae in the tail head cannot be distinguished. Pinbones cannot be seen. The withers are prominent but the structures under them, as well as those under the neck and shoulders, can't be seen.

SCORE 4 - MODERATELY THIN

The horse has a negative crease along the back and the outline of the ribs can just be seen. How prominent the tailhead is depends on conformation, however fat can be felt around it and the hook bones can't be seen. The withers, neck and shoulders no longer look obviously thin.

SCORE 5 - MODERATE.

The back is level, the ribs can be felt but not seen. Fat around the tailhead begins to feel spongy. The shoulders and neck blend into the body and the withers look rounded.

SCORE 6 - MODERATE TO FLESHY

Fat at the ribs feels spongy, at the tailhead it feels soft. The horse may have a slight crease down its back and the beginnings of fat deposits can be felt at the withers, behind the shoulders and on the sides of the neck

SCORE 7 - FLESHY

There may be a crease down the back and while the ribs can be felt, fat fills the spaces between them. Fat is also noticeable along the withers and neck and behind the shoulders.

SCORE 8 - FAT

The horse has a crease down its back and its hard to feel the ribs. The area around the tail head feels very soft. The neck is noticeably thicker and the area along the withers is filled with fat. The space behind the shoulders is filled in flush and fat is being deposited along the inner buttocks.

SCORE 9 – EXTREMELY FAT

The crease down the back is obvious. Fat appears in patches over the ribs and bulges around the tailhead, withers, shoulders, and neck. The inner buttocks may rub to-gether and the flank is filled in flush.

Some practical points of use include:-

A – any horse with a CONDITION SCORE below 3 virtually has no body reserves of fat to call upon for either work or body maintenance. If that horse needs extra energy for any reason, it will have to use energy derived from muscle tissue, losing weight and going down on the CONDITION SCORE scale.

B – a well conditioned and properly trained performance horse will probably be about CONDITION SCORE 5

C – at CONDITION SCORE 6 or 7, the horse will be carrying some excess weight but it may need the extra fat to produce energy for a coming lactation, cold weather or some similar reason.

D – Horses with CONDITION SCORE 8 or 9 are more likely to be affected by COLIC and LAMINITIS, are likely to be less agile performers than horses with a lower CONDITION SCORE and if brood mares, are probably going to have problems getting in foal.

E – this CONDITION SCORING system DOES NOT tell how fit a horse is.

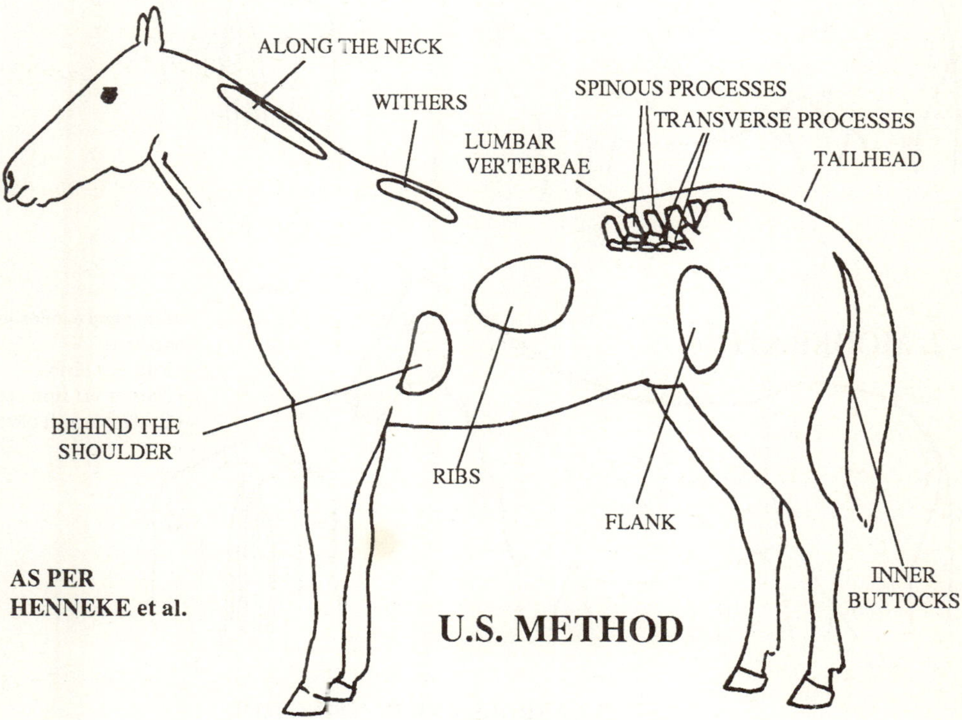

AS PER HENNEKE et al.

U.S. METHOD

AUSTRALIAN METHOD

0. VERY POOR

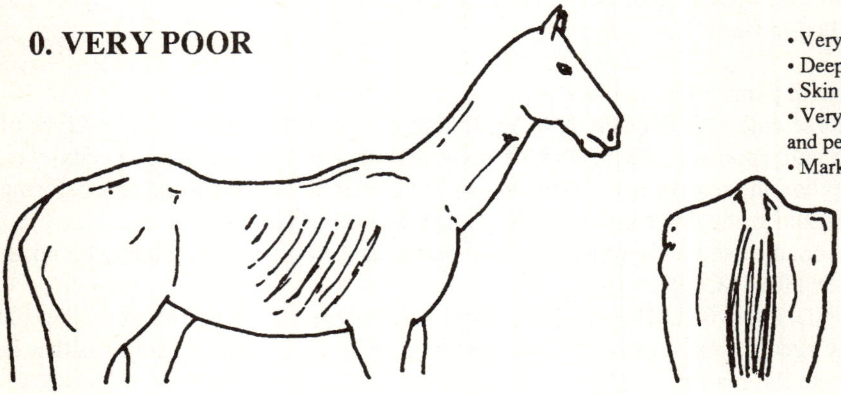

- Very sunken rump
- Deep cavity under tail
- Skin tight over bones
- Very prominent backbone and pelvis
- Marked ewe neck

1. POOR

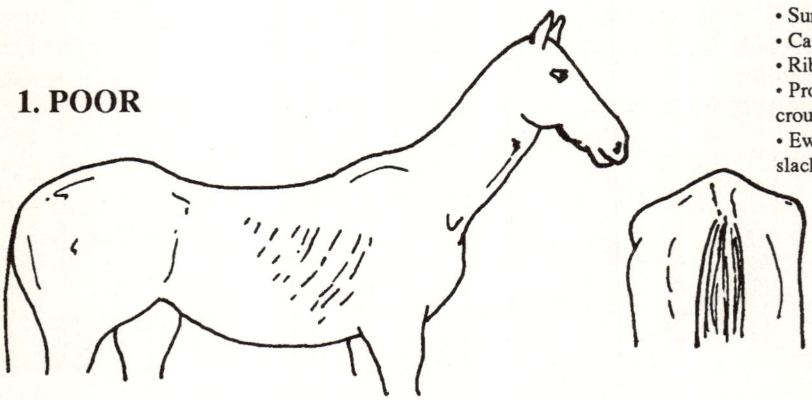

- Sunken rump
- Cavity under tail
- Ribs easilyvisible
- Prominent backbone and croup
- Ewe neck – narrow and slack

2. MODERATE

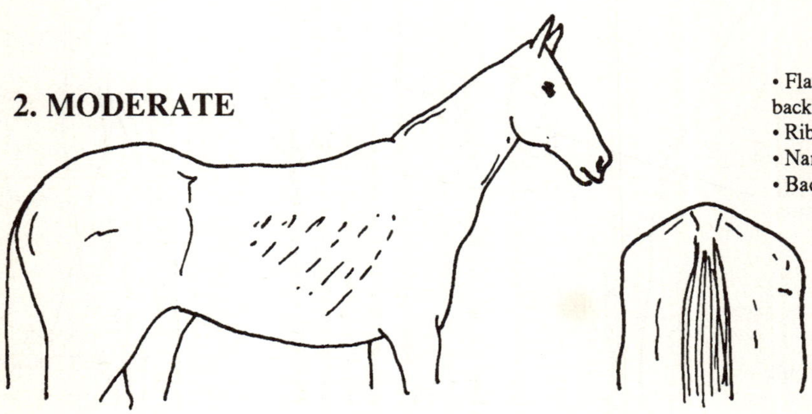

- Flat rump either side of backbone
- Ribs just visible
- Narrow but firm neck
- Backbone well covered

AS PER CARROLL AND HUNTINGTON

AUSTRALIAN METHOD

3. GOOD

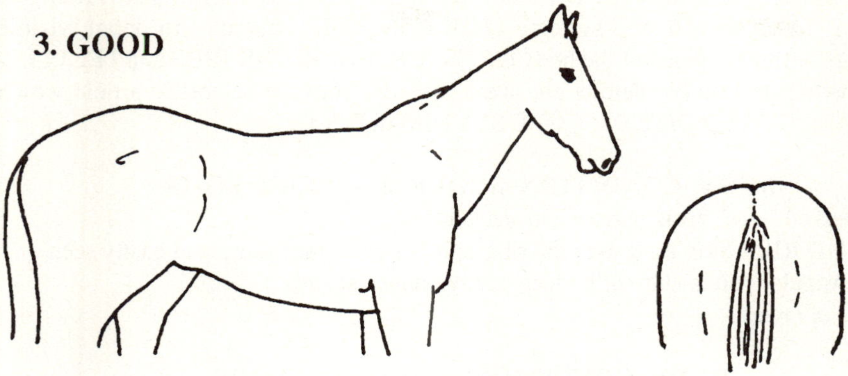

- Rounded rump
- Ribs just covered but easily felt
- No crest, firm neck

4. FAT

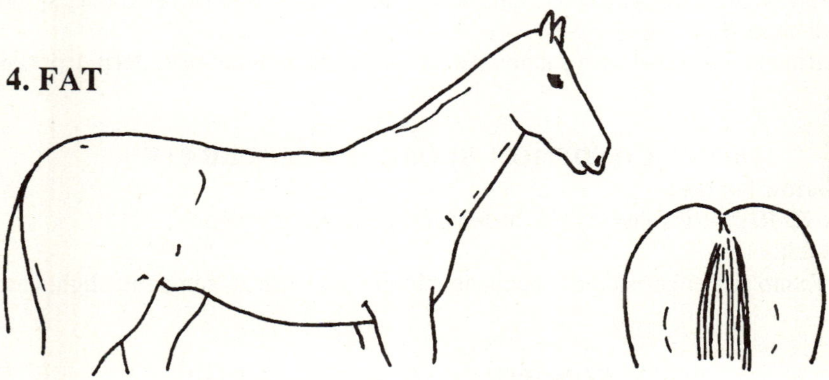

- Rump well rounded
- gutter along back
- Ribs and pelvis hard to feel
- Slight crest

5. VERY FAT

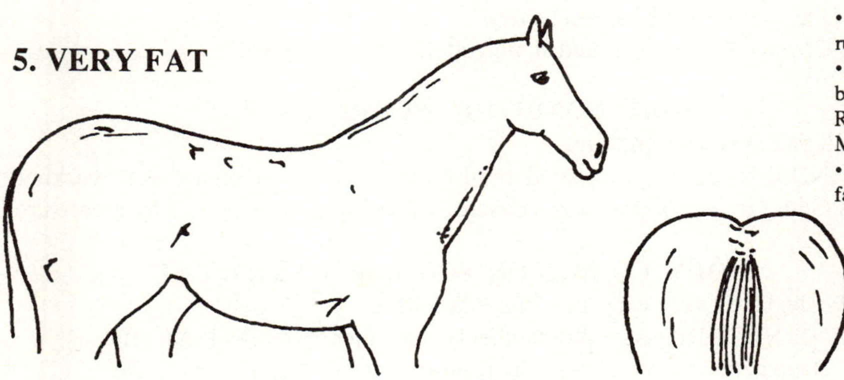

- Very bulging rump
- Deep gutter along back

Ribs buried•
Marked crest

- Fold and lumps of fat

AS PER CARROLL AND HUNTINGTON

THE AUSTRALIAN METHOD

The Australian CONDITION SCORING system, developed by Carroll and Huntington in Victoria, is based on a 6 step system, which individually describes in detail, visible specifications for three regions of the body only NECK, BACK AND RIBS and PELVIS.

The following descriptive details are taken directly from the scientific article which describes the BODY CONDITION SCORE SYSTEM in FULL

BODY CONDITION SCORE 0 - VERY POOR

NECK Marked "ewe" neck, narrow and slack at base.

BACK AND RIBS Skin tight over the ribs, spinous processes sharp and easily seen

PELVIS Angular pelvis-skin tight, deep cavity under tail and either side of croup

BODY CONDITION SCORE 1 - POOR

NECK "ewe" neck, narrow and slack at base.

BACK AND RIBS Ribs easily visible, skin sunken either side of backbone, spinous processes well defined.

PELVIS Rump sunken but skin supple, pelvis and croup well defined, deep depression under tail.

BODY CONDITION SCORE 2 - MODERATE

NECK Narrow but firm

BACK AND RIBS Ribs just visible, backbone well covered. spinous processes felt.

PELVIS Rump flat either side of backbone, croup well defined, some fat, slight cavity under tail.

BODY CONDITION SCORE 3 - GOOD

NECK No crest, (except stallions), firm neck

BACK AND RIBS Ribs just covered easily felt, No gutter along back, spinous processes covered but can be felt.

PELVIS Covered by fat and rounded, no gutter, pelvis easily felt.

BODY CONDITION SCORE 4 - FAT

NECK Slight crest, wide and firm

BACK AND RIBS Ribs well covered, need firm pressure to feel gutter along backbone.

PELVIS Gutter to root of tail. pelvis covered by soft fat, felt only with firm pressure.

BODY CONDITION SCORE 5 - VERY FAT

NECK Marked crest,very wide and firm, folds of fat.

BACK AND NECK Ribs buried cannot feel deep gutter back broad and flat.

PELVIS Deep gutter to root of tail, skin distended, pelvis buried, cannot feel.

The U.S. system of CONDITION SCORING assumes that all horses deposit fat and build muscle in exactly the same manner, the Australian system, on the other hand, does allow for the scoring to be used on a horse whose fat deposition and muscle bulking patterns are different from the majority.

Both systems do reach common agreement that CONDITION SCORING is very closely related to body fat content and that CONDITION SCORING can be used to monitor the change in body weight of horses as a result of feeding.

In the absence of any scales to provide accurate weight data and the inability of most people to judge with reasonable accuracy the weight of a horse, CONDITION SCORING does give a system of relative comparisons and also provides a common language for describing the amount of muscle and fat on a horse.

One of the major advantages of any body scoring system, no matter which one, is as long as two people are talking about the same system, it is possible to discuss body condition in absolute terms, e.g. the horse is a number 3 rather than in subjective terms i.e. the horse is a little too thin. The choice of which system to use will be left to the individual, it will be to their advantage to use one or the other, in conjunction with the programmes feeding of horses.

WORK LOAD ASSESSMENT OF HORSES

The terms AT REST, LIGHT WORK, MEDIUM WORK and HARD WORK have been used for some considerable time to describe the level of physical activity performed by a horse, and hence an estimate of the ENERGY REQUIREMENTS of the horse. These categories of WORK assessment originated in the days of draught horses and were defined in terms of the weight pulled for a given length of time at a given speed, (usually a walk). In 1971, subjective definitions were suggested to take into consideration the use of the horse, at that time.

With the modern day horse performing and competing in many different types of activities, about the only common factor is athletic performance.

Despite considerable advances in technical nutritional knowledge, there has not been any corresponding advance in the defining of the physical and or biological measures, indicators and or parameters which are common to all horses when physical effort is produced.

What may appear to be hard work for a dressage horse may, in fact, be light work for an endurance horse, simply because the two types of horse activities have vastly differing physical, physiological and metabolic requirements.

For the purposes of this book, the following definitions will apply. These definitions are based on observable physiological features of the horse, easily detected by the average horse owner. The definitions are in no way scientifically based as the average horse owner does not have access to all the equipment or expertise used in refined and advanced training and feeding programmes.

AT REST

When the work required or demanded, of the horse, is no greater in physical activity than similar activity expected of a healthy horse running freely in a paddock or field. Sweat MAY be observed in small amounts on the neck and in front of the forequarters in hot weather and the horses' breathing rate has not noticeably increased above normal.

Included in this category would be any horse which is spelling from past activities, a learner's or beginner's pony who would rarely get into a canter, the pleasure horse ridden carefully at a relaxing pace, for up to a maximum of 1 hour every day, the brood mare, weanling and yearling. These last three categories. BROOD MARE, WEANLING and YEARLING do however have some specific feeding problems, complicated by ENERGY LEVELS in the rations, which will be discussed in later sections of the book.

LIGHT WORK

When the work demanded of the horse is on a repetitive daily basis such as to cause increased and noticeable sweating on the neck, and a slight increase in breathing rate at the end of the exercise or training period. Expected gaits would be slow trotting and some cantering.

Included in this category would be active pony club and pleasure horses, the hack, western pleasure and bridle path hacks, the stock horse which does general work and any type of performance horse in the very early stages of a training programme. e.g. thoroughbred, standard bred, show jumper, eventer, endurance dressage, etc.

MEDIUM WORK

When the work demanded of the horse is on a repetitive daily basis, sufficient to cause sweating on the sides of the neck so as to be white in colour in some areas, due to salt and electrolyte excretion, where mild but observable sweating occurs under the flanks on the hindquarters and between the chest and the legs on the forequarters. Respiration rate at the completion of the exercise is increased to the extent that recovery back to normal takes at least 5 minutes after cessation of work. Expected activity would be fast trotting, cantering and some jumping.

Included in this category would be dressage horses at advanced levels of training, show jumpers competing about once a week, hunters, working stock and ranch horses, roping, cutting and barrel racing horses, and all other types of performance horses mid way through a training programme, e.g. endurance horses, eventers, standardbreds and thoroughbreds.

HARD or HEAVY WORK

Where the work demanded of the horse is of a repetitive daily basis, sufficient to cause active sweating to occur on the sides of the neck, flanks, under the forelegs,and over the body, with the noticeable presence of white salt and electrolyte secretions in all areas of sweat, but especially on the neck and body. Respiration rate is increased noticeably compared to normal and recovery to normal respiration rate takes at least 10 minutes after cessation of work. Expected activity would be cantering, galloping and jumping.

Included in this category would be any performance horse approaching or at the peak of a training and competition programme e.g. endurance horses, eventers, polo horses, standard breds and thoroughbreds and show jumpers who are actively travelling and competing.

MEASURING FEED

WEIGHT OF FEEDS

Very few people appear to have any idea of the weight of feed which their horse or horses are receiving. In the stables most feeds are measured by some form of container. Plastic ice cream containers, food tins, coffee cans, old saucepans, dippers and many other containers are used to measure horse feeds. However, because we vary rarely, if ever, measure horse volume, and or weight in old saucepans, coffee containers or ice cream containers, it is really essential that each feeder knows the weight of each feed which the appropriate container holds.

Instead of feeding an ice cream container of bran, the horse feeder should know that he is feeding 1 kg. of bran – the same approach should apply to all feeds. It is a simple matter to check what weight of each individual feed your own feeding utensils hold, by using a set of basic kitchen scales or similar weighing device and then write the exact weights, each feeding receptacle holds on the top of the feeding board in the feed shed, even if each horse's feed is still made up as 2 dippers of this and 4 dippers of that and one leaf of hay.

The following table relates to the common plastic 4 litre ice cream container but the principle remains the same no matter what type of container is being used.

FEED WEIGHT PER 4 LITRE ICE CREAM CONTAINER

FEED	KG	LBS
Oats (whole)	3.10	6.83
Barley (whole)	3.33	7.34
Maize (whole)	4.30	9.47
Sorghum (whole)	4.10	9.10
Bran	1.00	2.20
Pollard	2.00	4.40
Soybean Meal	3.00	6.60
Linseed Meal	3.33	7.34
Cottonseed Meal	3.33	7.34
Lucerne Chaff	0.77	1.69
Oaten Chaff	1.11	2.44

This Table is by no means comprehensive and certainly does not contain details of all feeds fed to horses. Neither is it intended to look at the weight of the various feeds which the many feeding utensils could hold.

The Table is meant to point out the VAST DIFFERENCES in weight of some feeds when compared on the basis of volume.

For processed feeds such as bran, pollard and the oilseed meals, the range of weights for the same feed from different sources will not show much variation whereas the weight of grains can vary considerably dependent on the soil fertility, availability of rainfall and or irrigation, the area grown and the seasonal conditions during the growing period. Oats have been known to vary by as much as 30% in weight when compared to the same volume.

This variation in volume weight is simply a function of the amount of ENDOSPERM, present or not present, in the grain. Grain with low volume weights will contain LESS ENDOSPERM and MORE CELLULOSE and therefore have LESS ENERGY/KG than will grain with high volume weights where the ENDOSPERM is a higher percentage and the CELLULOSE A LOWER PERCENTAGE of the total grain weight and therefore containing MORE ENERGY/KG.

Oats should weigh 18 kg (40lbs) per bushel, but oat samples collected from racing stables have been known to vary from 12.60 kg (27.7 lbs) per bushel to 23.40 kg. (51.6 lbs) per bushel. The heaviest sample of oats would have contained about 85% more ENDOSPERM and therefore ENERGY than the lightest sample

A bushel of grain is in fact a measurement of volume, equal to that of a cylinder, 8 inches (20 cms) deep and 18.5 inches (47 cms) in diameter, with a capacity of 2150 cubic inches or 35.24 litres and each grain has a different accepted bushel weight.

ENERGY DENSITY

The different volume (bushel) weights of grains related to the energy level of the individual grains provides an indication of ENERGY DENSITY or the amount of ENERGY in a specific volume of grain.

The following table, based on average values only, shows that OATS contains less energy for the SAME VOLUME than does any of the other grains.

GRAIN	DESIRABLE WEIGHTS	KG/10LITRES	DIGESTIBLE ENERGY MJ/10 LITRES
Oats	15.7 kg (40lbs)/bushel	5.2	51.7
Barley	22.3 kg (50lbs)/bushel	6.5	73.0
Sorghum	26.7 kg (58lbs)/bushel	7.2	89.7
Maize	35.0 kg (77lbs)/bushel	8.0	93.7

In relative terms, this is explained below.

ADDITIONAL PERCENTAGE OF ENERGY

OATS	BARLEY	SORGHUM	MAIZE	
OATS	100%	71%	58%	55%
BARLEY	140%	100%	81%	78%
SORGHUM	173%	123%	100%	96%
MAIZE	181%	128%	104%	100%

This table can be used in a number of ways to compare the ENERGY levels of THE SAME VOLUME of individual grains, all with DIFFERENT VOLUME WEIGHTS.

If you want to relate all the feeds to OATS, the same volumes of BARLEY contains 140%, SORGHUM 173% and MAIZE 181% more energy than OATS.

Similarly with MAIZE, the same volume of OATS will contain only 55%, BARLEY 78%, and SORGHUM 96% of the ENERGY content of MAIZE.

HAY AND CHAFF

Hay does not come packed in any standard size. It is generally accepted that 40 bales of good, well pressed hay weigh 1 tonne and most commercial transactions are done on this basis. This gives an average bale weight of 25 kgs. Hay however has been known to vary from 30 bales to the tonne giving an average bale weight of 33 kg. to 50 to the ton giving an average bale weight of 20 kg.

Careful hay buying, especially if buying on a per bale basis is to find a reliable supplier not only with the quality you wish but also with bales of commercially acceptable weight. It is not uncommon for commercial hay producers to produce hay bales shorter than normal, and hence lighter in weight than normal, if selling on a per bale basis, they get more bales to sell off each cut of hay.

Chaff is simply hay which is cut up into short lengths in the chaff cutter, is traded in accepted commercial quantities based on chaff bags and the general rule of a thumb is:

Lucerne (alfalfa) chaff 26 bags to the tonne or 39 kilos per bag.

Cereal chaff, wheaten or oaten, 22 bags to the tonne or 45 kg per bag.

The producers of chaff are far fewer in number than the producers of hay and are reliant on continually selling to retail outlets for survival so there is generally little variation in the per bag weights of chaff.

COMPONENT MEASUREMENT OF FEEDS.

Whilst it is very important to know the exact weight of each feed which the horse is eating each day, it is also necessary to be able to understand exactly what is in that feed.

FEED COMPONENT contents can be expressed in a number of ways.

1. ABSOLUTE WEIGHT

dependent on the country or state of feed registration, ABSOLUTE WEIGHTS can appear on the label in either METRIC UNITS or IMPERIAL UNITS.

METRIC UNITS are in predominant use and the terms commonly used, on stock feed labels and in stock feed terminology consist of

1000 MICROGRAMS (μG)	=	1 MILLIGRAM
1000 MILLIGRAMS (MG)	=	1 GRAM
1000 GRAMS (G)	=	1 KILOGRAM
1000 KILOGRAMS (KG)	=	1 TONNE (SHORT TONNE)

IMPERIAL UNITS (or AVOIRDUPOIS WEIGHT) are less commonly used

8 DRAMS (DMS)	=	1 OUNCE (OZ)
16 OUNCES (OZ)	=	1 POUND (LB)
28 POUNDS (LB)	=	1 QUARTER (QR)
4 QUARTERS (QR)	=	1 HUNDREDWEIGHT (CWT)
4 QUARTERS (QR)	=	112 POUNDS (LBS)
20 HUNDREDWEIGHTS	=	1 TON (LONG TON)

The use of METRIC UNITS allows much smaller levels of feed components to be calculated and described on the label.

2. PERCENTAGE

PERCENTAGE values can be worked out by most people, these are, by far, the easiest method of describing the actual contents of a ration.

If the ration contains a CRUDE PROTEIN PERCENTAGE of 10%, it is relatively simple to visualise that of the 10kgs being fed to the horse, 1 kg of that has to be protein. If one feed contains 60% energy and another only 40%, it is obvious that the 60% feed has more energy, in fact half as much again or 50% more than the 40% energy ration.

Some nutritional references refer to the amount of a feed component required by a horse in terms of a PERCENTAGE of total feed intake, i.e. SALT is fed at a level of 0.5% to 1.0% of the ration. Whilst this terminology may be of value to people trained in nutrition, it can be confusing to the average horse feeder.

The exact meaning of RATION needs to be spelled out as referring to the DRY MATTER content of the ration which, after excluding about a 10% water content, will be about 90% of the weight of HARD FEED. Pasture feeding is a different matter due to the much higher water levels in pasture.

The feeder then has to do a calculation as follows

RATION DRY MATTER. 9 KGS

1.0% OF 9000 GRAMS equals 90 grams so 0.5 % equals 45 grams.

Since most horse feeders do not have a set of scales accurate enough in the feed shed to weigh in grams, this weight then has to be converted back to the common measure used for this type of feeding, teaspoons or table spoons.

3. FRACTIONS

Very rarely are FRACTIONS used in technical horse feeding language. It is simple to say feed the horse, half and half hay and oats. It is also necessary to add whether the fraction refers to weight or volume. It is also difficult to relate fractions back to horses, have you ever seen half a horse ?

4. PARTS PER MILLION

Often abbreviated P.P.M. or p.p.m., this term is frequently used, especially with feed components, such as MINERALS and VITAMINS which are required by the horse in very small quantities or which are supplied in feed supplements in similarly small quantities.

PARTS PER MILLION can be related to a PERCENTAGE BASIS

1000 P.P.M.	equals	0.100 %
100 P.P.M.	equals	0.010 %
10 P.P.M.	equals	0.001 %

5. INTERNATIONAL UNITS

a recognised system of measuring the concentration of some vitamins, especially the FAT SOLUBLE VITAMINS, A, D and E.

In the case of VITAMIN A, 1 I.U. is defined as the VITAMIN A activity of 0.3 UG (pronounced MU GRAMS), or 0.3 MICROGRAMS of crystalline retinol.

With VITAMIN D measurement, 1 I.U. is defined as the VITAMIN D activity of 0.025 UG or 0.25 MICROGRAMS of crystalline VITAMIN D3.

For VITAMIN E measurement, 1 I.U. is defined as the VITAMIN E activity of 1 MG of synthetic racemic alpha tocopherol acetate.

In each instance, it is possible to relate INTERNATIONAL UNITS, via MICROGRAMS, to the METRIC system of ABSOLUTE WEIGHT MEASUREMENT.

All these definitions of INTERNATIONAL UNITS are often far too technical for the average horse feeder so he or she just has to accept a system, developed by scientists and in common use in all types of nutritional systems

FEED DRY MATTER

This is a technical term which means the weight of a feed, WITHOUT any water present. This situation does not exist in every day horse feeding, as all horse feeds contain some water content. Even if the feed was artificially dried to remove all the water, the feed would still take water up from the atmosphere, after complete drying and before feeding, due to the natural water content or humidity in the atmosphere.

If you wish to determine the DRY MATTER content of any feed, there are a number of simple ways in which you can get a reasonable result. Spread the feed out in the sunlight, after weighing and let the sun remove the moisture, over a period of days, exactly the same as if making hay. It will be necessary to regularly turn or re-organise the feed so that even drying is obtained. Weigh the feed again when dry and the weight of DRY MATTER, PLUS 12% MOISTURE is obtained. TOTAL DRY MATTER can then be obtained by making the necessary allowances for to 12% or so moisture still inside the feed. This basic technique will work with pasture but other feeds may be to dense to allow adequate drying from the sun.

The second method simply involves the use of the oven in the kitchen stove. Weigh any amount of feed, place in the oven at a temperature of 100-105 degrees CENTIGRADE (212-220 degrees FAHRENHEIT), until all the free water has evaporated. In practical terms, until the feed starts to burn and go black in colour. Then you have left the sample in too long so try again with a shorter oven time. Weigh the sample immediately out of the oven and this weight compared to the initial weight will provide you with the DRY MATTER content. This calculation of DRY MATTER doe contain some error, as all feeds contain some CARBOHYDRATES (sugars) and other volatile components, such as VOLATILE FATTY ACIDS (V.F.A.) which will be destroyed once the temperature exceeds 70 degrees CENTIGRADE (160 degrees FAHRENHEIT). To correctly assess DRY MATTER requires the use of a vacuum oven or freeze drying facilities, generally not available to the average horse feeder.

The third method involves the us of the microwave oven. The principles of use are the same as when the oven is used, EXCEPT temperature and length of time would have to be worked out for each feed and each microwave.

DRY MATTER can also be measured by moisture meters which have a probe which is pushed into the feed, accuracy depends on price, the cheaper ones are not as reliable as using the oven but the results are better than nothing.

Most if not all grains, hays, oilseed meals and similar "hard" or "concentrate" type feeds will have a WATER content of 12% or less. If the WATER content of these feeds are above about 12%, physical conditions of water and temperature in the feed will encourage the growth of mould and other organisms and the feeds will not be able to be stored for any length of time.

HENCE to get 10 KG (22 LBS) of DRY MATTER from "hard" feeds would require, at 12% water content, about 11.5 KGS of actual feeds.

RULE OF THUMB

FOR COMPLETELY HAND FED HORSES
TO CONVERT A "HARD FEED" RATION TO DRY MATTER CONTENT ONLY
DIVIDE THE WEIGHT OF THE RATION BY 1.15
OR
MULTIPLY THE WEIGHT OF THE RATION BY 8.7
TO CONVERT DRY MATTER TO "HARD FEED AS FED"

MULTIPLY WEIGHT OF DRY MATTER BY 11.5

A number of ration details are quoted in an "AS FED" basis which is DRY MATTER PLUS RESIDUAL MOISTURE. Whilst AS FED figures for all hard feeds and hays will be similar, there will be considerable differences between the DRY MATTER WEIGHT and the AS FED WEIGHT when the feeding of green pasture is taken into consideration.

HORSES GRAZING PASTURE

Water content and hence DRY MATTER content of PASTURE varies greatly, dependent on the stage of growth and maturity of the pasture. Young actively growing pasture can contain up to 85% moisture, whilst pasture approaching seed production reduces to 30- 40% and fully mature and dry pasture may only contain 15-18% moisture.

A 450 kg horse, obtaining all its feed requirements from young actively growing pasture, at about 85% water content, would have to consume some 66 KGS of pasture, comprising 10 KGS DRY MATTER and 56 KGS of water. It is quite possible that the horse would be unable to consume such daily amounts of young actively growing pasture so would suffer a DRY MATTER shortage in its daily diet.

The estimation of DRY MATTER intake in horses, expected to get most or all of their feed requirements from partial or complete grazing on pasture is NOT EASY, in fact in the practical situation impossible.

The one important practical difference between the completely hand fed stabled horse and the horse partially or completely grazing on pasture is that the horse at pasture is NOT RESTRICTED by human intervention in the amount of feed he or she eats and can eat as long as required to satisfy its needs. The stabled horse however MAY have a restricted physical weight of feed provided each day which MAY be insufficient to satisfy its daily feed requirements.

Daily DRY MATTER INTAKE is now examined in relation to three classifications of body weight:

450 kg (1000 lbs)	average thoroughbred 16 hands.
350 kg (790-800 lbs)	stock horse, galloway 14 to 15 hands.
250 kg (560 lbs)	thoroughbred weanlings, stock horse type yearlings, 13 to 14 hand ponies.

AVERAGE DAILY FEED INTAKE AS DRY MATTER

NOT "HARD FEED AS FED"

HORSE LIVE WEIGHT

	250 kg (550 lbs)		350 kg (770 lbs)		450 kg (1000 lbs)	
	kg	lbs	kg	lbs	kg	lbs
Horse at rest	3.82	8.42	5.35	1.80	6.88	15.20
Light work	4.33	9.50	6.06	13.40	7.80	17.20
Medium work	4.58	10.10	6.41	14.10	8.25	18.20
Hard work	4.95	10.90	6.93	15.30	8.92	19.70
Brood mares	4.58	10.10	6.41	14.10	8.25	18.20

It is generally accepted that there may be up to 20% variation above or below these figures dependent, on individual horse differences and work loads, the more work the greater the DRY MATTER intake.

From a practical angle, the daily DRY MATTER feed intake of a horse has been accepted as being between 2% and 3% of the individual horses' body weight. This estimate is applicable to a horse AT REST, but research work has shown that horses, performing physical work, can have quite considerable increases in the amount of DRY MATTER required/day to supply all the feed components required for both body maintenance and work or activity. One 500kg thoroughbred eventer, known to the writer, has an appetite of 26kgs HARD FEED/DAY, consisting of 14kgs oats and 12 kgs hay when competing. This works out at a feed intake AS FED of 5.20% of body weight or as DRY MATTER, at 4.6% of body weight, some 50% greater than the generally accepted standards.

GUT or DIGESTIVE TRACT FILL

The essential practical point is that the nature of the digestive process in the horse, requires the animal to receive feed continually throughout each and every day to maintain digestive tract volume. Studies of mobs of free ranging wild horses have shown that they spend from 16 to 20 hours per day feeding and, as such, have some feed passing through the digestive tract virtually ALL THE TIME. Nothing has happened since man came to domesticate the horse which has changed this biological need of the horse to have continual access to feed and a full gut all the time.

Two of the main problems in modern day horse feeding, especially with stabled fully hand fed horses are:-

1. provision of insufficient gut fill, i.e. the horse does not get enough physical quantity of feed to eat on a daily basis.

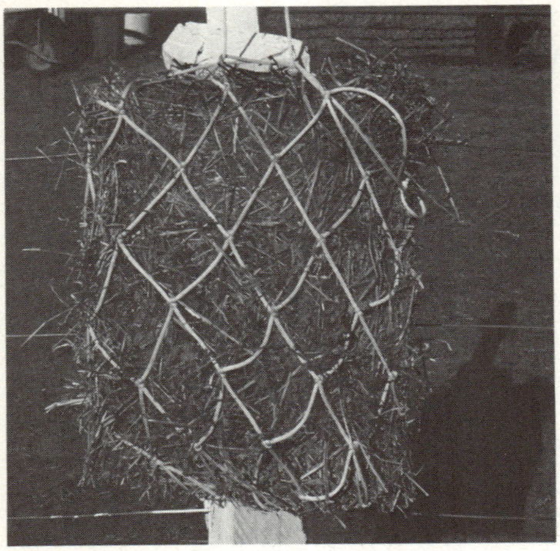

The handy hay net – very suitable when travelling

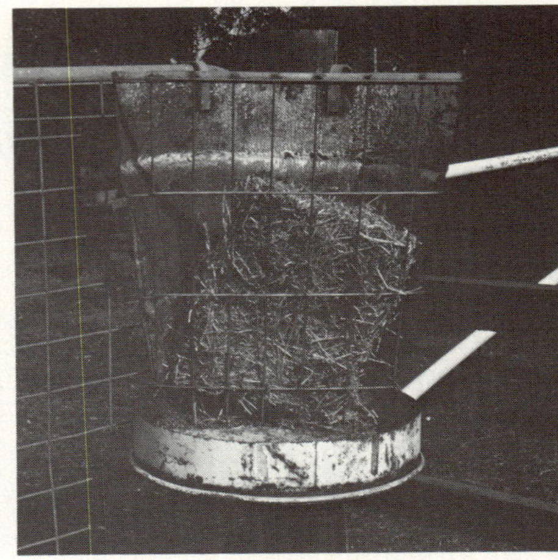

The handy hay net – very suitable when travelling

2. supply of sufficient weight of feed but the number of feeds are not spread over sufficient time to allow the horse to satisfactorily digest the nutrients supplied. The best example of this is the stabled performance horse fed twice a day only with no access to hay for the rest of the day or night. The horse will GULP or quickly eat its twice daily feeds and then has NOTHING but fresh air to consume in between.

The practical result of either of the above INCORRECT FEEDING practices is that the horse will have a digestive tract which will, at times during a 24 hour period contain insufficient food material and pockets of air, both of which will affect absorption, by the horse, of the feed nutrients present and this, in turn, will affect performance. In ponies, fed twice daily, there were definite cyclic changes or variations within the horse over a twenty four hour period of body water, electrolyte levels and electrolyte transport actions, all of which were due to the variation in VOLATILE FATTY ACID production, which was affected by cellulose breakdown in the large intestine which, in turn, was controlled by frequency of feeding.

Stabled horses require constant and adequate feeding and certainly should have access to hay 24 hours/ day, in a hay net, hanging in the stable. The horse can then regulate its own feed intake rather than having the feed intake regulated by humans who "think" they know what they are doing.

CLEAN FEED BINS

There exists a complete obsession by some people to see a horse CLEAN UP its feed bin. A clean and empty feed bin is supposed to indicate that the horse has eaten well and is therefore very fit and "doing" well.

Any horse will CLEAN UP its feed bin if it is UNDERFED in terms of the weight of feed it needs each day, it will be so hungry it will have no alternative but to clean up its feed bin. Being confined to a stable, the horse cannot regulate a lack of feed by eating more pasture and it cannot communicate with the feeder that it is still hungry and neither can it go to the kitchen or the fast food outlet to satisfy its hunger.

UNDERFEEDING OF COMPETITION HORSES, IN TERMS OF WEIGHT OF FEED IS ONE OF THE MAIN PROBLEMS CAUSING REDUCED PERFORMANCE.

The level of UNDERFEEDING does not have to be very much before performance is affected, maybe as little as 8-10% of daily needs.

A more preferred feeding practice is to have feed in front of the horse all the time.

Horses do have some funny individual habits as far as eating is concerned. Some do not like to eat alone, the company of another horse, at feeding time, can be all important. Other horses may not like eating, surrounded by activity, especially important in stabled horses where the stables fronts a busy working area or arena. Where does the horse go to get some peace and quiet? Some horses will eat more feed/day if the number of feeds are increased and the weight/feed is reduced. Still others need an "entree" of hay before commencing the main meal of hard feeds, especially if that hard feed contains a lot of concentrate and grain. Still others will NOT EAT sweet feeds or any feed containing any quantity of molasses, the taste of MOLASSES will make some horses go right off their feed. Feed consumption can also be affected by water taste and quality.

Because there are probably as many different horse feeding situations as there are horse owners, it is necessary for each horse feeder to be able to sort out exactly what the horse is capable of eating each day, and make sure that the horse DOES NOT SUFFER from lack of weight of feed, in simple words, the horse is able to satisfy the daily appetite.

DO NOT ADD MOLASSES TO DISGUISE THE OFFENDING TASTE. If the horse will not eat the feed without MOLASSES ADDED, the addition of MOLASSES will do nothing except satisfy the feeder that the horse has eaten what is basically unpalatable, and possibly offensive, feed. MOLASSES does not aid or assist the digestion of that "bad feed" in any way. Some horses also find MOLASSES unpalatable when mixed with feeds other than grain.

It is possible that the horse has some type of illness or problem which may be completely unrelated to the feed but should be diagnosed and treated before the horse suffers further.

Some of these problems could include:-

TOO MUCH GRAIN in the ration and NOT ENOUGH HAY
SHARP TEETH AFFECTING GUMS AND OR TONGUE
TEETH ABSCESS
CHOKING
PARTIAL DEHYDRATION
INTERNAL PARASITES
NEW HORSE-STRANGE SURROUNDINGS
"TRACK SOUR", possible VITAMIN B COMPLEX deficiency.
STRANGLES or some other BACTERIAL INFECTION

The only way to know what your stabled horse really needs in terms of feeds is to allow him or her free access to weighed amounts of feed and to weigh what is left at the end of the

24 hour period every day. You will then get a true and correct indication of what that particular horses' daily physical feed intake should be, and will then, be able to detect even the slightest change in feeding pattern which should be investigated.

Horse people are notorious for keeping records, they prefer to keep the details in their head, often forgetting the most important items. Those horse people who do keep records are always rewarded with information which allows problems to be clarified and corrected much earlier and easier than if records did not exist.

Horses on pasture suffer different problems to stall fed horses, whilst those horse which have access to pasture plus some form of concentrate feeding have different problems again.

These topics will be dealt with in detail in later parts of the book, especially in the Chapter on PASTURES.

PROXIMATE ANALYSIS OF FEED

This is a combination of ANALYTICAL techniques of feed, developed in Germany well over a century ago. Despite some faults, the system is still widely used in routine description of feedstuffs.

PROXIMATE ANALYSIS requires determination of:-

1. DRY MATTER and WATER CONTENT

as described above.

2. CRUDE PROTEIN

Determined by a long established and commonly used chemical process, known as the Kjeldahl method, which measures the amount of nitrogen in the feed, and this is then converted to CRUDE PROTEIN by a simple mathematical formula. CRUDE PROTEIN determination will provide a figure which is of value in RUMINANT digestion, but not necessarily for HORSE NUTRITION, as this method, of PROTEIN determination, does not distinguish between the various sources of protein, which is vital for the horse.

3. ETHER EXTRACT

This is the fraction or part of the feed which has high calorific or energy, or heating values. ETHER EXTRACT is a combined total of the amounts of FATS and related compounds, to-gether with any FAT SOLUBLE VITAMINS, vitamins A, D, E and K which may be in the feed.

4. ASH

This is the residue which remains after all the combustible material has been burnt off at temperatures of about 550 degrees CENTIGRADE (1000 degrees FAHRENHEIT). ASH represents a total amount of most of the MINERALS in the feed, IODINE and SELENIUM will not be included as they are volatile and will be burnt off in the high temperature.

5. CRUDE FIBRE

CRUDE FIBRE is composed of the structural materials of the plant, CELLULOSE and its related compounds, HEMI-CELLULOSE and LIGNIN. The CRUDE FIBRE result does

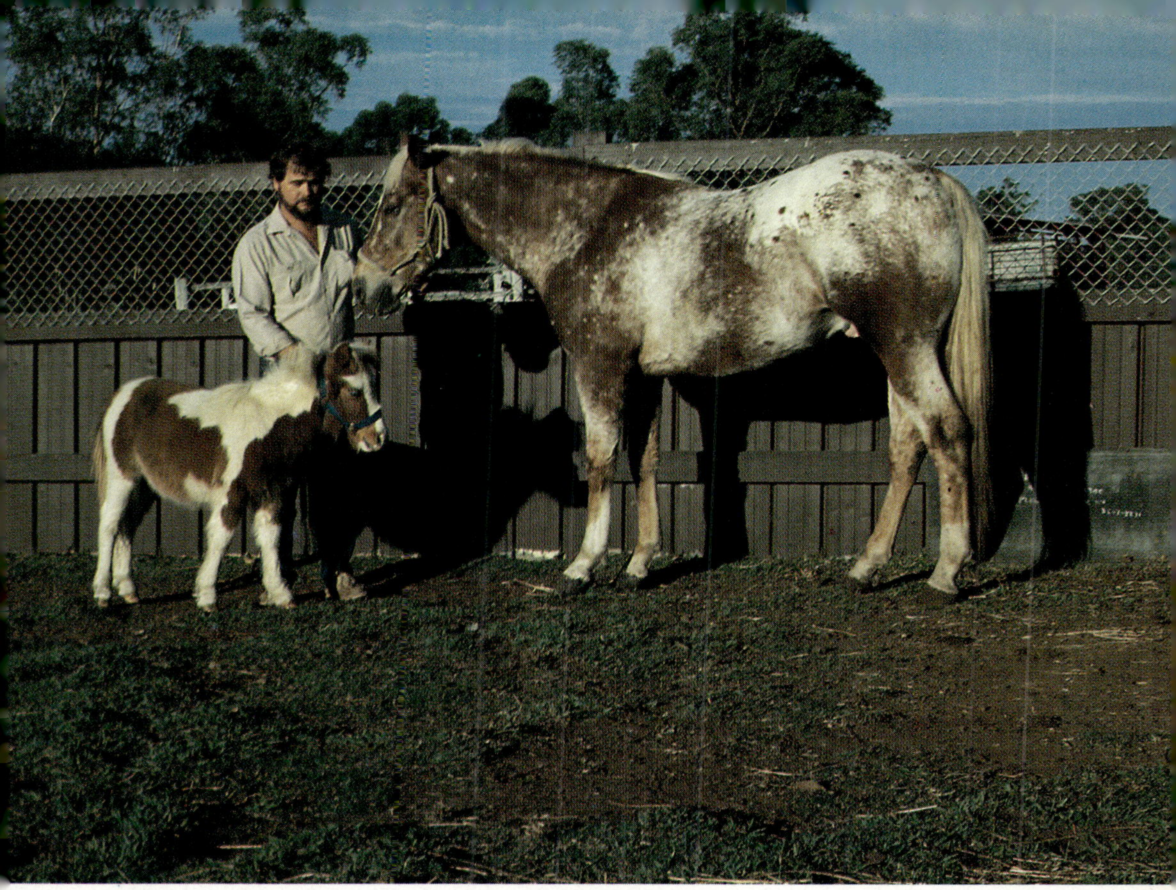

Different size horses should be fed in relation to their body weights.

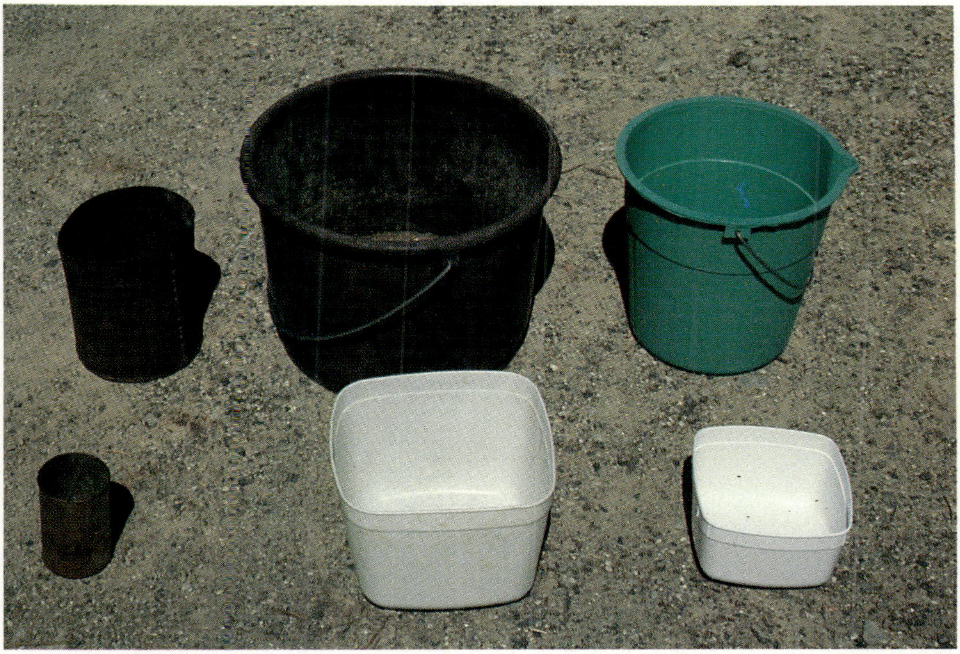

What weight of feed does each container hold?

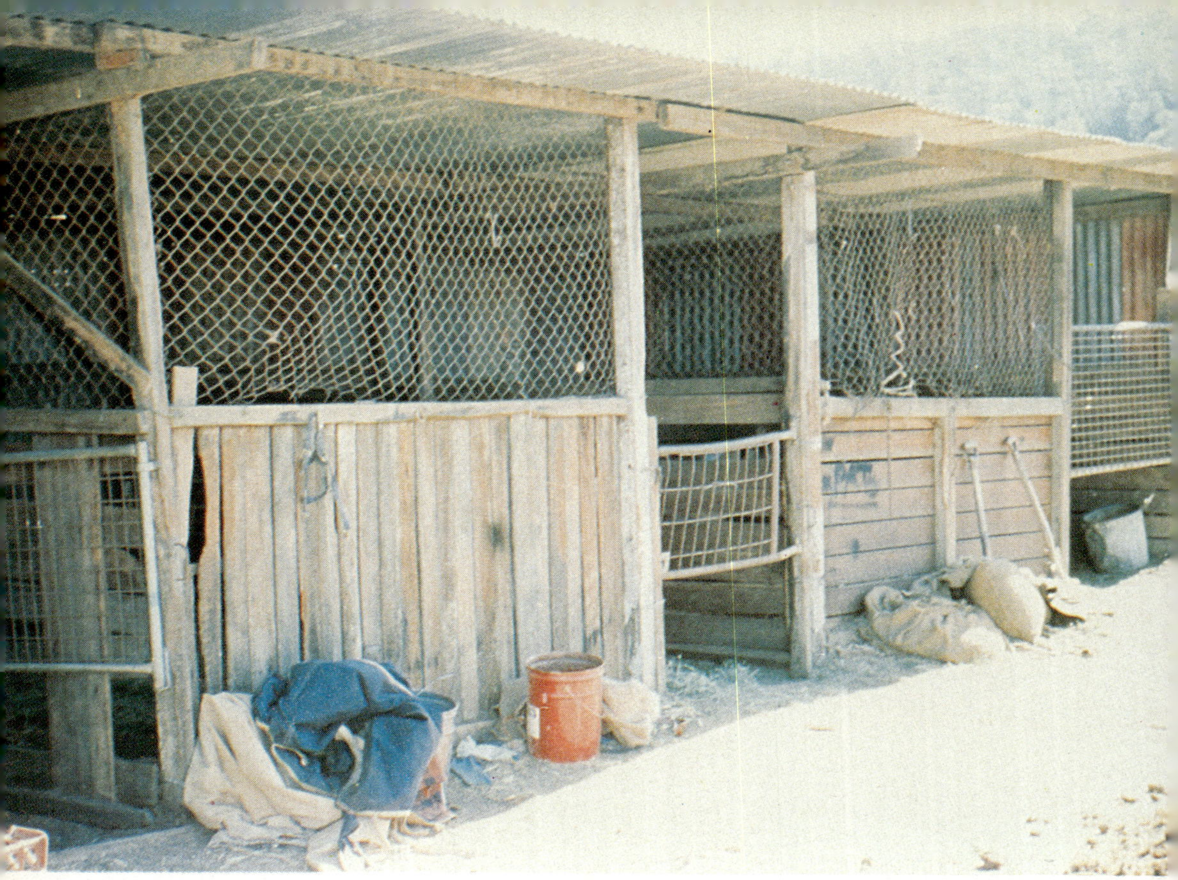

Unsatisfactory feed storage methods. Loss from weather, rodents and waste.

An ideal feed shed—weather and rodent proof and easily built.

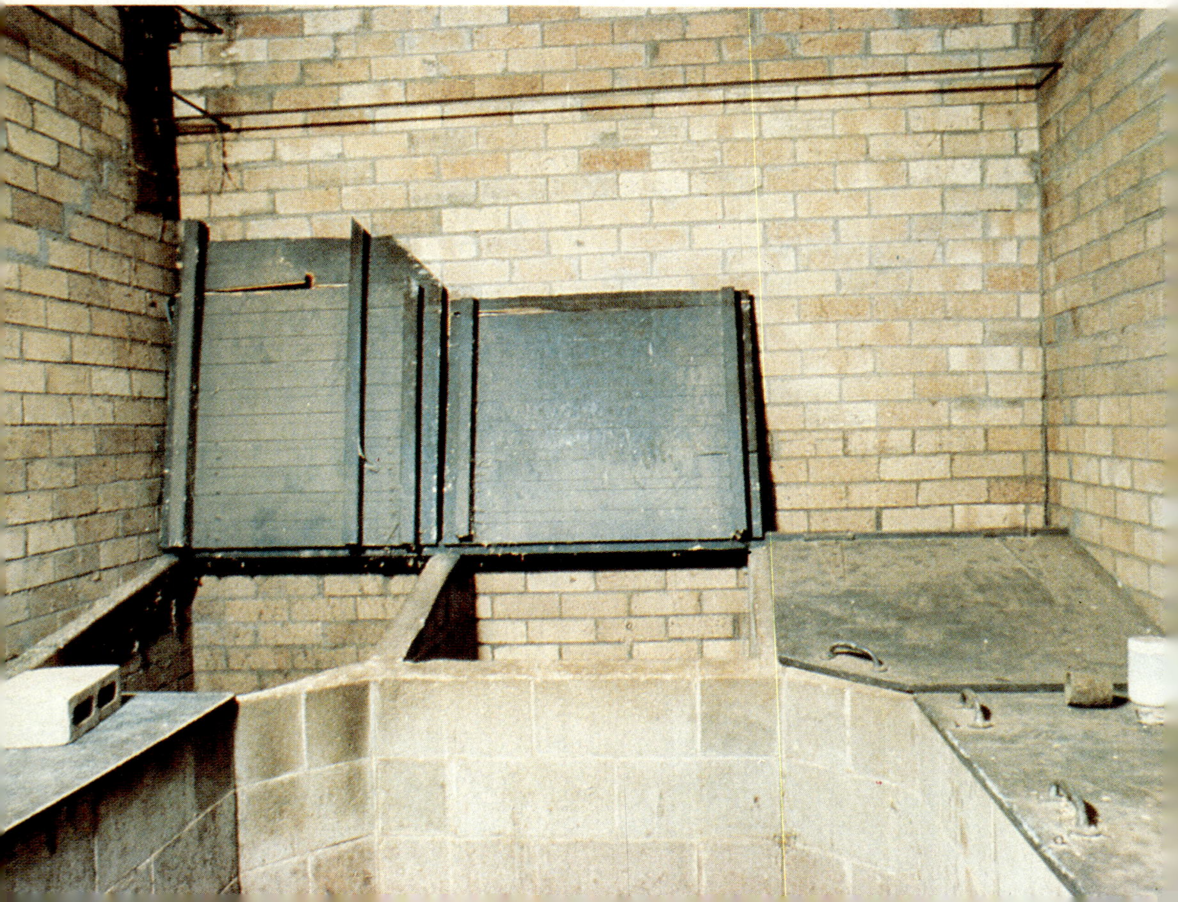

not include any measurement of the soluble fibres which may be in the feed. The content of SOLUBLE FIBRES will be included in the details for NITROGEN FREE EXTRACT.

6. NITROGEN FREE EXTRACT

this is a calculation of the amount of CARBOHYDRATE (sugars and starches) plus the soluble fibre portion of the CELLULOSE compounds. NITROGEN FREE EXTRACT is determined by subtraction of the above from total DRY MATTER and is the residue of the calculation.

PROXIMATE FEED ANALYSIS FIGURES are still appearing in technical details and on feed labels, advertising materials etc. Such information is of value for other domestic livestock species, especially RUMINANTS and as there is NO SPECIFIC FEED EVALUATION standard for horses, HORSE NUTRITION has to use what are basically ruminant figures and make modifications where research work and or experience suggests.

In summary, value of details from PROXIMATE ANALYSIS for horse feeding are:-

DRY MATTER	valuable
CRUDE PROTEIN	of some value but need to know AMINO ACID content
ETHER EXTRACT	OF NO VALUE
ASH	OF NO VALUE
CRUDE FIBRE	of some value
NITROGEN FREE EXTRACT	of limited value

Most labels on stock feeds and, sometimes, stock feed supplements are required, by law, to express the contents of the product in terms of PROXIMATE ANALYSIS results.

METRIC SYSTEM OF ENERGY MEASUREMENT

This is now accepted as the standard method of measuring the energy levels of any feed. The METRIC SYSTEM relates to the amount of HEAT produced by a feed or feed component.

There are a number of practical problems in relating ENERGY VALUES, measured under the metric system to horses.

JOULES OR CALORIES ?

There are two separate and individual sysrtems of measuring energy.

The use of the CALORIE is the most common in some countries and 1 CALORIE is defined as the amount of heat required to raise the temperature of 1 gram of water by 1 degree CENTIGRADE.

The term JOULE is also sometimes used on other countries to measure the ENERGY VALUE of feeds. 1 JOULE has the heating value of 0.24 calories.

To confuse matters even more, as the ENERGY VALUES or CALORIES are considered too small to be of practical use the term KILOCALORIES, which equals 1000 CALORIES is generally accepted as the common standard or measurement and expression of ENERGY VALUES.

Then, in some parts of the U.S., the term CALORIE is commonly used, when in fact, what is really meant is KILOCALORIE.

KILOJOULES are also used in some parts to express ENERGY LEVELS of horse feeds.

1 CALORIE	=	4.16 JOULES
1 KILOCALORIE	=	416.66 JOULES.
1,000.00 CALORIES		
1 MEGACALORIE	=	1,000.00 KILOCALORIES
	=	1,000,000.00 CALORIES
1 JOULE	=	0.24 CALORIES
1 KILOJOULE	=	1000.00 JOULES
	=	240.00 CALORIES
1 MEGAJOULE	=	1,000,000.00 JOULES
	=	240,000.00 CALORIES.

When trying to sort out energy levels of feed, quoted in the metric system, it is absolutely essential to determine which units are being used to describe the ENERGY CONTENT.

1. KJ/KG is the abbreviation of KILOJOULES of energy per KILOGRAM of feed.
2. MJ/KG is the abbreviation of MEGAJOULES of energy per KILOGRAM of feed.
3. KCal's/KG is the abbreviation of KILOCALORIES of energy per KILOGRAM OF FEED
4. MCal's/KG is the abbreviation of MEGACALORIES of energy/KG of feed.

15. FEED EVALUATION METHODS

PROTEIN and ENERGY are the two main feed components used in the technical evaluation of feeds for horses.

As all feeds cost money, and as we are always interested in feeding horses so that they will perform to our expected ability, it is in every horse feeder's interest to be able to select the best balance of feeds for the least cost.

Protein and energy are the two feed components that have been measured in various ways for some considerable time.

Measurement of vitamins and mineral components have been available over the past years and in fact a multitude of horse nutritional supplements are now available with the quantities of vitamins and minerals stated on the label.

PROTEIN is the most important ingredient in horse nutrition, it is the basis of the construction and maintenance of all living tissue, and if the level of PROTEIN in the ration is less than required, the horse will not have sufficient size, and or strength in its tissues to perform satisfactorily. ENERGY is the second most important ingredient in the horses' ration, ENERGY is the body fuel but energy cannot be used effectively if there is insufficient PROTEIN in the diet. It is absolutely essential that both PROTEIN and ENERGY levels in the diet be satisfactory for the requirements of the horse otherwise any addition of VITAMINS and or MINERALS to the diet will not be of any value.

PROTEIN MEASUREMENT

PROTEIN LEVEL CAN BE EXPRESSED IN ANY ONE OF TWO WAYS:

1. CRUDE PROTEIN – a measurement of the amount of protein in the feed or feeds as determined by an analytical technique performed in a laboratory.
2. DIGESTIBLE PROTEIN – a measurement of the amount of protein possibly digested by an animal. The digestible protein is equal to, or less than, the crude protein of the feed of ration.

NOTE: Emphasis on the word POSSIBLY in the definition of DIGESTIBLE PROTEIN. The reason for this phrase is that very little research work has been carried out on the horse to provide DIGESTIBLE PROTEIN FIGURES directly applicable to that animal. Virtually all the DIGESTIBLE PROTEIN figures quoted for feeds are derived from studies on ruminants, pigs or poultry and as we have seen elsewhere in this book, the horse DOES HAVE quite different nutrient needs and digestibilities of feeds, compared to these other domestic animal species.

Soybean is one feed where the crude protein level is close to the digestible protein level, i.e. most of the protein in the feed is accepted as being available to the horse. Soybean meal has a crude protein of 50% and a digestible protein of 40% giving a protein digestibility of 80%.

At the other end of the scale, dry mature standing pasture of mixed composition, grass and legume, may contain 6% crude protein and only 1% digestible protein, a protein digestibility of 16%.

Protein evaluation is further complicated by the water content of the feed concerned.

Soybean meal only has a water content of about 10%, whereas dry mature standing pasture may have a water content of 30- 40%.

The effects of this PROTEIN DIGESTIBILITY, on nutrient intake, by horses will be discussed in more detail in the section on pasture feeding of horses.

DESIRABLE PROTEIN LEVELS IN RATIONS

These figures are provided as CRUDE PROTEIN (C.P.) i.e. that protein level present in the feed as determined by laboratory analysis. CRUDE PROTEIN is not necessarily the same as DIGESTIBLE PROTEIN (D.P.) which is the level of protein in the ration which the animal actually absorbs in the digestive tract. DIGESTIBLE PROTEIN figures are available for SOME feeds for SOME other animals, namely poultry, pigs and ruminants. Very few, if any, DIGESTIBLE PROTEIN figures are currently available for horses and those which are available DO NOT cover enough feeds, to allow the complete ration to be calculated in one single standard. It is also unwise to attempt to translate data from other forms of livestock to horses as we know, from other nutritional work, that the horse has quite different feeding requirements from pigs, poultry and ruminants.

No definite figure can be given for the ABSOLUTE PROTEIN level to be fed to each horse. Firstly very few people would have every days' ration for the horse analysed to determine protein levels being fed, secondly, there will be, in practice, a continual daily variation in protein levels of most common horse feeds and thirdly, there will be individual horse differences re protein requirements.

It is however possible to indicate a range of CRUDE PROTEIN values that the horse feeder should aim for.

DRY ADULT HORSES

1. Dry adult horses at rest, such as spelling horses or adult animals with little work requirements. These animals have little protein needs for growth and generally only need protein for maintenance of body tissues. These animals can exist on feed protein levels of 6-8%. This can also be described as a CRUDE PROTEIN requirement of 1.3 grams of C.P./KG body weight/day or if considered in conjunction with the energy levels of the ration of a resting adult horse 40 grams C.P./MCal of DIGESTIBLE ENERGY.

2. Dry adult horses in some form of activity, but not in full training. Included in this category would be the working stock horse, performance horses in the early stages of training, the active pony club horse and animals subject to similar work loads. Protein is required in these horses not only to support the normal body functions such as heart, lungs, liver etc. but is also needed to maintain muscles in correct order as the animal is working and this involves muscle use, wear and tear and hence protein needs to be available to muscle repair and rehabilitation. Protein level 8-10%

3. Dry adult horses in full work. Included in this category is any performance horse in the latter part of a training programme, including eventers, endurance horses, standardbreds, thoroughbreds, showjumpers, polo and polo-crosse horses and similar animals. Muscle wear and tear will naturally increase due to the extra demands of the training and performance programme. These animals need a ration protein level of about 12%.

EXCESSIVE LEVELS of PROTEIN in the rations of these types of horses can have the following adverse effects:-

1 – increased blood ammonia concentration.
2 – increased sweating.
3 – increased electrolyte demand.
4 – early fatigue in performance horses.
5 – reduced speed in thoroughbred horses.
6 – increased urinary output.
7 – increased water consumption.

GROWING HORSES

4. Growing horses up to 4 years of age. As protein is responsible for the growth and maintenance of all body tissues. these animals have higher protein needs, than any horse fully grown and over 4 years of age, to be able to grow to their full genetic potential. A minimum protein level in the ration of 15% is required and in fact feeding rations with higher levels of protein MAY be of advantage to this type of animal.

Growing horses have been shown to respond to the addition of the amino acid, LYSINE, to normal rations. Added to a weanling ration of 14.5% C.P., at the rate of 0.7% of ration weight as LYSINE and to a yearling ration of 12% C.P., at the rate of 0.45% LYSINE, produced increased growth rates in weanlings and yearlings, over the same rations which did not include LYSINE. LYSINE does not have to be added to a ration which contains about 500 grams of SOYBEAN MEAL/day as this feed contains very high natural levels of lysine.

5. Growing horses in training – specifically 2 year old trotters and/or pacers and gallopers in full training. This type of horse is the most DIFFICULT to feed as the animal is still growing and at the same time is being asked to perform at its physical best. Protein is therefore needed for BOTH growth and also performance.

CRUDE PROTEIN levels of at least 18% are needed for this type of horse and response has been obtained from feeding rations with higher protein levels that 18% to 2 years old in training. It is essential, in order to get the best from this type of horse that not only is the overall levels of protein at a desirable value but also that all the 10 ESSENTIAL AMINO ACIDS are present in the protein being fed.

Whilst these young growing horses in training need higher than normal levels of protein in the ration, problems may well be encountered from palatability of the ration and this can be accentuated if the young horse is receiving a supplement of Vitamin B Complex or has an undiagnosed specific ELECTROLYTE problem. Individual horse variations need to be carefully analysed to clarify the exact nature of the problem.

BROOD MARES

6. Brood mares. The mare needs protein for three reasons:

a) to maintain its own body tissues
b) to produce sufficient milk to satisfactorily rear a foal
c) to conceive and produce a healthy foal

These matrons when dry and pregnant require a protein level of about 10% in the ration. LACTATION and a further PREGNANCY combined can, however, increase the brood mares' ration protein requirements to about 14% during the suckling period

Protein DEFICIENCY in the feed, available to a brood mare, generally restricts the genetic potential of the mare to produce milk, causing a reduction in milk production, so that the foal at foot will not get the possible supply of milk, that could have been available, if the mare was properly fed.

The end result of this may be a foal which does not grow as well as it is genetically capable. Secondly, if the protein level is still low the mare generally dries up completely and at the same time starts to lose body weight or condition, a result of the mare using muscle protein to complement her reduced daily intake for survival of herself and the developing foetus.

If protein deficiency continues, the mare will come to the stage she is so poor that the foal being carried will be aborted so that the mare may survive on the limited feed available. It is also important to remember that adequate exercise is just as important for brood mares as is protein level in the ration.

ENERGY MEASUREMENT

ENERGY LEVELS OF FEED CAN BE MEASURED IN THE FOLLOWING WAYS:

1.STARCH EQUIVALENT or S.E.

The starch equivalent system of measuring energy levels was developed many years ago using cattle and pigs. It is a simple and easily understood system. Animals were fed pure starch and their growing and fattening performance measured. Other feeds were then fed and the animal's performance on other feeds compared to that performance obtained from the feeding of starch.

Maize (corn) with an S.E. value of 80-85 means that 10 kgs. of maize (corn) will produce 80-85% of the energy available from 10 kgs of starch. Oats with an S.E. value of 60 means that 10 kgs. of oats will produce 60% of the energy from 10 kgs of starch.

The higher the S.E. value of a feed, the more energy that feed contains, the lower the S.E. value of the feed, the lower the energy content of that feed.

2. CALORIFIC SYSTEM OF NET ENERGY

This system uses the measure of the energy values of feeds in terms of the METRIC nomenclature, in CALORIES, as an estimate of the energy or heating value of a food. As one calorie is a very small unit of heat, the system generally expresses energy values in terms of Kilocalories (KCAL) or Therms. Sometimes the term JOULE, as in KILOJOULE will also be used, one JOULE being equal to 0.24 CALORIES.

This method of energy assessment then relies on measurement of GROSS ENERGY in the feed similar to crude protein and also the actual or NET ENERGY, in the feed similar to digestible protein.

Maize has a net energy value of 46 compared to hay at 24 and straw at 5. The system works exactly the same as the S.E. system in that the feed with the highest value contains the greatest amount of energy.

Various modifications of the calorific system of measuring net energy are also now being used in advanced nutritional assessment for animals other than horses.

THEORETICAL ASSESSMENT OF CALORIFIC ENERGY

The CALORIFIC ENERGY NEEDS and or CALORIFIC ENERGY CONTENT OF SPECIFIC FEEDS for most "commercial animals", cattle pigs, poultry etc. have been carefully evaluated by scientific research.

The procedure is simple to do but very time consuming and expensive to perform. Determination of ENERGY NEEDS and or ENERGY AVAILABILITY involves placing the animal or bird, in the case of poultry, in an enclosed chamber where every thing which goes into the animal is measured. These measurements include URINE and FAECES output as well as any variation in temperature within the enclosed area which is used to determine the heat loss from the animal's body, both by faecal and urine output and also by body heat.

The ENERGY needs of or use by the animal or the ENERGY VALUE of a particular feed can then be assessed as follows:-

GROSS ENERGY

Abbreviated to G.E. – represents the total amount of ENERGY obtained by the complete burning of any feed in the laboratory. A strictly theoretical figure which does not consider any different digestibilities of various animal species for the same feed.

DIGESTIBLE ENERGY

Abbreviated to D.E., the level of any feed is reasonably closely related to FIBRE or CELLULOSE level, PROVIDED THAT feed DOES NOT contain FATS or related compounds. The higher the FIBRE or CELLULOSE level, the lower is the amount of DIGESTIBLE ENERGY. DIGESTIBLE ENERGY levels of feed are further complicated by volume weight, the bushel weight under the Imperial system of measurement. MAIZE (CORN) will have a higher DIGESTIBLE ENERGY level than will OATS, simply because the same volume of maize weighs about 40% more than oats.

To calculate the DIGESTIBLE ENERGY LEVEL of any feeds which contain a FAT fraction requires very careful consideration of the amount of FAT in the feed and the amount of ENERGY required to break that fat down to a compound which can be absorbed by the horse.

DIGESTIBLE ENERGY VALUES are as close as it is practically possible to get figures which actually indicate how much energy in the feed an animal is able to use.

DIGESTIBLE ENERGY + ENERGY LOST IN FAECES = GROSS ENERGY.

METABOLIZABLE ENERGY

Abbreviated to M.E., is that energy remaining after energy losses are considered in URINE and any gas which is produced and or lost during digestion.

NO CURRENT INFORMATION IS AVAILABLE ON ANY METABOLIZABLE ENERGY LEVELS OF ANY FEEDS FOR HORSES.

METABOLIZABLE ENERGY + ENERGY LOST IN URINE AND DIGESTION GASES =DIGESTIBLE ENERGY.

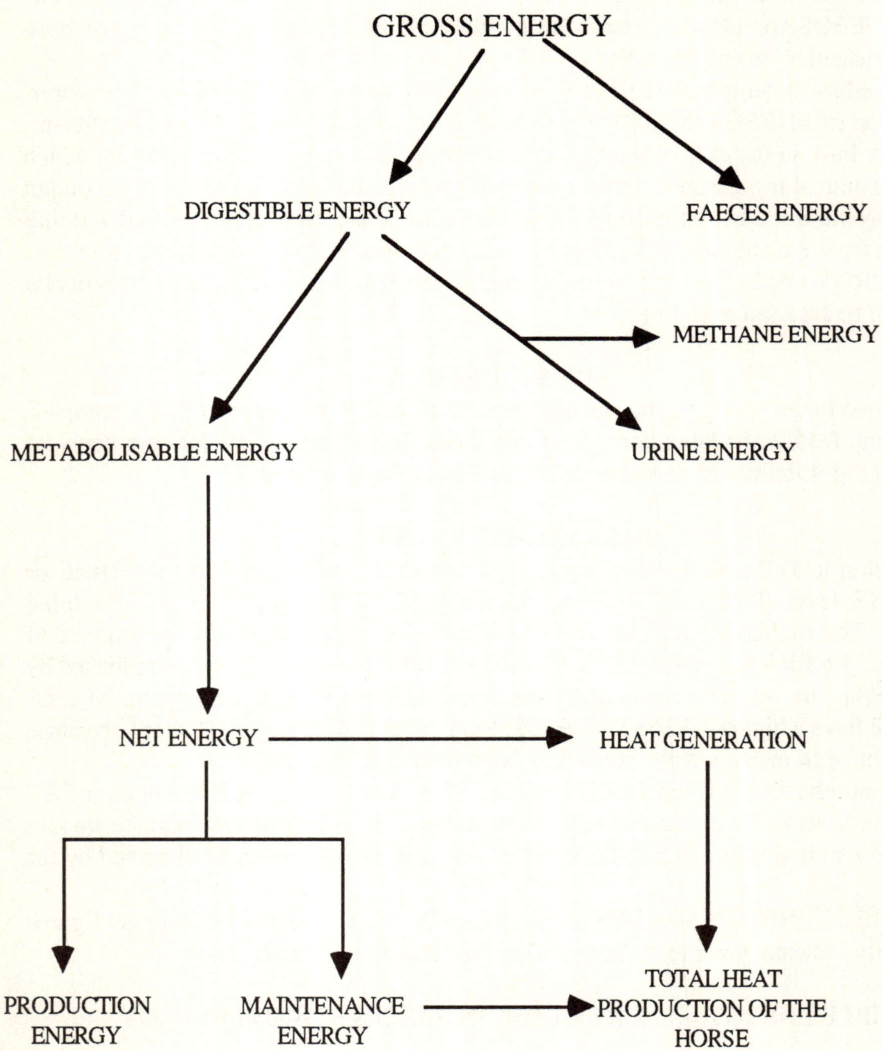
GROSS ENERGY
DIGESTIBLE ENERGY
FAECES ENERGY
METHANE ENERGY
METABOLISABLE ENERGY
URINE ENERGY
NET ENERGY
HEAT GENERATION
PRODUCTION ENERGY
MAINTENANCE ENERGY
TOTAL HEAT PRODUCTION OF THE HORSE

NET ENERGY

Abbreviated to N.E., is that ENERGY which is used by the animal for maintenance and production, in the horse, this relates to the energy which is available for all the functions which are asked of the horse by man, including growth, performance and reproduction.

In order to get a NET ENERGY value, consideration has to be taken of the energy which has been lost as HEAT in the processes of DIGESTION and METABOLISM, or that energy which is needed and is part ofthe MAINTENANCE systems inside the horse.

NET ENERGY + ENERGY LOST IN MAINTENANCE = METABOLIZABLE ENERGY

THEORETICAL PROBLEMS OF ENERGY DESCRIPTION

The problems with the practical use of this system of ENERGY description for horses are:-

1. VERY FEW VALUES are available for any feeds for NET ENERGY, but NET ENERGY is readily used in feedlot beef and dairy cattle where a mathematical measurement of production can be obtained, in weight gain/day or litres milk produced/day.
2. NO VALUES are available for any horse feeds for METABOLIZABLE ENERGY, this is used strictly in the pet food industry.
3. The values which are available for DIGESTIBLE ENERGY are mostly for animals other than horses and are therefore NOT DIRECTLY APPLICABLE to horse feeding.
4. The phrase METABOLIZBLE ENERGY, as used in the U.K. for ruminant feeding and sometimes transferred to horse nutrition refers to NET ENERGY, under the system described above.

PRACTICAL PROBLEMS IN DEFINING ENERGY NEEDS

1. DEFINING EACH HORSE'S ACTUAL ENERGY REQUIREMENTS

The main problem, from a practical viewpoint, is for the horse feeder to be able to determine the CORRECT ENERGY level in the ration and to do so to able to quantify or describe in mathematical terms, the amount of energy the horse requires. Since the horse is able to produce so many different products, in terms of energy requirements, this is currently a very difficult, if not, impossible task. These energy derived products are in the many different forms of exercise and physical activity which the horse is expected to produce. Two diverse examples would be the energy product, or energy used of the learners' pony compared to the energy used by an endurance horse.

From a theoretical viewpoint, based on the present academic systems of measuring ENERGY in feeds and animal use, the following criteria need to be known to be able to calculate the ENERGY NEEDS of a horse

SPECIFICATION	AVAILABILITY
1. AGE OF HORSE	possible if birth date known.
2. WEIGHT OF HORSE	needs access to scales.
3. RATE OF GROWTH	needs access to scales.
4. AMOUNT OF WORK	requires serious definition and continual recording by trainer of a number of physiological features of the horse.
5. TEMPERAMENT	difficult to define in numbers and may even be a function of the attitude of the horse feeder to the horse.
6. DAILY TEMPERATURE	records available.
7. INTERNAL PARASITES	able to be detected and treated.
8. GUT FILL	only possible if horses are being fed on weight of feed and to full appetite, NO MORE EMPTY FEED BINS.
9. PREGNANCY	records should be available.
10. LACTATION	anyone can tell when a mare is suckling a foal.
11. MAINTENANCE ENERGY	no one, apart from research organisations are going to have available facilities to be able to measure, for each horse at each stage of training the amount of ENERGY which is used by the horse as HEAT in the body processes of DIGESTION and METABOLISM.
12. ENERGY LOST IN URINE	comments as above.
13. ENERGY USED IN DIGESTION	comments as above.
14. ENERGY LOST IN FAECES	comments as above.

Of these 14 criteria which are required to assess the THEORETICAL ENERGY needs of a horse,

DETAILS OF 5 ONLY – 36% – are likely to be available
AGE, TEMPERATURE, INTERNAL PARASITES, PREGNANCY, LACTATION,

DETAILS OF 4 ONLY – 28% – are possibly available, if the horse feeder is aware of the correct records to keep.
WEIGHT, GROWTH, WORK, GUT FILL,

DETAILS OF 5 ONLY -36%-are NOT LIKELY TO BE AVAILABLE AT ALL, simply because the average horse owner does not have access to the facilities for measurement.

TEMPERAMENT, MAINTENANCE ENERGY, ENERGY LOST IN URINE, ENERGY USED IN DIGESTION, ENERGY LOST IN FAECES,

In addition, the details of DIGESTIBLE ENERGY available for feeds are generally only applicable to animal species other than the horse, e.g. cattle, sheep, pig and poultry.

FOUR problems immediately arise when transferring nutritional data from other species to the horse.

1. the horse digests food vastly differently from other animals.
2. the data for other species is based on the measurement of an economic factor, e.g. milk yield, growth rate etc. Apart from growth rate in the horse, most of the ideals which people are trying to attain with their horses CANNOT be defined in quantitative terms. Horse people know what they want with their animals but are unable to define, in numerical terms, just what that requirement is.
3. the ENERGY requirements of the one horse can change continually, dependent on the eventual use of the horse. No reasonable horse trainer would ever feed the same amount of grain to a racehorse at the start of a training programme as he would at the peak of the programme.
4. Horses are generally fed as individuals, each with its supposed specific nutritional needs, most FEED ENERGY VALUES are based on application to large numbers of animals all being fed basically the same, e.g. steers in a feedlot, meat chickens in a broiler shed.

COMBINED PROTEIN AND ENERGY MEASUREMENT

TOTAL DIGESTIBLE NUTRIENTS

Abbreviated to T.D.N., TOTAL DIGESTIBLE NUTRIENTS are the total of all the digestible organic nutrients – protein, fibre, nitrogen free extract and fat, these results being derived from the PROXIMATE FEED ANALYSIS system described earlier in this chapter.

This form of nutrient measurement is sometimes used but its use is decreasing as the T.D.N. system COMBINES and totals the value for protein and energy into one figure and does not allow separation of the value of PROTEIN and ENERGY in the feed. T.D.N. actually measures the approximate heat or energy value of the feed.

T.D.N. PERCENTAGE IN A FEED is the TOTAL of:

% NITROGEN FREE EXTRACT	X	DIGESTIBILITY
% CRUDE PROTEIN	X	DIGESTIBILITY
% CRUDE FIBRE	X	DIGESTIBILITY
% CRUDE FAT X 2.25	X	DIGESTIBILITY

However the T.D.N. system of measurement of feed components is based on the assumption that the protein level of the ration is adequate or in excess of the animals needs. Excess protein over and above an animals needs for growth and tissue maintenance is converted, in the majority inside the animal to energy. Practically the T.D.N. system does not separate the levels of the protein and energy components of the ration.

Some of the most controversial problems in horse nutrition are the levels of protein, fed in the rations, of young growing horses. Protein is also the most expensive nutrient used in horse feeding and hence we need to know the individual protein levels of the feeds so that the least expensive or cheapest ration can be fed, at the same time allowing optimum growth and performance to be achieved. As such, the use of the T.D.N. system of nutrient measurement is not ideally applicable to ration compilation for young growing horses

To those who still evaluate horse feeds in terms of T.D.N. 1 kg of T.D.N. is equal to approximately 4400 KILOCALORIES (1 lb T.D.N. is approximately equal to 2000 KILOCALORIES.)

N.R.C. RECOMMENDATIONS

N.R.C. is the abbreviation for the NATIONAL RESEARCH COUNCIL, an American organisation which produces information on many matters relating to science. One of their publications is entitled NUTRIENT REQUIREMENTS FOR HORSES. This publication provides a considerable amount of scientific information on the feeding of horses and is used as a standard reference by many horse nutritionists

The N.R.C. recommendations are based as follows:-

"The requirements stated herein indicate the minimum amounts needed to sustain normal health, production and performance of horses. The numbers are not averages of all the data available but are selected values based on published research, calculations designed to extrapolate information over the total population and the subcommittee's experience in applying information to field situations."

Nevertheless, N.R.C. recommendations are an excellent base set of data to start from in formulating rations for individual horses.

The problems which occur in individual horse ration formulation include:-

1 – individual ability of each horse to use food nutrients, i.e. the fat horse you cannot get thin etc., due to individual digestive and or physiological functions of each animal.

2 – the many different types of activities which horses are required to perform.

3 – the need to consider changed feeding, for the one horse, undertaking different activities.

4 – variability in nutrient values in the feeds.

5 – the effect of one feed nutrient on the use, availability and or toxicity of any other food nutrient.

6 – previous feeding history of the horse.

7 – climatic and environmental conditions which the horse is subjected to.

8 – the general health status of the horse.

9 – the expectations, aims and ambitions of the owner.

A.F.R.C. RECOMMENDATIONS

A.F.R.C. or sometimes shortened to A.R.C. stands for the English AGRICULTURAL AND FOOD RESEARCH COUNCIL, the English equivalent of the N.R.C. All their publications on feeding data is based on livestock other than horses. A.R.C. also has a different definition of METABOLIZABLE ENERGY to that used by the N.R.C. and also uses information relating to PROTEIN levels in terms of BY PASS PROTEIN, which is that protein which by-passes the RUMEN. As the horse does not have any rumen, BY PASS PROTEIN is of no interest to the horse owner.

PRACTICAL PROBLEMS WITH FEEDING STANDARDS

For the nutritionist, FEEDING STANDARDS provide a base level of information from which INDIVIDUAL feed requirements can be estimated and diets can be formulated for each animal.

The N.R.C. requirements are formulated to be MINIMUM REQUIREMENTS for a population of animals of a given species, age, weight and exercise or pregnancy status.

Problems, concerning the interpretation and use of such general population data immediately becomes relevant when considering the application of standards such as these to the feeding of the horse.

1. By far the greater majority of hand fed or partially hand fed horses are considered as individuals, either correctly or incorrectly, by their owners. As such, each horse is perceived to have individual and specific feed needs, often markedly different from the general horse population.
2. MINIMUM REQUIREMENTS make no allowance for the individual horse who has nutritional demands in excess of the minimum, the causes of any excess demand can cover a multitude of reasons.
3. Most feeding standards for horses do not consider changes in feeding methods and or composition as a horse increases its work load as in a long training programme.
4. Individual human management techniques are known to have an effect of feed intake by individual horses.
5. There is no allowance for the horse with the unusual feed problem, sometimes caused heredity, individual horse differences or by a training schedule.

METHODS OF EXPRESSING FEEDING STANDARDS.

Unfortunately, for the practical horse feeder, there is no one accepted method of expressing the amounts of PROTEIN and ENERGY to be fed to any horse.

Even if agreement is reached by scientific people on some points, there are a number of other points in which the use of different methods of measurement can only confuse the situation for the practical horse person.

PROTEIN

PROTEIN standards or feeding levels can be expressed in the following ways:-

1. PERCENTAGE OF THE DIET.

In this form of expression, the horse can be said to require 12% PROTEIN, by weight, in the ration. If the horse is eating say 10 kgs/day, then 1.00 KG of that ration needs to be protein. Generally with horses, the value used for each feed is that which measures CRUDE PROTEIN in the ration, NOT DIGESTIBLE PROTEIN, yet some recommendations are provided in terms of DIGESTIBLE PROTEIN.

The use of PERCENTAGE VALUES of CRUDE PROTEIN has been accepted for some considerable time and a lot of practical people are able to relate to the use of PERCENTAGES in feed formulation.

2. GRAMS/KG FEED

This form of PROTEIN MEASUREMENT requires a reasonably accurate knowledge of the amount of DRY MATTER which the horse is eating each day. Most practical horse people would probably not know the horses' daily DRY MATTER consumption, so the use of this measurement can only be of value where such information, re daily DRY MATTER intake is available.

3. GRAMS/KG OF HORSE.

The use of a PROTEIN measurement as GRAMS of PROTEIN/KG of HORSE is commonly accepted in the scientific world and a number of research articles use this system of measurement.

The problem in translating this information, back to the practical situation, is that initially the weight of the horse needs to be known and secondly the DRY MATTER intake of the horse needs to be known so that the required amount of PROTEIN can be supplied in the correct amount of DRY MATTER.

4. GRAMS /MCal DIGESTIBLE ENERGY.

This system of PROTEIN measurement relates the horses' daily protein needs to the amount of energy being used. There are considerable practical problems in defining and measuring the actual ENERGY NEEDS of the horse and any error which will be made in ENERGY measurement will be reflected in PROTEIN needs.

ENERGY

ENERGY can be measured in any of the following ways:-

1. STARCH EQUIVALENT

ENERGY levels of the feed, nominated as STARCH EQUIVALENT, is the method of expressing ENERGY in PERCENTAGE TERMS. Oats, for instance is generally stated as having a STARCH EQUIVALENT value of 60, or 60% of the feed, on a weight basis, is composed of energy. This is an old yet simple system of describing the energy levels of feedstuffs. The STARCH EQUIVALENT value represents the DIGESTIBLE ENERGY portion of any feed as the S.E. values were obtained using animal tests and not laboratory results. Most STARCH EQUIVALENT values are estimates, derived from the data provided by a series or original tests and DO NOT take into consideration any energy value of FATS.

2. FAT

The measure of FAT in a horse ration is an interesting example of two systems being used for the one purpose.

For stock feed registration purposes, FAT levels of any ration have to appear on the label in PERCENTAGE terms. i.e. FAT content of the ration is 3%.

In ration formulation terminology however, FAT is measured in terms of DIGESTIBLE ENERGY in MEGACALORIES/KG of feed.

3. DIGESTIBLE ENERGY/KG FEED

The most common method of expressing ENERGY content of feed is by the use of DIGESTIBLE ENERGY values. The problem arises however in that DIGESTIBLE ENERGY can be expressed completely in metric terms as MCals/KG (Megacalories/kilogram) OR in a combination of metric and imperial measurement as in MCals/LB (Megacalories/pound).

Added confusion can then exist when KILOCALORIES, MEGAJOULES or KILOJOULES are used, instead of MEGACALORIES, again on a KILOGRAM or a POUND basis and then further confusion can occur when the term CALORIES are used to mean MEGACALORIES and not CALORIES as are commonly defined.

Having sorted out what units you actually want to work in, it is then necessary for this method of ENERGY MEASUREMENT, to work effectively, to have some idea of the DRY MATTER intake of the horse on a daily basis. This need to know daily DRY MATTER intake is more important with energy than with protein measurement, as all sorts of problems can happen to a horse which is overfed energy in relation to work load.

4. DIGESTIBLE ENERGY/KG HORSE

The problems described above with clarifying the exact method of measuring DIGESTIBLE ENERGY/ KG of feed still apply, except in this method of ration calculation, you need to know the weight of the horse and then work back to the DRY MATTER INTAKE.

PROTEIN AND ENERGY COMBINED

The T.D.N. or TOTAL DIGESTIBLE NUTRIENT system of measuring feeds is really a combination of the PROTEIN and ENERGY levels of the ration, expressed as one figure. The T.D.N. system has been used for a long period of time and is of value, provided the level of PROTEIN in the ration is not limiting for the proposed purpose. This is important, as the T.D.N. SYSTEM, combines the effects of PROTEIN AND ENERGY content in the ration. T.D.N. figures may be of value in formulating rations for mature adult horses, which have reasonably low protein requirements which can be satisfied by most horse feeds. However, for lactating mares, foals, weanlings, yearlings and two year olds, where the desirable PROTEIN level of the ration is probably in excess of the protein content of a number of horse feeds, the use of T.D.N. values in ration formulation may lead to the preparation of rations which are deficient in protein for the purpose required.

FEEDING STANDARDS assume that the ration, i.e. the "recipe", being eaten by the horse is correctly balanced, in relation to the horses' individual and varying workload for all the essential feed components. Any deviation from this balanced ration, as happens, very frequently, in practice, can affect the whole approach to feeding individual horses.

FEEDING STANDARDS should be used as a reservoir of information from which BASE levels can be determined, then allowing a ration or rations to be formulated to make allowance for any separate and different requirements which that horse is either perceived to have, is known to have or because of personal preference of the horse owner.

The definition of management goals, in a physical sense, i.e. what do we really want this horse to do physically, instead of in a emotional sense i.e. to win a championship ribbon, is highly desirable and most advantageous necessary in the formulation of correct feeding programmes.

The horse feeds to be described in detail in later chapters of this book will have the AVERAGE VALUES for CRUDE PROTEIN, DIGESTIBLE ENERGY as MCals/KG and T.D.N. provided.

It is up to each individual to decide which system is to be used as all systems are still being widely used in horse feeding, select the one which you can understand the best.

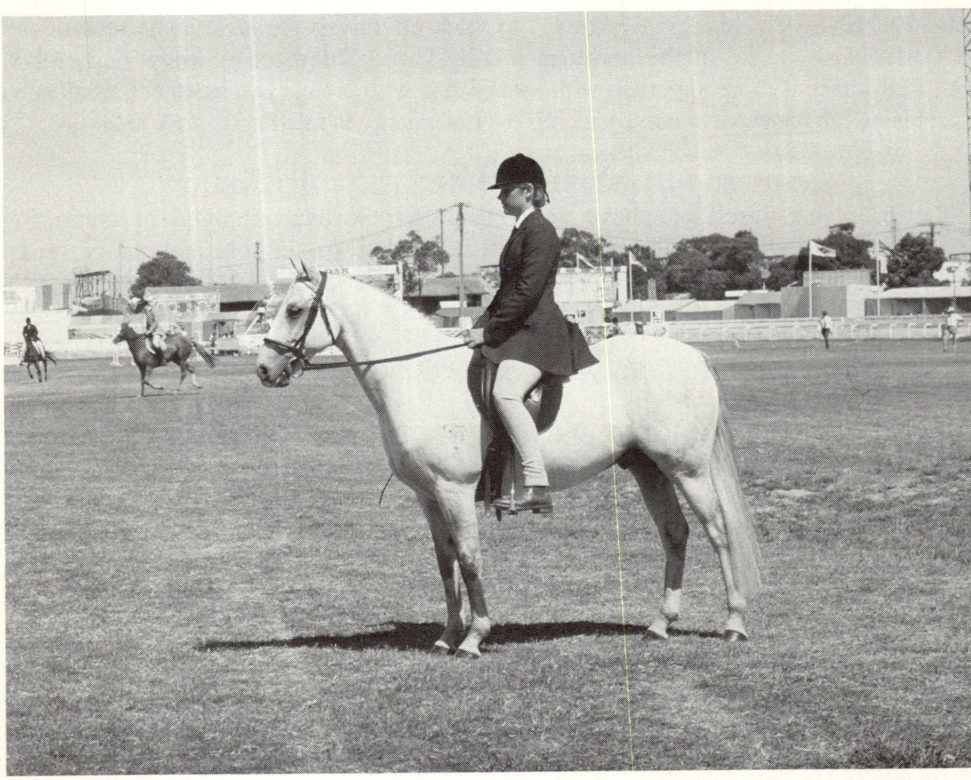

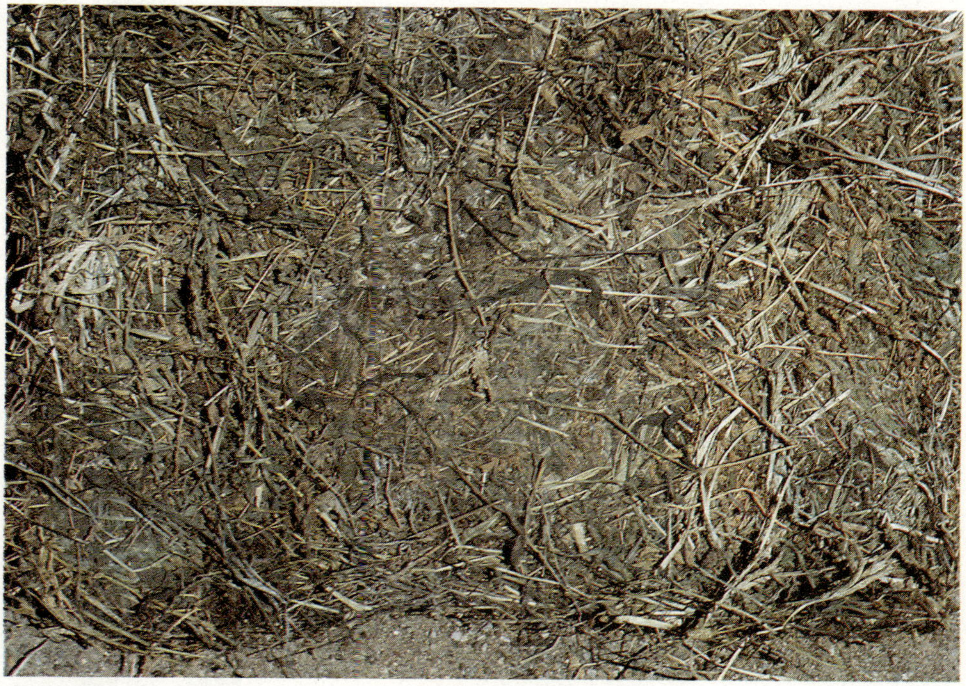

Mouldy hay—unsuitable for horses—note grey mould on the right hand side.

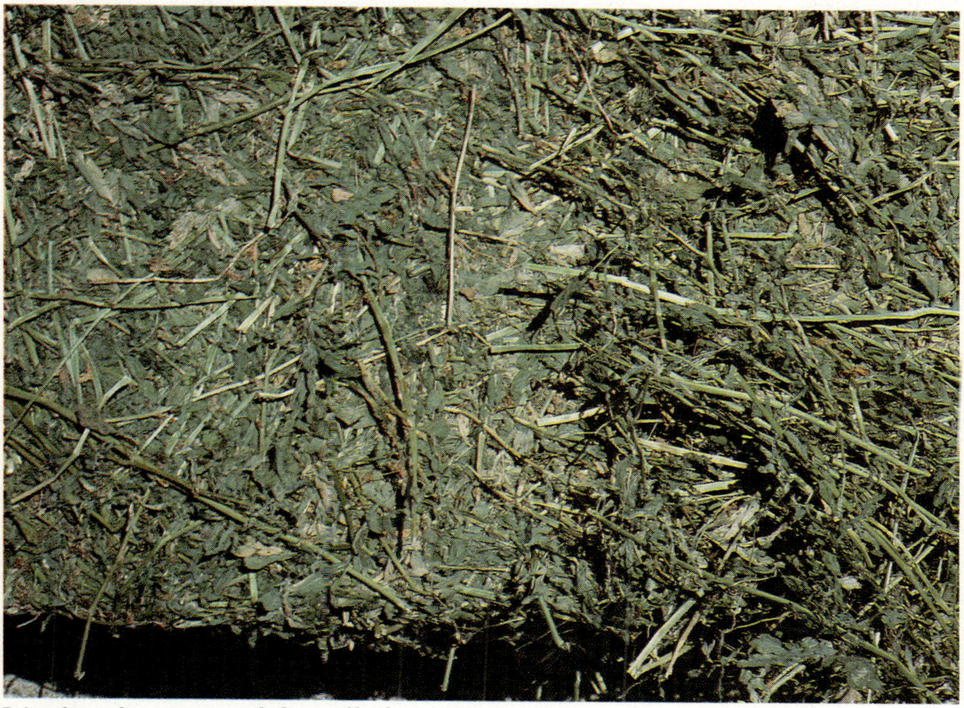

Prime horse hay—green and plenty of leaf.

What supplement are you feeding? Are you adding vitamins and minerals already in the feed? Does your horse really need any supplements at all?

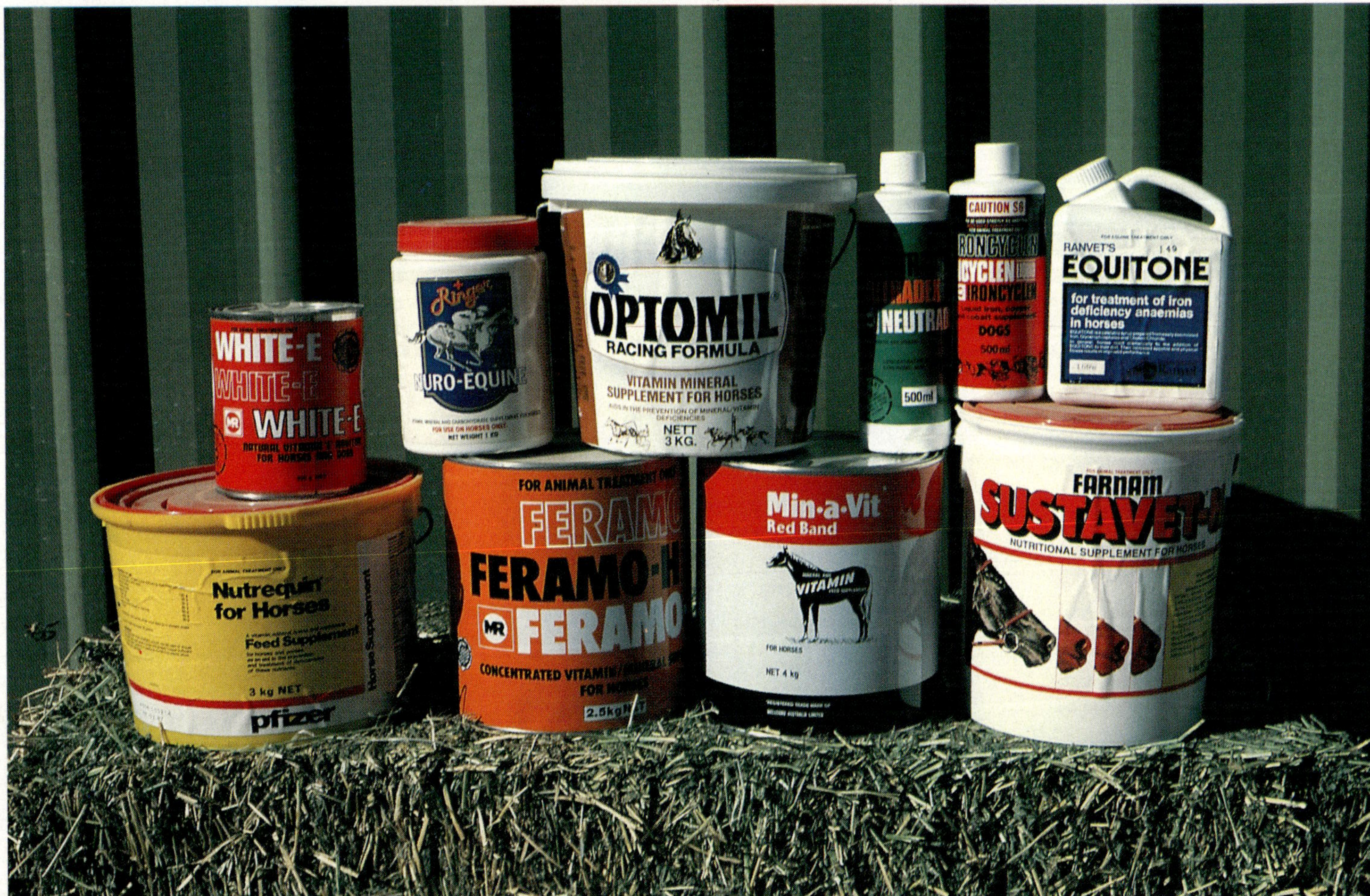

16. LABELLING REQUIREMENTS OF HORSE FEEDS

Have you ever carefully studied the label on a bag of horse feed or on a container of feed supplement? To most people, they have the same feeling after reading a feed label as they have after they have missed the point of a joke, a feeling of ignorance and lack of intelligence. FEED LABELS, often detailing long, complex, indecipherable names, which nevertheless appear impressive, APPEAR to contain quite a lot of information. Possibly they do but most of the information, except daily dose or feeding rates, is not of the type which can be used for every day horse feeding.

LABELS are not supposed to be equine nutrition textbooks, they are required to reveal SOME of the feed components in the product, the purchaser then is supposed to be able to assess and or calculate, whether the details on a particular label are what his horse requires.

LABELS ARE REQUIRED TO BE A DESCRIPTION OF WHAT THAT PRODUCT CONTAINS, BUT ARE NOT REQUIRED, OR MEANT TO BE A DESCRIPTION OF THE QUALITY OR VALUE OF THE PRODUCT.

Throughout the world, anyone mixing or making a feed or feed supplement, which is to be sold for addition to horse rations, under the law of the particular country or state, normally has to have the product approved for registration by the controlling government body. Once this registration approval has been obtained, the product is then required to carry a label, clearly visible to the buyer, on the outside of the product.

This need for registration of prepared and mixed feeds will vary slightly, from area to area, but basically the need for registration, applies to any feed which has been physically changed from its natural shape, has been modified in any way, has had another feed added to it or is a mixture of various feeds and or feed additives.

Hence CLIPPED BARLEY, where a physical process has removed the AWN from the top of the grain, and nothing else, has in some places, to be a registered stock feed. The same principles can apply to CRACKED CORN, ROLLED OATS, PREPARED MIXED FEEDS of grain and CHAFF and to any preparation which contains one or more vitamins and or minerals which is added to horse rations.

LABELS ARE NOT REQUIRED BY LAW TO BE PLACED ON PASTURE, HAY OR ANY OTHER FEED WHICH HAS NOT BEEN PHYSICALLY CHANGED, MODIFIED AND OR MIXED.

The legal requirement, for registration of such feeds, applies to all feeds which are commonly called "OPEN SELLERS", that is any product which is freely available to the public to purchase "off the shelf" and use according to the directions on the label. The requirement to register a stock feed or feed supplement DOES NOT generally apply where the product is made for a specific use on a specific property.

All stock feeds, whether for cattle, sheep, pigs, dogs, cats, poultry and or horses, usually comes under the one registration act in the particular area or region. To the best of current knowledge, there is, apparently, no specific set of regulations anywhere in the world, which relate directly and only to horse feeds.

The basis for the original requirements of these stock feed registration requirements are NOT VERY RELEVANT to modern methods of horse feeding. What is relevant is the various ways in which these registration requirements are controlled and administered and the information, OR LACK of information, on the labels which affect the horse and or horse owner.

Most labels on registered feeds DO NOT CONTAIN sufficient information to allow the conscientious horse owner to be able to determine whether that feed or feed supplement is of advantage to any particular horse.

BULK FEEDS

This category comprises pre-mixed commercial rations, which are supposed to provide all the horses' daily requirements in the one bag. They are generally based on some type of grain, grain by-product such as bran, oilseed meals, chaff, molasses and other common feeds.

ACTIVE INGREDIENTS

Active ingredients, also termed INGREDIENTS, sometimes shortened to A.I.-not ARTIFICIAL INSEMINATION-is a list of the various feeds or feed components which are POSSIBLY in the registered feed. The interpretation of the administration of the ACTIVE INGREDIENT requirements will vary considerably, from authority to authority.

Often you will see a label of a prepared BULK horse feed, comprising grain plus chaff plus additives, which will have sometimes up to 30 different feeds and or feed components on the label. This list will include a description of the grains, OATS, BARLEY, MAIZE, SORGHUM, GRAIN BY-PRODUCTS, such as BRAN, WHEAT MIDDLINGS and or POLLARD, generally some oilseed meals, SOYBEAN MEAL, COTTONSEED MEAL, LINSEED MEAL, often other product such as COTTON SEED HULLS, SUNFLOWER BRAN, GROUND LIMESTONE etc.

There are a number of administrative interpretations of ACTIVE INGREDIENTS.

A – the feed producer is allowed to put on the approved label ALL the possible feeds which are ever likely to go into that product, BUT DOES NOT NECESSARILY have to have all those feeds in every bag of that product, sometimes known as CATCH-ALL labeling. This administrative attitude is taken so that the feed producer is able to change and alter the contents of the mixture, at will, so as to be able to produce a product, even if one or more than one of the listed ingredients are unavailable, say due to drought or are too expensive too use. So if the label states the feed contains MAIZE and you cannot find any maize in the mix, you probably are buying feed registered with an authority which allows this attitude to prevail.

Comparisons of two labels from the same product, manufactured a short time apart showed the early label to read:-

"crimped oats, steam rolled corn, soybean meal, wheat middlings, dried whey, alfalfa meal, soybean hulls and cane molasses".

The later label was changed to read :-

"grain products, plant protein products, processed grain by-products, animal protein products, forage products, roughage products and molasses products".

Whilst the use of CATCH-ALL terms of horse feed labels does allow the feed manufacturer, the ability to change feed ingredients, within general feed classifications, at will, it is generally not a very good approach from a practical feeding angle, to be continually changing the components of a mix. Horse people may not be able to notice a change in performance, using the same product but with different ingredients. Dairy farmers are quick to notice any effect in milk yield, due to a variation in ingredient change in dairy cow concentrates, as milk production will react overnight to changes in feed composition. The reason for changed ingredients in each mix is usually one of price, the feed manufacturer attempting to get the cheapest mix. Maybe being price conscious DOES NOT PAY when feeding horses. I certainly know some dairy farmers who are just as much interested in the technical specifications of the feeds as they are in price, they suffer too much of a financial loss if the cows drop down in milk production.

B – in some areas there is no requirement for the feed producer to place any details on the label of ACTIVE INGREDIENTS so there is in fact no way that the purchaser is going to know what he or she is buying. Some of these registration authorities require that the feed mills supply, at the time of registration, details of the feeds and or feed components that are going into the feed BUT DO NOT REQUIRE such information to be displayed on the label. Neither, in some instances, is it possible for any purchaser of such feed to able to obtain, from the appropriate feed registration authority, details of what the feed is supposed to contain. There is absolutely nothing in this situation to prevent the feed manufacturer from getting a product registered and then deleting one or more of the ACTIVE INGREDIENTS before manufacture, it has been done before.

REMEMBER
THERE ARE NO BARGAINS IN THIS WORLD, ONLY VALUE FOR MONEY
and
YOU ONLY EVER GET WHAT YOU PAY FOR.

If you want cheap pre-mixed commercial horse feed, that is exactly what you will get but, do not expect your horse to perform as well as on better quality but more expensive feed.

2. Some registration authorities DO NOT REQUIRE any indication, on the label, of the MINERAL and or VITAMIN content of pre-mixed bulk commercial feeds. This attitude may be satisfactory, if the pre-mixed feed is made entirely from individual feeds, each of which the horses would eat if each feed was fed separately. However, in the price conscious horse feed market, some pre-mixed feeds are based on components which the horse would not eat if presented as individual feeds. One such feed is based on COTTON SEED HULL, SUNFLOWER SEED HULLS, flavoured with MOLASSES and with a mineral mixture added. Horses, unless starving, will not eat cotton seed hulls or sunflower hulls, both of which have a nominal horse feeding value of zero. Add a flavouring of MOLASSES and the mix is eaten by the horse. The owner may as well feed his horses sawdust, it is about as

valuable. Nevertheless the feed is registered as a stock feed in the appropriate state of manufacture.

EMOTIVE OR DESCRIPTIVE LABELLING

3. Requirements concerning the use of various emotive words on the label vary considerably between registration authorities. In some situations, the use of the word COMPLETE is required to indicate that the feed contains everything the horse will need on a daily basis, except for water. The label is not required to tell you that if you only need to feed say 5 kgs of this COMPLETE PRE-MIXED FEED/DAY for the average 450 kg horse to obtain all its nutrient requirements, that this horse will need to be supplemented with about 5 kgs of hay per day to satisfy appetite, maintain digesta flow and stop the horse from becoming bored and a likely candidate to develop the vices of windsucking and weaving. Neither is the label going to tell you that if you feed more of this feed/ day than advised on the label, that there is a chance that the horse may become affected by overdoses of some vitamins and or minerals.

BALANCED is another term which can have different meanings to different people. It is generally accepted that BALANCED refers to any feed where all the known nutrients are in the correct amounts for the purpose stated on the label or bag, e.g. for growing horses. Where as a COMPLETE FEED is also expected to provide bulk and in theory be the only feed the horse receives, a BALANCED FEED is normally fed in conjunction with something else, such as hay and or access to pasture. As hay and or pasture also contains all the vitamins and minerals that the average horse needs, the use of a BALANCED FEED COULD LEAD to toxicities from overdoses of some vitamins and minerals. This will depend on each individual feeding situation but should be carefully considered.

Some stock feed registration authorities ban completely the use of words such as HIGH, BETTER, INCREASED etc. on labels whilst others allow the use of such words, without any qualification. The complete banning of the use of such words is preferred as they all refer to relative rather than absolute levels. It is simple to have an increased level of something in a new feed supplement when its predecessor had nothing at all.

HIGH PERFORMANCE is another word which needs to be carefully considered on a feed label. What it should mean, in those areas which allow its use on stock feed labels, is that the feed will provide enough energy for strenuous or hard work. What the label does not say, is that the horse has to be trained and conditioned to use such energy effectively, otherwise it could suffer from any one of the problems resulting from the oversupply of energy in a feed and insufficient exercise in the horse, refer chapters on ENERGY and NUTRITIONAL DISORDERS.

GUARANTEED ANALYSIS

For bulk feeds, the GUARANTEED ANALYSIS normally consists of the following details, based on the PROXIMATE ANALYSIS method of determining feed composition:

MINIMUM PERCENTAGE OF CRUDE PROTEIN

Protein is the most expensive part of a ration, so there is little chance of the level of protein exceeding the minimum level. No reference is made at all about protein quality, generally in the price competitive market of mixed feeds, the protein source will be the cheapest available and therefore most unlikely to be of reasonable quality for horse feeding.

Some stock feed registration authorities require that the PROTEIN content be displayed as from NATURAL SOURCES and ADDED SOURCES.

Protein from natural sources refers to the protein in natural feeds of vegetative origin, pasture, grass, legumes, grains, oilseeds etc. Natural protein can also include protein of animal origin e.g. fish meal, liver meal, meat meal, skim milk etc. although most of these are not fed to horses, either due to the high cost or due to palatability problems.

Protein, from added or artificial sources, refers to those compounds which can be converted to protein in the animals' digestive tract. UREA is a common nitrogen containing compound, in this category. Urea is commonly used as a fertiliser but is also of value in increasing the potential protein level of the ruminant feeds, i.e. sheep, cattle and goats. Ruminants are able to satisfactorily convert the urea into protein, inside the digestive tract, and can be fed reasonably large quantities of urea before any toxic symptom may appear.

Urea feeding to horses however, is a different matter. Whilst some research work has shown that the horse is able to consume urea in reasonable quantities, without problems, the practical experiences have not followed the research results. There have been toxicities occurring, in horses, following the feeding of feeds containing urea. The problem may well be due to inadequate mixing of the urea present in the feed with the result that one animal may get all the urea in the bag, in one feed. Death may result. It is advisable to delete urea completely from rations being fed to horses for this reason. Some authorities even require the amount of urea in the ration to be stated as such and in some areas, the use of UREA in horse rations is not allowed at all.

There is currently no requirement to indicate the contents of any of the AMINO ACIDS on feed labels. Despite PROTEIN QUALITY, and therefore AMINO ACID content, being vital for efficient horse nutrition, there is the problem of the general availability of equipment to analyse for AMINO ACIDS.

MINIMUM PERCENTAGE OF CRUDE FAT

Of little application in horse feeding. Fat is now a recognised feed for horses, be it a possible expensive feed. Of a number or pre-mixed or prepared feeds analysed, the minimum percentage of crude fat in pre-mixed feeds is generally of the order of 2% to 3 % with the highest level being about 5%. As fat converts to CARBOHYDRATE energy inside the horse, this amounts to a CARBOHYDRATE energy level in the ration from fat of 5% to 11%. Fat, in the form of vegetable oil, is commonly added to most prepared horse rations, not for the energy producing ability within the horse but, to act as a binder for the feeds and to provide a shiny appearance to the feed which makes it look good to the owner. One must ask the question, does the owner eat the horse feed or does the horse?

MAXIMUM PERCENTAGE OF CRUDE FIBRE

Crude fibre or CELLULOSE is the most indigestible part of horse feed. It is usually much cheaper than the protein and or fat contents of the ration and is generally used as a "filler" in pre-mixed or bulk horse feeds. Horses require a certain level of fibre in the ration, a minimum of 25% of daily DRY MATTER feed weight. Crude fibre can in fact be related to the roughage needs of the horse. The horse has a daily roughage need of at least 0.5% of body weight. A 400kg. horse therefore has a roughage need of 2kgs. The same horse would have an appetite of about 8-9kgs. of total feed. Hence any horse ration should have 2 divided by 8 or 25% crude fibre in the feed.

Virtually all feed labels DO NOT provide any indication of the source and or the quality of the fibre. Clover would have the most digestible fibre content of any feed, followed closely by lucerne whilst at the other end of the scale, containing fibre, which is mostly INDIGESTIBLE by the horse, would be cottonseed hulls and sunflower hulls, all of which are used as fibre sources in horse rations. Once the CRUDE FIBRE level of a pre-mixed horse feed exceeds 8%, any such feed will contain only average levels of energy or less compared to grazing feeds. HIGH FIBRE feeds will contain LESS ENERGY than LOW FIBRE feeds as fibre produces very little available energy in the horse.

PERCENTAGE OF SALT

Salt is an important component of daily horse rations and the normal daily needs are in the range of 0.5% of the total ration.

Not all authorities require the salt level to be stated but often a MAXIMUM LEVEL has to be indicated.

MAXIMUM PERCENTAGE OF FLUORINE

Fluorine, in only small quantities in the ration, can have adverse affects on bones and bone growth, the maximum level of fluorine in any ration is generally required to be less than 0.005% which is the common natural level of the frequently used horse feeds.

OTHER COMPOUNDS AND OR ADDITIVES

Various authorities will have individual lists of compounds, additives and or substances which are to be SEPARATELY and INDIVIDUALLY detailed on a stock feed label. These lists can vary tremendously but the following are a list of the specific items which have to be stated in MINIMUM QUANTITIES in N.S.W.

Phosphoric acid	Lime	Magnesia
Iron	Sulphur	Iodine

In addition, if the stock feed manufacturer desires to claim product content of any other mineral and vitamin, not included in the above list, this product content must also be stated on the label, to-gether with the actual levels of the vitamin and or mineral in the feed.

ENERGY LEVELS

There appears to be no legal requirement, in any of the stock feed registration legislations investigated, for the level of ENERGY, in the feed, to appear on the label. The feeding of energy in relation to work load and training programme is one of the most important items to be considered in feeding horses, yet details of the energy content of feed are ignored for labeling purposes. FAT can be converted to energy within the horse but there is no reference on the label to CARBOHYDRATE type energy.

LABELLING REQUIREMENTS OF HORSE FEEDS

The CARBOHYDRATE type energy level, in a feed, can be calculated from the details already supplied on the label, if you are aware of the following method.

e.g. MINIMUM PERCENTAGE OF CRUDE PROTEIN	say 10%
MINIMUM PERCENTAGE OF FAT	say 5%
MAXIMUM LEVEL OF FIBRE	say 25%
MAXIMUM LEVEL OF WATER	say 10%
(the product will go mouldy if water content was much higher)	
TOTAL	50%

Therefore the balance of the ration, 50% must be energy of the CARBOHYDRATE type.

FEED SUPPLEMENT LABELS

FEED SUPPLEMENTS, as opposed to pre-mixed bulk commercial feeds, consist of products which contain one or more of the micro-nutrients, principally MINERALS and or VITAMINS and which are administered to the horse in relatively small daily amounts, often at 30 grams/horse/day or 1 teaspoonful. FEED SUPPLEMENTS are NOT designed to replace any of the bulk feeds in a horses' ration.

ACTIVE INGREDIENTS

There is very rarely any legal or administrative requirement to use standard names to describe MINERALS and or VITAMINS in a supplement. The minerals and vitamins, necessary for horse nutrition, are well known but it is possible to use a number of different names to indicate the addition of a mineral or vitamin to a supplement. The following table will give an indication of SOME of the names which can be used.

ALTERNATE NAMES FOR ACTIVE CONSTITUENTS IN FEED SUPPLEMENTS.

MINERALS

CALCIUM

also known as
CALCIUM CARBONATE
CALCITE
OYSTER SHELLS
GYPSUM

PHOSPHORUS

also known as
AMMONIUM POLYPHOSPHATE
DIAMMONIUM PHOSPHATE
MONOAMMONIUM PHOSPHATE
MONOSODIUM PHOSPHATE
DISODIUM PHOSPHATE
SODIUM TRIPOLYPHOSPHATE
PHOSPHORIC ACID

CALCIUM AND PHOSPHORUS

also known as
DICALCIUM PHOSPHATE,
BONE MEAL
MONODICALCIUM PHOSPHATE
TRICALCIUM PHOSPHATE
CALCIUM PHOSPHATE
ROCK PHOSPHATE

IRON

also known as
FERROUS SULPHATE
FERRIC SULPHATE
FERRIC IRON +++
FERROUS IRON ++
IRON SULPHATE
IRON CARBONATE

MAGNESIUM

also known as
MAGNESIUM SULPHATE
MAGNESIUM BI-CARBONATE
MAGNESIUM OXIDE
EPSOM SALTS

POTASSIUM

also known as
POTASSIUM SULPHATE
POTASSIUM BICARBONATE
POTASSIUM CHLORIDE
POTASSIUM IODIDE

SULPHUR

also known as
FLOWERS OF SULPHUR
SULPHATE OF MAGNESIUM
SULPHATE OF POTASSIUM
SULPHATE OF IRON
SULPHATE OF ZINC
SULPHATE OF COPPER
SULPHATE OF MANGANESE

ZINC

also known as
ZINC SULPHATE
ZINC OXIDE

COPPER

also known as
COPPER SULPHATE
BLUESTONE
COPPER OXIDE

COBALT

also known as
COBALT CARBONATE
COBALT SULPHATE

MANGANESE

also known as
MANGANOUS OXIDE
MANGANESE SULPHATE

SELENIUM

also known as
SODIUM SELENITE

IODINE

also known as
ETHYLENEDIAMINE DIHYDROLATE or POTASSIUM IODIDE

LABELLING REQUIREMENTS OF HORSE FEEDS

VITAMINS

VITAMIN A

also known as
RETINOL
CAROTENE
ALPHA CAROTENE
BETA CAROTENE

VITAMIN B1

also known as
THIAMINE
THIAMINE MONONITRATE
VITAMIN B COMPLEX
BREWER'S YEAST

VITAMIN B2

also known as
RIBOFLAVIN

VITAMIN B6

also known as
PYRIDOXINE

VITAMIN B12

also known as
CYANOCABALAMIN

FOLIC ACID

also known as
FOLATE
FOLACIN

NIACIN

also known as
NICOTINIC ACID
NICOTINAMIDE

PANTOTHENIC ACID

also known as
CALCIUM PANTOTHENATE

BIOTIN

also known as
VITAMIN H

CHOLINE

VITAMIN C

also known as
ASCORBIC ACID

VITAMIN D

also known as
ERGOCALCIFEROL
CHOLECALCIFEROL
CALCIFEROL

VITAMIN E

also known as
TOCOPHEROL
TOCOL
ALPHA TOCOPHEROL
BETA TOCOPHEROL

VITAMIN K

also known as
MENADIONE or PHYLLOQUINONE

Of some 26 minerals and vitamins listed above with their accepted common names, it is possible to obtain some 77 alternate names of similar or related compounds which have appeared on labels of feed supplements, as being ACTIVE INGREDIENTS. To the average person feeding horses, most of these names would have little meaning on a label, they would look impressive and would probably convey to some that it is a "new" product and possess some magical, indefinable, sought after quality. IT IS PROBABLY THE SAME OLD THING DRESSED UP IN DIFFERENT names. So much for MARKETING BY CONFUSION.

Some registration authorities require that the list of ACTIVE INGREDIENTS be presented on the label in descending order of concentration, commencing at the top with the component present in the largest amount and working down.

NO REQUIREMENT TO NAME FLAVOURINGS.

A considerable number of combined MINERAL/VITAMIN supplements are unpalatable, to horses, as mixed. There is considerable use of artificial flavourings in these products, ANISEED, STRAWBERRY and BANANA being the most popular. Very few feed registration authorities require any indication of the addition of artificial flavouring to any product.

PRODUCT STABILITY

In most areas requiring registration of stock feeds and supplements, very rarely is any consideration given to product stability, i.e. the fact that what is put in the mix will still be there, at some reasonable time in the future. The following two practical examples illustrate the point.

VITAMIN E is only stable when kept isolated from all other vitamins and minerals until immediately before feeding. E will decompose rapidly in contact with minerals in particular. Despite this, inspection of product labels on stock feed outlet shelves will indicate a number of products containing VITAMIN E mixed with other vitamins and minerals. The VITAMIN E may have been placed in the original mix but little, of any value to the horse, would have been left after a day or two. Where ever VITAMIN E appears in a mix with VITAMIN A present, the E is not there for the horse, it is generally there to reduce oxidation of VITAMIN A, the E being destroyed before the A.

LIMESTONE or CALCIUM CARBONATE is sometimes used as a base or carrier for vitamin/mineral mixes. CALCIUM CARBONATE will rapidly destroy any vitamin added to it.

LABELLING REQUIREMENTS OF HORSE FEEDS

NO USE BY or EXPIRY DATE

There is no legal requirement, in the majority of countries, to have expiry dates on HORSE FEED supplements. Apart from any loss which occurs in the preparation, due to instability of the mixture, detailed above, there will deterioration and reduction in concentrations of some components of the mixtures, especially vitamins, so that some time after manufacture, there will be virtually no vitamins left in the product. Recently a vitamin mineral supplement product was purchased in an English speaking country with a foreign label. After translation, the wording which was most striking was the statement that the product had a shelf life of 3 months, after manufacture. It really did not take much to work out that this product had not sold in the non English speaking country, was shipped considerable distances and re-sold in a country where expiry dates were not applicable. The product would have had to be shipped, rather than flown by air, due to the low value/high weight factor which would have meant that the product, when purchased was at least 7 months old and 4 months out of expiry. Anyone buying that product would have been paying considerable sums of money for nothing.

ADMINISTRATION or DOSE RATE

Whilst some authorities require registration of feed supplements, the following two examples of registered feed supplements, in one area, indicate that no attempt was made, in these instances, to check the practical details or effectiveness of label dose rates administration.

One product had directions for administration of 0.1 grams of product/50kgs of horse. This meant that a normal 450 kg thoroughbred or similar horse would require 0.9 grams of product/day, recommended to be given in the feed. Most feed supplements are administered in the feed at the rate of 25-30 grams/ day or about 1 teaspoonful. How the average horse feeder is going to be able to measure 1 gram of supplement and then practically incorporate that in the feed so that it does not end up in the bottom of the feed bin is an interesting question.

Most feed supplements have alongside the names of the ACTIVE INGREDIENTS, the concentration of that ACTIVE INGREDIENT in the product, usually in GRAMS/ KILOGRAM or GMS/KG. One particular feed supplement had the ACTIVE INGREDIENTS in GRAMS/TONNE. When the actual amount of each ACTIVE INGREDIENT, in the recommended dose was calculated, the horse was basicely receiving nothing except the carrier or the bulk of the supplement into which all the other ingredients are mixed. The carrier, in this instance, was starch. The product was a very expensive way of the horse feeder buying starch, yet the product was registered for public sale.

The problems with the current labeling of pre-mixed bulk feeds and feed supplements are as follows:-

1. labels are only required by, law, to give limited information on the actual contents of the labeled bag or container.
2. one of the reasons for the limited amount of information required to be on a label is that laboratory techniques have not yet been developed to do reliable testing for a number of the important feed components in horse rations. This statement DOES

NOT APPLY to the ENERGY LEVEL of PRE-MIXED FEEDS. Laboratory analysis of ENERGY is relatively simple, and there is considerable information available on the energy contents of most horse feeds, yet the registration authorities choose not to recognise this very important horse feed component when labeling horse feeds.

3. The use of CRUDE PROTEIN levels on a label provides NO INDICATION of protein quality in the feed.
4. Some feed registration authorities DO NOT require any indication of MINERAL levels on pre-mixed feeds.
5. There is NO requirement to indicate CARBOHYDRATE energy levels on the label, one of the most important horse feeding components.
6. There is generally no standardised system of indicating weights or amounts of feed components on a label.

Quantities of VITAMINS can be indicated as anyone of the following:-

METRIC SYSTEM GRAMS
MICROGRAMS
μ GRAMS
MILLIGRAMS
either as PER KG to PER TONNE.

PARTS PER MILLION

INTERNATIONAL UNITS

A possible total of 10 different methods of expression for VITAMINS A, D, and E and 9 different methods of expression for the other vitamins.

MINERAL content is able to be presented as either:

METRIC SYSTEM GRAMS
MICROGRAMS
μ GRAMS
MILLIGRAMS
either as PER KG to PER TONNE

PARTS PER MILLION

A possible total of 9 different ways to express levels of any one of the 13 or so minerals which are sometimes used in feed formulations.

7. Most feed labels use terms which are either unfamiliar to the average horse owner or in some instances possibly designed to confuse.

In summary, if the feed labels, as required by law, are UNABLE to provide sufficient information of the content of the feed, how is the horse feeder to know exactly what the horse is eating and, therefore, if it is being properly fed.

Maybe, it is the trade name, or the label design, or colour, or the advertising brochures which attract the use of such feeds, but in most instances, the use of such feeds appear to have nothing to do with correct horse feeding.

The same comment can however be made to people who feed their horses on pasture and or hay. They DO NOT have any label at all.

HEREIN IS ONE OF THE MAJOR PROBLEMS OF HORSE FEEDING.

Stock feed registration requirements and the use of labels have caused the average horse feeder to believe that all the "goodies" are only available from anything in a bag or a tin with a label on it.

NOTHING COULD BE FURTHER FROM THE TRUTH.

If we were to put a label on green pasture or hay, made from such pasture, we would get a list of feed components which would make any pre-mixed bulk feed or any MINERAL/VITAMIN supplement redundant. All the feed components, not only PROTEIN and ENERGY, but also all the essential MINERALS and VITAMINS would appear on the label and, generally, at levels which satisfy the horses' daily needs, without the problem of toxicities from excess levels etc. After all, the horse survived and lived for many years very satisfactorily on pasture, before the advent of feed supplements.

The advertising and promotion of PRE-MIXED FEEDS and FEED SUPPLEMENTS have diverted the attention, of a considerable number of horse owners, away from understanding and appreciating the benefits of pasture and pasture products as an excellent source of horse feeds. Furthermore, there is no cheaper supply of horse feed than from pasture, often some 20 times or more cheaper than most HARD FEEDS and certainly up to 50 times cheaper than most MINERAL/VITAMIN mixtures.

17. PRACTICAL HORSE FEEDING

VISUAL HORSE PROBLEMS

Horses present a number of individual and different feeding problems which often are quite distinct from the average.

FAST EATERS

Sometimes called BOLTERS, because they "bolt" their feed or eat at a much faster rate than most other horses. The end problem of this condition can be some type of attack of COLIC or LAMINITIS as rapid eating of feed, especially if there is any grain in the ration, will lead to an intermittent and rapid uptake of energy from the digestive tract, possibly at a rate which the horse cannot handle satisfactorily for normal uses and the excess energy in the bloodstream can cause COLIC and or LAMINITIS.

BOLTING or FAST EATING may be due to:-

1. insufficient feeds/day.
2. insufficient total quantity of feed available/day.
3. roughage hunger, too low a level of roughage in the ration.
4. no hay available for AD LIB or unrestricted access feeding, especially of a night.

Practical solutions include:

A. reducing the concentrate portion of the ration and increasing the roughage content.

B. feed more frequently each day with more weight/feed.

C. provide hay in a hay net at all times.

D. place some round smooth river stones on top of the feed and make the horse muzzle them out of the way before the feed can be eaten. Make sure the stones are smooth, then no teeth can be broken and the stones need to be at least the size of a large orange or small grapefruit so that the horse cannot swallow them.

FEED SIFTERS

This is the horse who will separate out some feeds and or feed supplements from the ration and leave them in the bottom of the feed bin. The problem is one of individual taste and palatability and needs to be sorted out for each horse. However, the following principles will help.

1. if the residue left behind is one of the major feed components, something is wrong with the sample you have. Soybean meal has been overcooked before to-day, changing a palatable feed in to rejected mess. Check this aspect first and if this is the reason for feed rejection, go straight back to the supplier and seek answers.
2. if the residue happens to be part or all of a supplement which you are trying to give to your horse, try a little supplement preparation. Moisten some bran, about two handfuls, DO NOT OVERWET, add a little BENTONITE to the barn plus the feed

supplement plus a little sugar. MIX well to-gether and then mix again well into the grain and chaff. Trial and error will quickly allow you to determine the best mix. This technique has worked well to stop FEED SIFTERS. BENTONITE swells to about 6 times its normal size when wet and holds the feed supplement and sugar onto the bran. The moist bran, in turn, binds and attaches to the balance of the ration.

3. if that does not work, try the flavouring department. Most feed supplements are flavoured these days, strawberry, banana and apple being the horse's preferred choice. Go to the local supermarket and buy some flavouring, used for human cooking, and determine your horses' individual choice.

REMEMBER some feeds and feed supplements will be unpalatable no matter what you do. NEGUVON given as a drench for BOTS will be rejected by virtually every horse if mixed with the feed.

QUIDDING

QUIDDING, sometimes known as SLOBBERING, occurs when the horse only partially chews its feed and then allows partially or semi-masticated food to either drop from the mouth or else be spat out.

Quidding is always due to some problem within the mouth of the horse. Thorough examination of the mouth should take place to determine the cause. Whilst abscesses, ulcers and similar problems, within the mouth can cause the horse to spill feed, the most common cause is TEETH which need attention.

The incidence of QUIDDING is generally directly related to the amount of "convenience feeds" in the ration. In natural conditions and when grazing, the horse has to thoroughly chew and masticate the pasture, before the digesta can be swallowed. This chewing of the feed, before swallowing, can sometimes take considerable time and in doing so the horse moves the feed from one side of the mouth to the other, this action causing slow but constant and continual wear on the MOLAR TEETH, also known as GRINDERS or CHEEK TEETH.

In stabled horses, on CONVENIENCE FOODS, which can include chaff, grain, oilseed meals, pellets, commercial pre-mixed rations etc.

There is generally little need for chewing of the feed to take place before the digesta enters the stomach. All of these feeds are in a form which does not need much physical breakdown for the digestion process to commence.

As there is much reduced feed movement across the molars, when the horse is eating convenience foods, there is much less wear on the molars. Dependent on the level of convenience foods in the horses' ration, the development of the sharp edges on the inside and outside faces of the molars will eventually become so sharp that they will initially rub against and later cut into the tongue and the inside of the cheeks, causing pain which is reflected in QUIDDING or SLOBBERING of semi masticated feed occurring.

The cure is simply attention to the teeth of the horse, to physically remove those sharp edges on the sides of the teeth. The frequency of this dental attention will vary from horse to horse and with feeding regimes. If your horse obtains all, or the greater proportion, of its feed from pasture and or hay, then attention to the teeth may never be needed, some horses have kept their molar teeth in order, for years, on this type of feed. If however the horse is fed predominately convenience feeds, attention to the teeth may need to occur every 6 to 8 weeks.A simple practical test to determine whether the teeth need attention or not is to get the horse used to passing the hand on the outside of the cheek, in the region of the molar teeth on both top and bottom jaw, at the same time gently pressing the cheek against the molar teeth. Once the horse becomes accustomed to this hand movement, he will only react adversely when the inside of the cheeks, touch the sharp edges of the molar teeth, causing pain. If and when this happens, it is time to get the teeth attended to.

STABLE BED EATING

The horse which insists on eating stable bedding, especially barley straw can be a problem. The answer is very simple, just give the horse a plentiful supply of good quality hay in a hay net, available, at all times, as eating STABLE BEDDING or LITTER as it is sometimes called is generally a roughage problem, possibly both in terms of weight of feed the horse is getting each day and the quality of that feed. It may also pay to check the quality and palatability of the ration contents, there may be a problem with one or more individual feed components.

If after attention to the present ration, both in terms of quality and quantity, STABLE BEDDING consumption still persists, change the type of bedding. Replace the type of straw, you have three choices OATEN, BARLEY and WHEATEN, or change to SHREDDED PAPER, SAWDUST and or WOOD SHAVINGS are used.

Do not as suggested by some authorities, muzzle the horse to prevent STABLE BED EATING, that is an easy and quick solution but ignores the main problem, which is ROUGHAGE HUNGER.

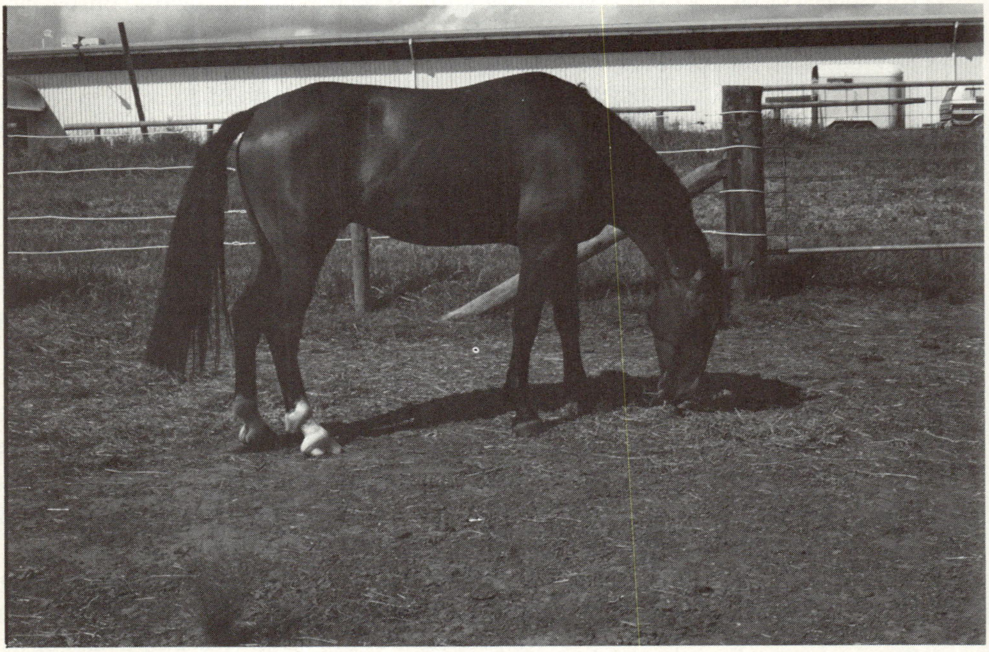

Ground feeding – loss of feed may lead to ingestion of dirt and possible internal infection.

DIRT EATING

Some horses are often seen licking or eating DIRT and this habit can cause considerable concern. It is very difficult for the owner to really know exactly what amount of dirt the horse is consuming i.e. is it only licking and ingesting small amounts or is the horse really eating large amounts for some unknown reason, unless of course a 24 hour watch is kept on the horse and then the assessment will only be subjective, as there will be no practical way of knowing the weight of dirt eaten.

Consumption of small amounts of dirt, by licking should not be taken as much of a problem, the horse is probably playing or is attracted by something different, as a result of a appetite control reflex, known only to the horse.

If however the horse is actually eating large quantities of dirt, there may well be a mineral deficiency of some description in the feed which the horse is trying to correct.

The problems, in sorting all this out, are as follows:-

1. how do you determine if the horse is eating large amounts of dirt in the first place?
2. remember horses are incapable of self correction in the diet in everything except, water, energy and salt.
3. if the supposed mineral deficiency has occurred from feed grown in the same paddock, then that feed reflects the minerals available in the soil, so if the feed is deficient in something, so is the soil.

Any supposed mineral deficiency can be clarified. Various techniques are available which will allow any know mineral deficiency to be scientifically evaluated.

BARK EATING

In some parts of the world, horses will, on occasions, eat the bark, often in significant amounts from trees growing in grazing paddocks. There have been all sorts of reasons put forward as to why horses eat bark including boredom, unspecified mineral requirement, lack of fibre, etc. One report from Queensland detailed the results of an actual study of bark eating horses. The activity increased markedly when the horses were grazing on improved lush irrigated pasture as opposed to the alternate grazing of dry native pasture. Analysis of pasture showed that the irrigated pasture contained 86% water and only 14% dry matter. For an average sized horse, about 15 hands, needing about 7.5 kg D.M./day, some 54 kg of pasture would have had to be eaten to supply the 7.5 kg of D.M. Included in this 54 kg of total feed would have been some 46.5 kgs or litres of water. The fibre level of improved irrigated pasture was only 50% the fibre level of the dry native pasture. It would appear that the habit of eating bark from the trunks of trees is to satisfy a fibre deficiency in the pasture feed, which at the time contained too little fibre and too much water for the horses' digestive tract to function properly.

FAECES EATING

The reader is referred to Chapter 3 – WATER AND FAECES where a full description is given of this subject.

TAIL CHEWING

Some horses often develop the nasty habit of chewing and or eating the tails and manes of other horses. The problem can appear suddenly, generally with one animal in a mob and the exact cause or causes are not known. It has been suggested that TAIL CHEWING is due to a fibre and or mineral deficiency in the diet, but the practice tends to occur in horses which are grazing in mobs on pasture, yet only affect one horse. One would think that more than one horse would be affected if the problem was due to lack of fibre and or minerals. Practical experience has shown that the problem of TAIL CHEWING MAY be due to a SALT HUNGER problem and the provision of salt to the horse for AD LIB or unrestricted access has sometimes cured the problem. In other situations, analysis of the ration, has lead to the possibility of deficiencies of PHOSPHORUS and COPPER as being the cause. It is possible that weight loss and deaths may result from horses which ingest hair, the hair actually forms a ball in the stomach and restricts the normal passage of food.

PAWING

Some horses have an annoying habit of PAWING at the ground with one front feet whilst eating, often digging a hole in the one spot. This problem will become more evident when the horse is fed in bins or receptacles placed on the ground. The problem appears to be one of the horse following natural, instincts in that, in the grazing situation, the horse is continually moving all the time whilst eating. The natural movement pattern, whilst eating is generally BITE/CHEW/STEP, repeated many times. However when the horse is eating from a stationary receptacle or feed bin, there is no physical need to STEP but there may well be a psychological desire to STEP, hence the continual PAWING of the ground. Probably the only answer to this problem is to re-educate the horse by reprimand, even if this does mean someone having to be alongside the horse every time it is fed until the problem is cured.

BOREDOM

BOREDOM or nothing to do appears to be correlated with or identical to what some people see as a lack of DIETARY FIBRE in the feed. BOREDOM in horses is a probably a combination of both nutritional and psychological problems.

The horses' natural instincts are to be able to graze all day in company with other horses.

When the horse is individually confined to stables or small yards, man has imposed on the horse a behavioural pattern which is foreign to everything the horse expects. Add to this the habit of some people of either not feeding the horse enough weight of feed to satisfy daily gut fill and or not allowing the confined horse continual access to roughage in the form of hay and you have a horse who becomes bored and seeks something to do.

BOREDOM is shown, by the horse, as one of the following problems.

WOOD CHEWING – when the horse will scrape and or eat with its teeth any piece of wood which happens to be around. Stable doors, wooden yard rails etc. are all fair game for a horse which starts to adopt this habit. Apart from damaging any timber, there is always the chance of the horse puling out one or more teeth by adopting this habit. On particular stud, feeding twice a day on pellets, stopped wood chewing by making all the yard rails out of steel pipe. With no feeding change e.g. hay in the hay net at night etc., the horses quickly learnt a new trick, to suck the steel pipes with their tongue.

WINDSUCKING – also known as CRIB BITING or AEROPHAGIA, generally follows on from WOOD CHEWING and or PIPE SUCKING. The horse learns the particular annoying habit of grabbing hold of any object with its teeth , mouth open and sucking in air, through the mouth, into the digestive tract. WIND SUCKING is incurable, once the horse has the habit it has got it for life, and it will reduce the expected performance of the horse in that it is impossible to get enough feed into a windsucker, due to the continual presence of air, in the digestive tract. The habit is also readily spread amongst horses by imitation, an unaffected horse very quickly learning how to windsuck from a horse with the problem.

WEAVING – when the horse has nothing to do to keep itself occupied, it will stand at the door of the stable or in the one spot in the yard, continually swaying sideways, crossing one front leg over the other, at the same time the head and neck move in a semi circle. WEAVING can be so severe that horses have been known to wear large holes in the spot where the habit is practised.

GENERAL PROBLEMS

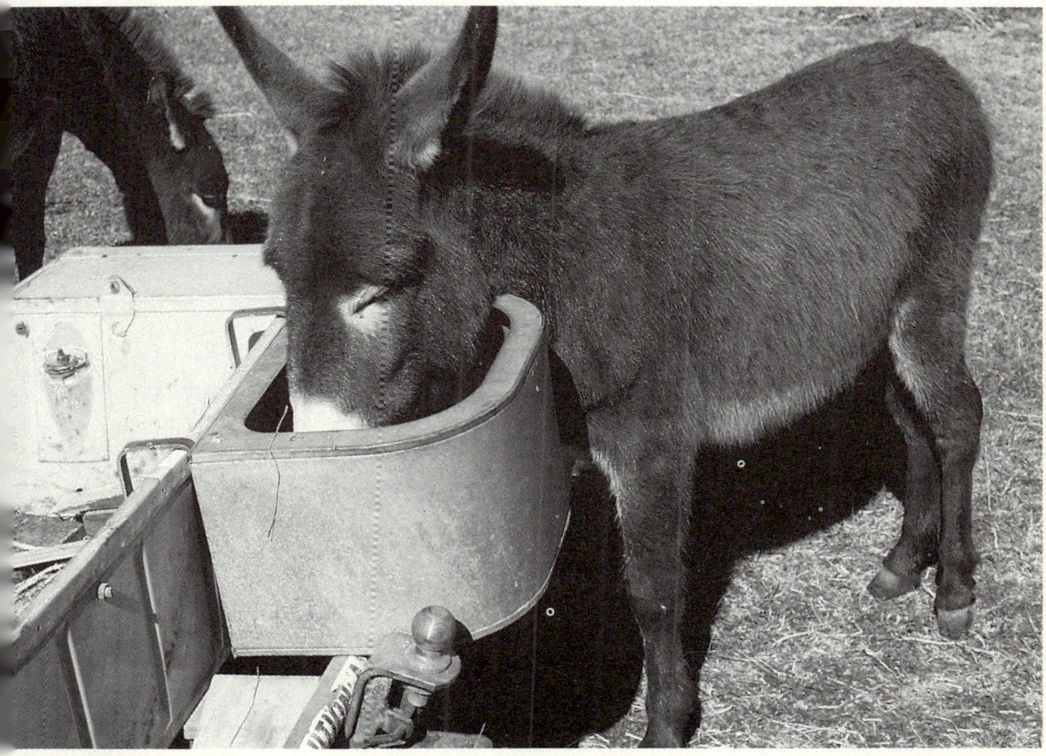

Convenience feeding—mobile, safe and little possibility of leg injuries.

FEEDING HEIGHT

Some people get very concerned about the height at which feed bins have to be placed.

There are two schools of thought, ON THE GROUND and UP IN THE AIR, generally at about HORSE chest height.

FEED BINS ON THE GROUND

FOR

1-it allows the horse to eat in the same physical attitude at which the animal grazes.

AGAINST

1 – when hand feeding, much easier for the horse to knock the feed bin over and waste feed. The horse then has the opportunity to ingest soil and possibly pasture infected with the eggs and larvae of the internal parasites which most horse people attempt to keep out of their horses, by worming and drenching.

2 – Feed bins on the ground, in the stable, means that the horse, when eating, is breathing in air in a part of the stables where there is little air circulation and increase the chance of the horse inhaling dust and associated organisms, which may cause HEAVES.

3 – the horse is able to kick the bins and possibly suffer some type of leg or hoof injury.

FEED BINS UP OFF THE GROUND

FOR

1 – the horse cannot knock the bin over and waste feed.

2 – Feed bins, off the ground, at about horse chest height will be in that part of the stable where there is some air movement and this will reduce the chance of the horse inhaling dust and associated micro-organisms which may cause HEAVES.

3 – the horse is unable to kick the bins and so the possibility of lower leg and hoof injuries, within the stable, is considerably reduced.

AGAINST

1 – the horse is in an unnatural physical position when eating.

There does not appear to be any answer one way or the other as to which is the preferred method. It is sufficient to say that the problem cannot be considered of any consequence as there does not appear to have been any research work done on the subject and reported in any of the scientific literature.

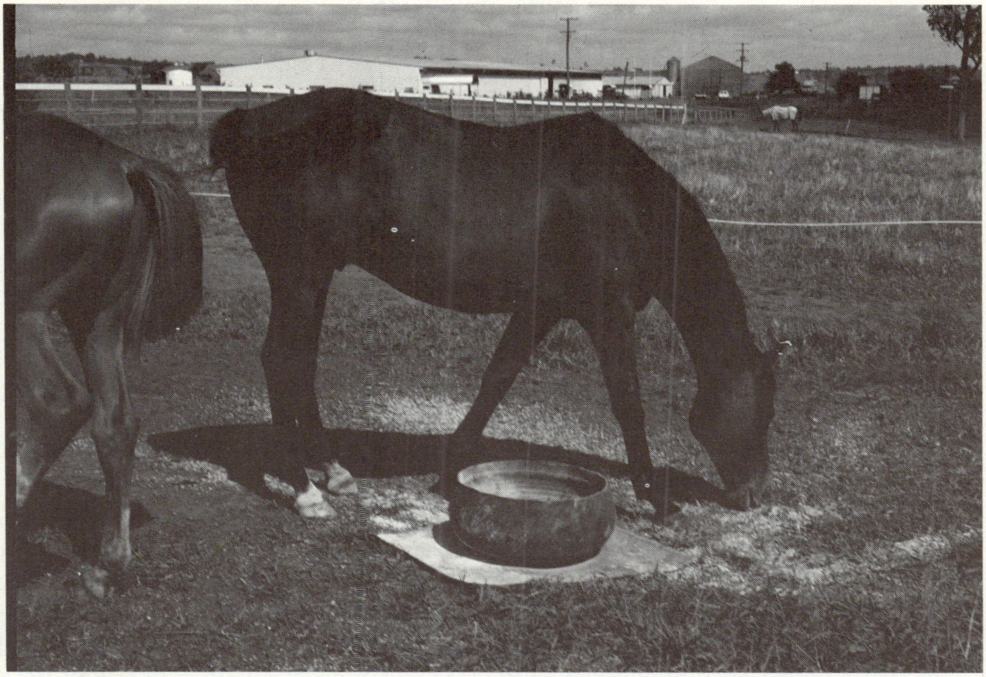

Be careful of feed wastage in the paddock. This could be due to a playful horse or too much feed in the feeder.

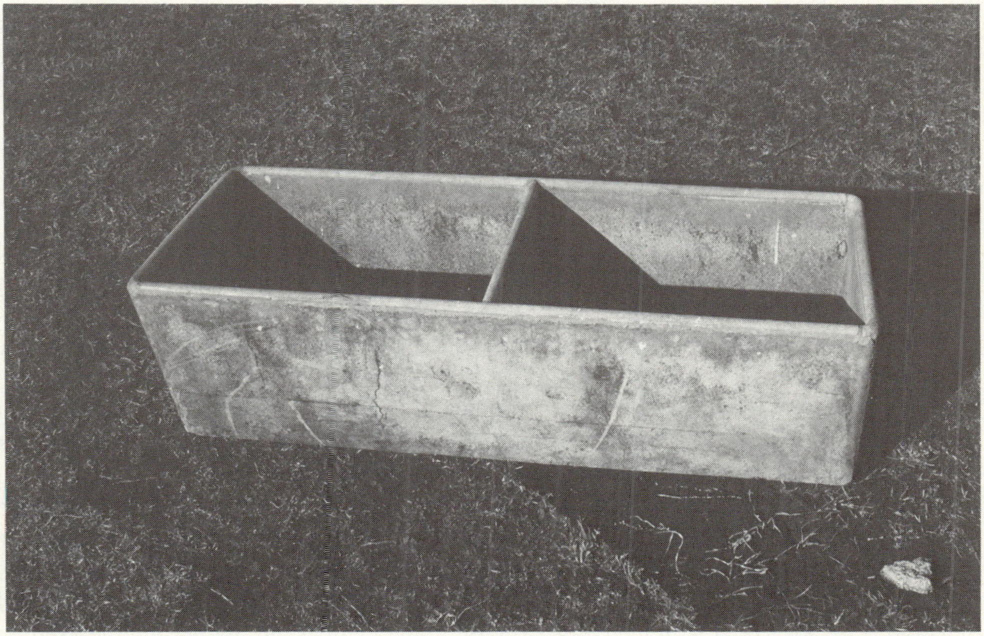

Young horses especially kick this type of feeder and may get lower leg problems.

FATTENING HORSES

Many people want to know the easiest way to FATTEN a horse. What they really mean is what is the easiest way to make the horse put on weight and or appear bigger or larger than before.

The problem can be looked at from a number of ways.

1. firstly make sure the horse has treated, by drenching, to remove all internal parasites
2. is the horse capable of getting "fat"? To use a human comparison, some people will for ever remain thin no matter what they eat whilst some people will remain fat no matter what they eat. This is a function of the hormonal output, controlling feed uptake and utilisation by each individual and generally cannot be changed. Be careful that the thin horse, which you wish to fatten does not have a hormonal control system which is very inefficient in converting feed energy to muscle bulk and internal fat deposits, ensuring that that the horse will for ever remain thin.
3. To get a horse "FAT" requires building up the horses' muscle bulk and fat reserves and this requires additional supplies of energy in the ration.
4. Horses, on natural grazing, are able to self regulate the amount of energy which their bodies use and store. Very rarely do you hear of or see a horse in the wild with any of the nutritional disorders associated with hand fed horses receiving too much energy in the ration.
5. Provided the energy level in the new ration, combined with the horses' increased work output is co-ordinated ENERGY SUPPLY equates with current ENERGY NEEDS plus a little extra energy for any expected weight increase, the horse will build up as follows.

A – Initially FAT will be deposited within the abdomen in the internal fat depots, invisible to the human and only measured if regular weighings are made of the horse. Once these internal fat depots reach a certain level of fat, the horse then starts to lay down FAT within and between the muscles, known as INTRAMUSCULAR FAT.

B – initially the muscles of the body will increase in bulk. They cannot increase in length, that is already determined by the skeleton of the horse which cannot be changed but the muscles can increase in bulk.

C – Intramuscular depots of fat will be deposited at some time shortly before the muscles attain their greatest bulk which will be determined by a number of factors including skeletal size, hormonal output and previous feeding history.

Both phases B and C are obvious and the results can be measured and visually appreciated by the owner.

The aim then in feeding ENERGY to put bulk on a horse is to adjust the ration, so that the muscles "bulk up", but once the muscles cease to increase in size, then reduce the energy level of the ration so that the muscles maintain the desired size.

Associated with the feeding of additional energy to build muscle bulk, there should be some increased exercise and or training programme for the horse, this will ensure that more of the additional energy being fed goes into muscle bulk than into abdominal fat deposits. Your horse should be likened to a human bodybuilder, increased bulk comes from increased nutrition ASSOCIATED with increased exercise in the gymnasium. Increasing the exercise programme may also benefit the rider. It is remarkable the number of people who want to FATTEN a horse without any extra work being involved.

The reader is referred to the section on BODY SCORING in Chapter 14 for more information.

POOR PERFORMANCE SYNDROME

The term POOR PERFORMANCE SYNDROME is sometimes used to describe a condition, in horses, where performance is not as expected and the answer to the problem does not appear to be obvious. The problem is rarely confined to any one horse but is generally obvious in stables etc. where a number of horses are in close contact with each other.

SYMPTOMS INCLUDE:-

1. occasional coughing.
2. poor appetite.
3. rough coat.
4. possible intermittent nasal discharge.
5. sub standard performance.
6. possible mild TYING UP effects, such as increased sweating, muscle twitches, unco-ordinated gait etc.

The problem is most common in groups of horses, as in racing stables, and is generally caused by a VIRAL infection of varying intensities. The condition can be initially assessed from the use of BLOOD TESTS, in particular looking at the results for the following; changes in WHITE BLOOD CELL number, especially lymphocytes and neutrophils, and reduction in the A;G RATIO, indicating increased anti body production and rises in the level of the enzymes which reflect any possible muscle damage.

HOT OR HEATING FEEDS

The expression HOT FEEDS or HEATING GRAINS are terms often used by horse feeders, who do not appear to understand the basic principles of nutrition.

The HEATING VALUE of a feed and hence the use of the term HOT FEED is related to the ENERGY DENSITY OF THE FEED as well as the level of FIBRE in the feed.

Maize (corn) has a reputation in some places of being a hot feed. Maize is, in fact a high energy feed, with a relatively low fibre content, about 2% compared to 12% on average in oats, and there is no evidence to suggest that the energy and fibre component of maize is any different, chemically, from the energy and fibre components of any other grain or similar source of energy for the horse. The problem probably arises in that the energy level of a given weight, called ENERGY DENSITY, of maize will be at least 33% higher than the energy level of the same weight of oats.

One kilogram of maize will contain at least 800 grams of energy, whilst 1 kg of oats will contain only 600 grams of energy. If the horse feeder is to substitute maize for oats on a weight basis, then the horse will immediately receive an increase in energy in the ratio of 33%.

However maize is a heavier grain on a volume basis than oats, and if the feed is measured in ice-cream containers, old saucepans, coffee tins or whatever, the same volume of maize will contain at least 85% more energy than the equivalent volume of oats.

The calculations are very simple and are discussed in the chapter on feed measurement.

In fact if volume feed measurements are being used, such as coffee tins, saucepans etc., the maize weight should be 2.3 kgs to provide the same energy as 3.1 kgs of oats, or in volume terms, about half the volume of maize will provide the same energy as oats.

Most likely the reason that some feeds have gained the reputation of being HOT FEEDS is that the feeds are measured on a volume basis, not a weight basis. If this is so, then the straight substitution of maize for oats on a volume basis to any horse will immediately increase the energy level of the ration by at least 80%,

The immediate reaction of the horse will be either to get sick – colic, founder, tying up etc., or else to be so full of energy as to misbehave and possibly become very difficult to control.

In such situations there is nothing at all wrong with the horse, the animal is only reacting to the high level of energy in the diet. The problem lies with the horse feeder who does not understand the principles of energy feeding.

The breakdown of fibre in the large intestine of the horse produces all the heat. Hence if the feed has a lower level of fibre as maize has compared to oats then maize is a less heating feed than oats. Similarly FAT when used as a source of energy will be less heating again compared to maize as FATS do not contain any fibre at all.

Claims have also been made that some feeds are not as fizzy or hot as other feeds. No reasonable scientific evidence exists to prove these claims, and such advertising statements should be treated with caution until evidence becomes commonly available to prove the statements.

PRE-PERFORMANCE FEEDING

The timing and amount of feed, given before a race or event can have a considerable effect on the performance in that event.

Roughage, generally in the form of hay can be fed within reason at any time, but GRAIN or CONCENTRATE feeding should be carefully controlled.

If any high energy feed is added to the ration of a performance horse, within 6 hours before the race or event, there will be a rise in BLOOD SUGAR, leading to a rise in INSULIN which in turn causes a drop in compounds called CORTICOSTEROIDS which then decrease the ability of the muscles to mobilise and use the stored energy reserves in the body.

In a nutshell, FEEDING ANY ENERGY FEEDS TO ANY PERFORMANCE HORSE WITHIN 6 HOURS OF COMPETITION IS COUNTER PRODUCTIVE.

ACTUAL HORSE FEEDING MISTAKES

The feeding of horses, for all types of activities, is now a science, where it is possible to correctly determine feed and ration formulation, specifically for each horse and or each horse activity.

Over the past years, whilst advising on the feeding of horses of all types, a number of ACTUAL PRACTICAL PROBLEMS, concerning feeding have been diagnosed and corrected, in all instances with results which have had one or more of the following visible effects.

1. reduction in ration cost for the same level of performance.
2. increased performance.
3. better mare conception rates.
4. better foal growth.
5. less breakdowns as two year old racehorses.

The interesting point, with this list of problems, is the continued repeatability with which the same problem is occurring in different stables and also the same problems are spread across all types of equine activities.

Some of the actual specific technical reasons for these improvements are detailed below

PRACTICAL PROBLEMS COMMON TO MANY HORSES

1 – Inadequate internal parasite control programmes.

2 – Overfeeding of supplements, leading to toxicity problems, particularly of VITAMINS A and D when horses have access to pasture plus sunlight as well as a supplement containing these two vitamins.

3 – "SHOTGUN" mineral and vitamin supplements where the vitamin and mineral content had no value, for horses, on the particular property, as all the vitamins and minerals in the SHOTGUN mix were already present in sufficient quantities in the pasture and other available feeds.

4 – The feeding of two or more proprietary vitamin mineral supplements to-gether, "just in case", leading to toxicity problems by the cumulative effect of the components of the two supplements plus what was naturally available in the feed.

PASTURE GRAZING

5 – Soil and pasture nutrient problems which were reflected in the growth and production of the horses, particularly soil deficiencies of both PHOSPHORUS and MOLYBDENUM.

6 – Inability to understand the variation in feed nutrient composition of pasture and to compensate for seasonal shortages, especially in PROTEIN.

STABLED HORSES

7 – Underfeeding of horses, by weight, horses simply do not get enough to eat.

8 – Frequency of feeding not adequate to get all the feed required into a performance horse, e.g. should be fed 4 times/day instead of twice a day.

9 – Roughage hunger, no supply of hay for the horse to eat between feeds.

10 – Changing feeds and ration composition too quickly.

11 – HIGH LIGNIN content of the diet due to content of oaten or wheaten hay or chaff in the ration, reduces overall digestion of all the other feed components.
12 – Partial dehydration of performance horses, due to nil or incorrect electrolytes.
13 – Inadequate water intake, often linked to electrolyte problem.
14 – INSUFFICIENT daily salt supply, especially in hot weather.
15 – CALCIUM and PHOSPHORUS problems in the ration, often extreme.
16 – TOO MUCH FAT in the ration
17 – FAT being fed to horses which have AEROBIC muscle activity, so cannot effectively use fats as a source of energy.
18 – AMINO ACID balance not present, affects performance.
19 – STABLE SOUR or over feeding of B VITAMINS
20 – EXCESS SELENIUM, given without professional advice.
21 – FAILURE to recognise symptoms of mild TYING UP and to clarify why the horse has suffered such symptoms.

GROWTH PROBLEMS

22 – Poor quality hay being fed to young horses, up to yearling stage, affecting growth, due to insufficient protein and or energy content of the hay.
23 – Imbalances in CALCIUM and PHOSPHORUS supply to growing horses, shown as vast variations in CALCIUM intake and also high PHOSPHORUS diets, especially when supplementary feeding.
24 – Feeding excess energy and not enough exercise to growing horses, often associated with CALCIUM and PHOSPHORUS problems in the feed, causing abnormal leg development and a number of METABOLIC BONE DISEASES.

BREEDING PROBLEMS

25 – Reduced conception rates, mares not gaining enough weight prior to mating or mares too heavy at mating.
26 – Reduced milk production from mares, lack of sufficient energy in the mare's diet.

18. NUTRITIONAL DISORDERS

Most people would call the following conditions "diseases" but, in fact, they are all MAN MADE, caused completely or partially by lack of attention to the feeding and conditioning of the horses. Over feeding, in relation to the horse's workload, especially with grain, failure to exercise the horse properly, failure to reduce the grain content of the ration on days of rest or little exercise, incorrect mineral levels in the rations and over feeding of some vitamins as well as other feeding practices, under the direct control of the feeder, are the likely cause of nutritional disorders.

These nutritional disorders produce, in various ways, horses which need some form of veterinary attention, leading to reduced usage of the animal for some period of time, even of a permanent nature and always involving a financial cost to the horse owner, both in terms of veterinary treatments and inability to use the horse for the desired purpose.

DIARRHOEA

DIARRHOEA, also known as SCOURS or PURGE, in Australia TULLOCH'S DISEASE after a well known racehorse, in foals WET TAIL, in severe cases DYSENTERY and incorrectly called ENTERIC FEVER, is an external symptom of another problem in the horse rather than a disease.

DIARRHOEA is the result of changes in the basic mechanisms, in the digestive tract of the horse, which affect fluid and electrolyte movement in the digestive tract, but especially in the bowel or large intestine, intestinal smooth muscle activity and perfusion or blood flow and results in some change in the colour, consistency and texture and frequency of output of faecal material.

DIARRHOEA can be caused by any of the following:-

1. internal parasite infestations.
2. ingestion of weeds and other plants which can cause digestive tract upsets.
3. bacterial infection.
4. sudden changes to the ration composition and or feeding schedules.
5. various drugs and other chemicals.
6. mouldy feed.
7. training stress in performance horses.

An affected horse is generally suffering an immediate ELECTROLYTE and WATER deficiency, especially in cases where the faeces increase in liquid content, as these abnormal liquid faeces rapidly reduce the level of the both WATER and associated electrolytes in the body. The horse will rapidly become lethargic and listless, will dehydrate, suffer loss of appetite, possible abdominal pain and increased thirst.

Immediate treatment of DIARRHOEA involves reducing the increased rate of digesta movement, back to normal, by administration of BENTONITE, JUNKET TABLETS, human DIARRHOEA remedies etc., administration of electrolytes to restore body hydration or water content, elimination of the concentrate and or lush pasture portion of the ration and feed only hay.

Having stabilised the faecal output of the horse then clarify exactly what is causing this problem and treat accordingly.

Some horses will suffer from CONTINUAL and PERSISTENT DIARRHOEA, often due to some damage to the walls of the intestine, which can have been caused by incorrect feeding practices and or excessive use of some drugs at some stage in the past. Horses, showing this persistent and continual DIARRHOEA, which will not respond to normal treatments, should have the feeding schedule changed to allow more feeds of lesser weight per day, reduction in concentrate and or grain level of the ration, specific electrolyte supplementation and the addition of increased quantities of BENTONITE to the ration.

LAMINITIS

Commonly called "FOUNDER" – inflammation of the sensitive laminae that covers the pedal bone, inside the hoof.

Predisposing causes are many but are generally involved with the horse eating too much feed and at the same time getting insufficient exercise.

1. Overfeeding of grain, especially wheat, in relation to work load and exercise, can cause laminitis. Wheat should NEVER be fed to horses, unless under professional direction and care should be taken with the amount of other grains used (refer to later section on Horse Feeds).
2. Grazing on fresh young pasture, especially if that pasture contains clovers and similar species. This type of feed contains excessive levels of protein and plenty of energy and as the horse has little need to use energy to graze, because there is plenty of feed available, the excess energy, and or excess protein in the fresh young pasture appears to cause laminitis in the horse.
3. Consumption of large amounts of water, especially very cold water by the horse when the animal is hot, can be another cause of laminitis. The golden rule for restricted water intake is – do not allow a hot horse to drink large quantities of water until it has cooled down. Hot horses allowed large water intakes before they cool down are very likely to get a bad attack of laminitis or colic.

   Horses generally always drink in two separate motions. If a hot horse has to be given a drink of water, allow him only the initial short drink which all horses appear to take. Once he lifts his head and before he commences the second drink, normally only after 20 to 30 seconds after the first, take the horse away from the water. Allow the horse to have the balance of his water needs at least 45 to 60 minutes after the initial drink, and preferably, after he has completely cooled down. This approach will reduce considerably the possibility of a hot horse getting ill from drinking too much water immediately after exertion.
4. Other suspected causes of LAMINITIS are irregular but severe exercise on hard surfaces, e.g. tar roads, diarrhoea and other digestive tract dis-orders, and possibly the retention of the afterbirth by foaling mares.

Symptoms of LAMINITIS are generally confined to the front feet of the horse, the hind feet are very rarely affected, but do not be surprised if hind feet show the symptoms of founder, especially, in horses which have foundered previously in the front feet only.

The most obvious symptoms generally start with a fat pony – LAMINITIS is much less frequent in larger horses.

Chronic or first stage LAMINITIS generally appears with the horse being lame occasionally, and generally changing gait so that the heels hit the ground first, instead of the full sole of the foot.

The feet are often warm and the sole drops. Instead of the sole having a convex shape, it becomes concave and drops below the natural sole level. This DROPPED SOLE is the result of destruction of the lamellar bed and sinking of the PEDAL BONE below its' normal level. As a result, the heel of the foot grows faster than the toe, due to internal pressure being generated by the swollen sensitive laminae, and possible pedal bone rotation, due to the simultaneous destruction of the laminae. The effect of the pressure from the pedal bone rotation may eventually be such as to cause the horse to walk continually on its heels, in an effort to relieve the pain.

Cure of the problem at this stage is very simple. The condition is generally due to overfeeding and restricted exercise, or possibly too much wheat or other grains in the ration. Change the ration to delete wheat completely and reduce the level of other grains and maybe delete these other grains altogether. Failure to do this could worsen the problem. The horse is probably too sore at this stage to be lunged or exercised so the excess energy can only be controlled by removing it completely from the ration. This does not do the horse any harm, this type of horse will already have more than adequate internal fat reserves and the founder is probably hurting the horse more than the removal of the energy source will.

All forms of exercise should be restricted for horses suspected of having LAMINITIS, the horse should be confined in a small an area as possible. Any type of exercise can increase destruction of the laminae, especially the bed below the pedal bone, causing it to change texture and possibly completely preventing a full recovery from the problem. It is virtually impossible to determine the amount of damage to the LAMINAE in the early stage of LAMINITIS. DAMAGED LAMINAE, under the PEDAL BONE, will allow the PEDAL BONE to sink below its normal level and generally once the pedal bone starts to sink, it does not stop until it has penetrated the sole of the hoof and become exposed to the outside. Even in horses where the pedal bone sinks below normal level but does not protrude through the sole of the hoof, only 5-10% of such affected horses ever completely recover. Once this exposure of the pedal bone, through the sole of the hoof, happens the horse is beyond any sort of help.

Provided the pedal bone HAS NOT penetrated the sole, recovery from LAMINITIS will be slow. Dependent on the severity of the condition, recovery could take any where up to 6 months before the horses' feet get back to normal. Where founder occurs in pasture fed horses, move the horse to a paddock with less volume of feed and preferably one with poor grass pasture only. LAMINITIS will occur less frequently on grass pasture alone than on mixed pastures containing legumes or pure legume stands of clovers, lucerne etc. If a poorer quality pasture is not available for grazing, lock the horse up in the yard and feed only grass hay until some improvement is seen. Do not feed clover or lucerne hay as you will only slow down the rate of recovery. Again it is being kinder to the horse to adopt this type of approach than to let the condition continue.

The easiest way to determine whether the horse is overcoming the founder problem is to look at the growth lines on the wall of the foot. Most horses have growth lines of some type on the wall of the foot and, in normal horses, the growth lines will be parallel all the way from one side of the heel around the toe and back to the heel on the other side. In horses with founder the growth lines will diverge at the heel, and this increase in space between the individual growth lines will be very obvious. Once the growth lines become parallel at the heel, after treatment for founder, it is a reasonable assumption that the condition has been cured. Remember that it takes about 6 months for the hoof wall to grow, from the coronary band to the heel, and about 9 months to grow from the coronary band to the toe and the position of any divergent growth lines in relation to the depth of the heel will provide some indication of when the horse may have suffered founder. Careful observation of these growth lines MAY detect a horse which has previously suffered LAMINITIS but no longer shows the lameness symptoms, usually associated with the condition.

In severe cases, ACUTE LAMINITIS is produced. The horse will suddenly become extremely lame, often finding difficulty in moving its front feet. It often shifts from one leg to another in an effort to ease the pain by redistribution of weight from one front hoof to the other. The affected feet are always hot and the horse stands with the hind legs up under the body, again to transfer weight off the affected limbs.

The horse often refuses to eat and to drink. The animal will show advanced stages of long toes and low heels, with very obvious diverging growth lines at the heel.

Acute founder involves the inflamed laminae pushing the pedal bone forward and down. This will, in turn, put pressure on the sole and, in very advanced cases, the pedal bone has, in fact, penetrated the sole and is exposed. Rotation of the pedal bone is also likely to occur in ACUTE LAMINITIS, often in conjunction with sinking of the same bone. PEDAL BONE ROTATION CANNOT BE CORRECTED and once it has occurred, the horse will be of no further value.

If acute founder is observed, hose or saturate the horse's legs and feet,with cold water, to cool the area down, and call your veterinary surgeon. The condition has progressed too far for every day management treatments to work. The horse will need anti-inflammatory agents and other treatments which will reduce the swelling in a reasonable time and provide some pain relief to the horse.

These treatments are only of value if the horse has not suffered a rotation of the pedal bone. If this has occurred, or if the pedal bone is about to break or has broken through the sole, then you horse may well be past the stage of any help.

LAMINITIS should not occur. The symptoms are easily recognisable and the horse person has only themself to blame if the condition proves a problem.

TYING UP.

Formerly known as AZOTURIA and now sometimes known as CARBOHYDRATE OVERLOAD, CORDING UP, SET FAST, PARALYTIC MYOGLOBINURIA, EXERTION MYOPATHY, CAPTURE MYOPATHY, PARALYTIC HAEMOGLOBINURIA, MYOGLOBINURIA and EXERCISE RHABDOMYOLYSIS, the condition is a complicated one, affecting the use of the major muscle masses in the horses' body and generally involving the OVERFEEDING OF ENERGY, in relation to work load and training and competition programmes, but this can also be complicated by specific electrolyte problems in some horses.

In the days when horses were the main form of movement of goods and transport, this condition was known as "Monday Morning" disease. This was the name given to the condition after the horses had been working for about an hour, on the first day of the week, after two days of rest and little change in diet, during the days of rest. It is reported that the astute veterinary surgeon, of the time, established his business on the main traffic routes, about one hours distance from the main stables of the period.

TYING UP was, for some period of time, thought to be a different but somewhat related condition to AZOTURIA. Recent research however has shown that the two disorders are now the same. In fact TYING UP appears to be the common name at the moment with AZOTURIA being deleted from the general veterinary vocabulary.

The condition was generally associated with high grain diets and insufficient work and or failure to reduce the grain content of the diet, in hard working horses on their days of rest.

SYMPTOMS OF TYING UP

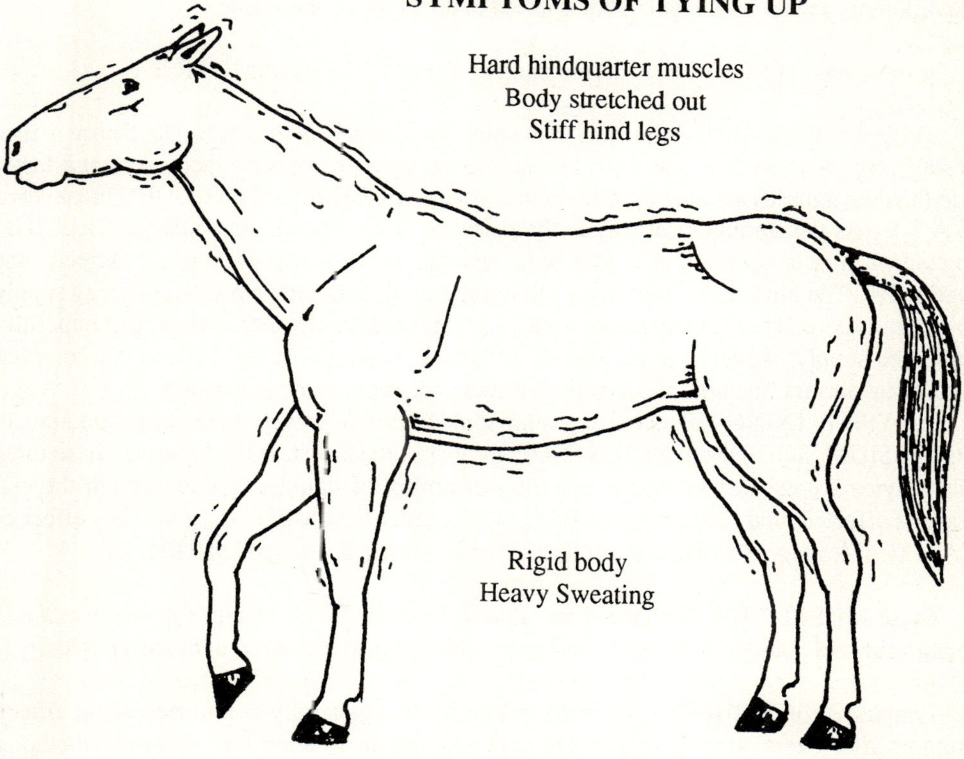

LACTIC ACID accumulation in the muscles during the lay period or periods of light work, was originally thought to be the reason for TYING UP, LACTIC ACID accumulation leading to the CLASSIC SYMPTOMS of muscular weakness, pain, stiffness at the limbs with resultant limb inco-ordination and stumbling, and in more advanced stages, profuse sweating and trembling of the large muscle areas, especially in the rump and shoulder regions.

Continuation of exercise with horses with these symptoms increased the severity of these signs and permanent muscle damage often occurred. Muscle masses of affected horses were often tight to feel and pressure applied to these areas generally caused pain to the horse.

If the horse with these symptoms was exercised or worked without any type of treatment, complete physical collapse generally occurred with the need for immediate veterinary attention.

TYING UP has similar and somewhat related symptoms. This condition occurs, not only as described, above in performance horses but, also in young fillies, nervous horses, very fat animals and sometimes in certain horses during floating and travelling. TYING UP has also been observed in horses which have had a sudden change in work or been overloaded or stressed too much, without an appropriate change in feeding and or training and conditioning, as in a barrel racing horse asked to do a long distance ride.

In some areas TYING UP, is divide into two forms TYPE A and TYPE B.

TYPE A TYING UP is defined as that which occurs early in exercise. The theory is that, during early exercise, the signals to the muscles, asking them to contract, come at a faster rate than the muscles are able to re-build the energy supplies from GLYCOGEN breakdown to A.T.P.. As the amount of energy in the muscle cell is reduced, the ability of CALCIUM to control muscle contraction is affected, causing the muscles to become "cramped" and ineffective. The muscles will not return to normal until, either the amount of energy supply to the muscle cells is increased, by reducing the work load (rest) and or, the hopefully increased supply of energy to the muscle cells acts on the CALCIUM to cause it to revert back to its normal function of controlling muscle contraction and expansion.

In TYPE B TYING UP, occurring after some period of steady work, large amounts of POTASSIUM, SODIUM and CHLORIDE are lost in the sweat. If the losses of these three electrolytes are excessive, the permeability or ability of liquids to pass through the cell walls is affected, and CALCIUM "LEAKAGE" occurs from within the cell. This effect of CALCIUM leakage is to cause the cell to remain contracted, cramped or TIED UP.

These MUSCLE CELL changes are able to be detected by changes in the levels and relationships of some of the specific enzymes which can be measured in blood samples.

Symptoms, of TYING UP, in performance horses, generally commence about fifteen minutes after exercise commences. There is no distinct dividing line between whether a horse has TYPE A or TYPE B TYING UP, one grades into the other. These symptoms include, sudden muscle rigidity, especially over the hindquarters, lameness, muscle pain, profuse sweating, increased heart rate, possibly up to sixty or seventy beats/minute and difficult in getting the animal to move. In some cases, brown or coffee coloured URINE may be passed, indicating muscle breakdown, hence the brown colour, and the possibility of

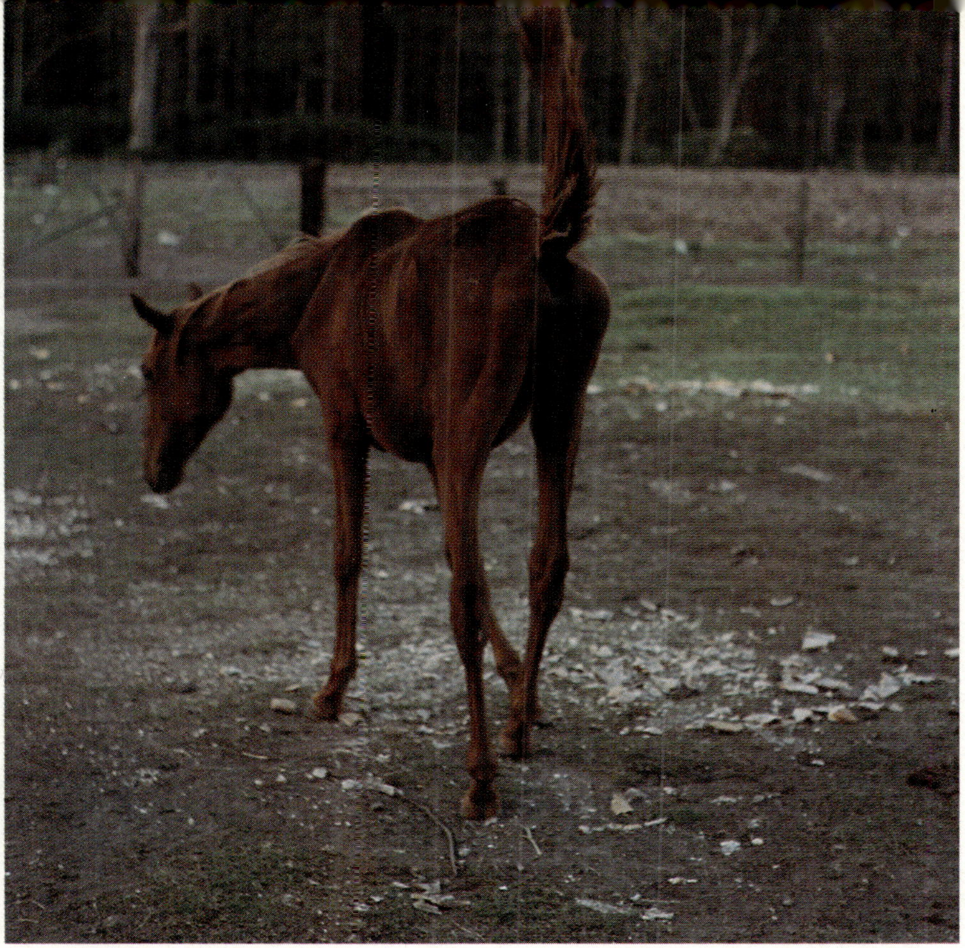

The extremes of horse nutrition.

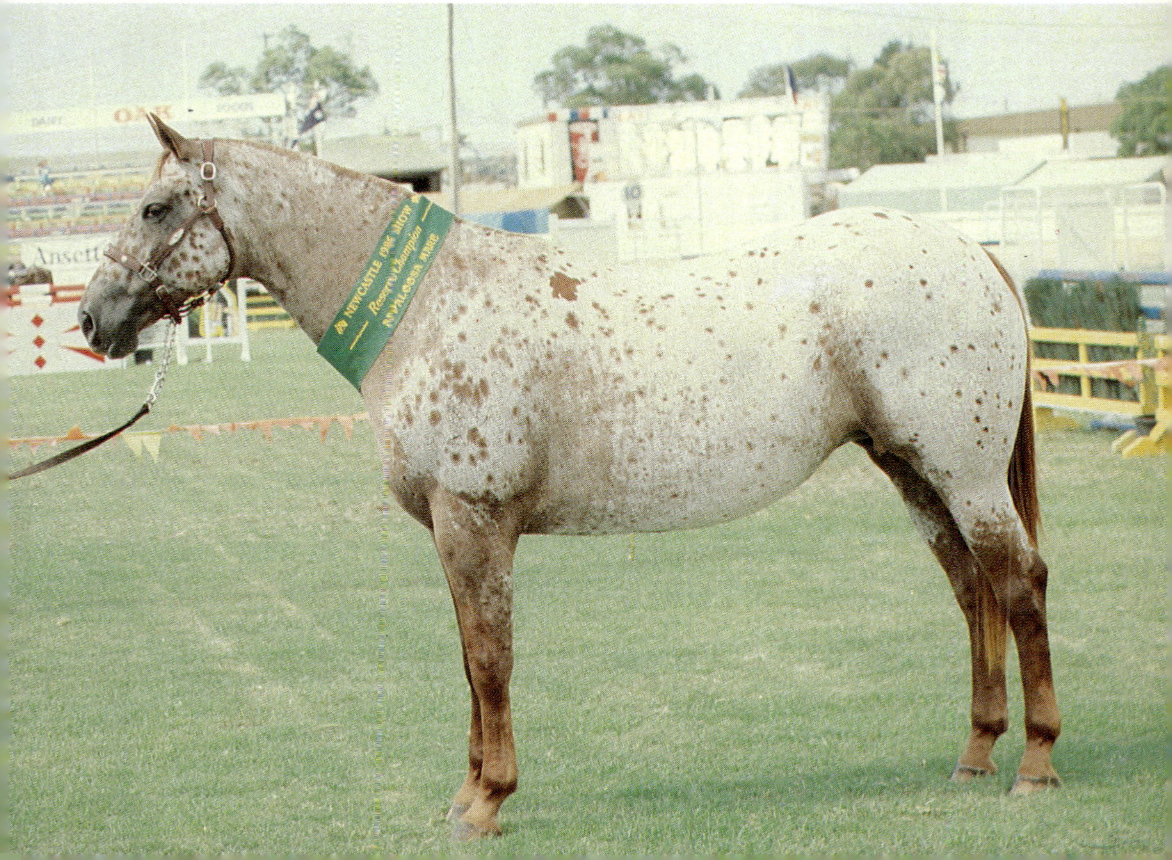

Torsion colic. Arrow points to the "sausage twisting" of the intestine.

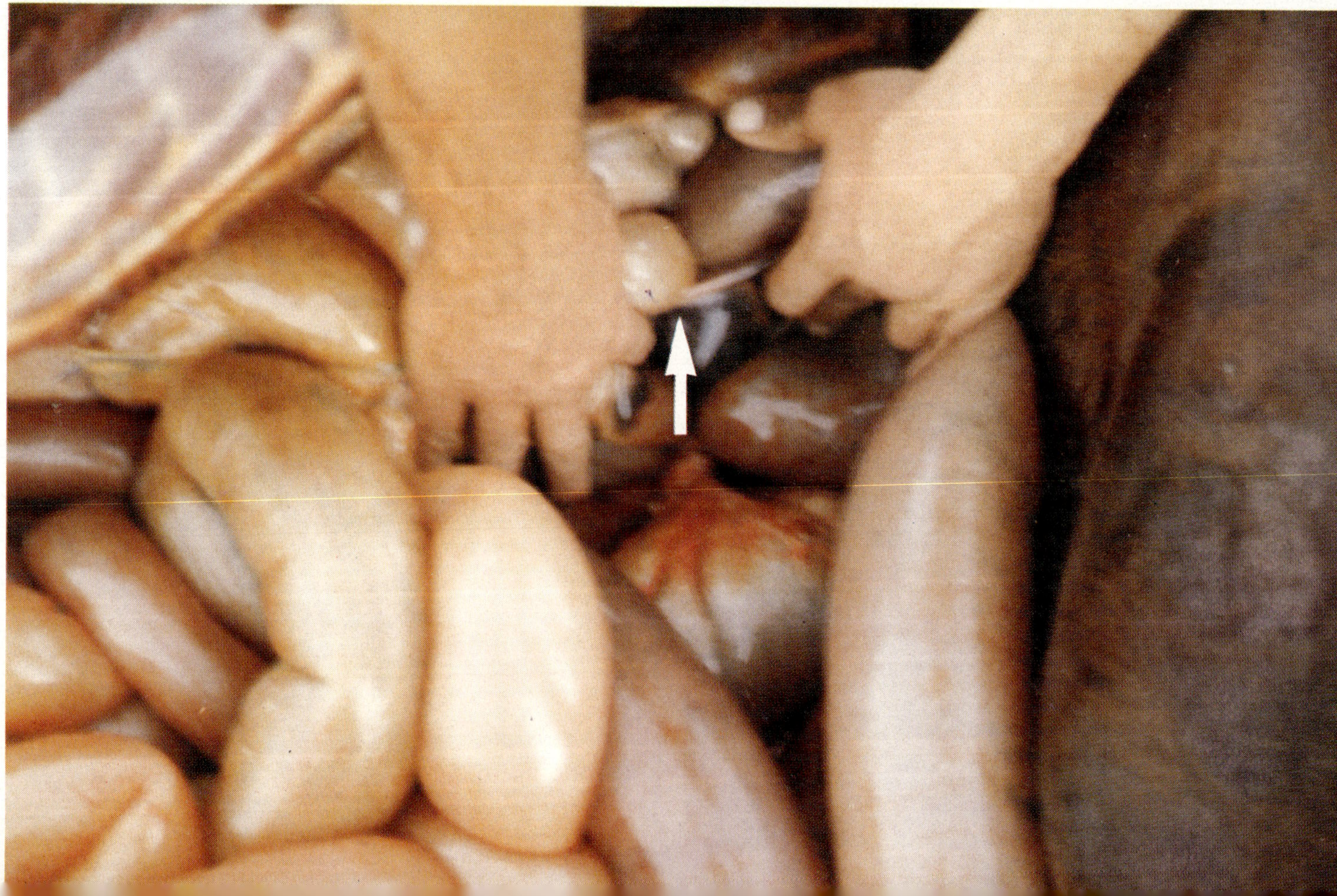

permanent muscle and kidney damage occurring, unless exercise is prevented and veterinary attention immediately sought. In the interim ensure that the horse is able to drink plenty of water to assist to flush the brown urine out of the kidneys and so reduce the possibility of kidney damage occurring.

ANY ATTEMPT TO CONTINUE TO EXERCISE A HORSE WHICH HAS EVEN THE MILDEST FORM OF TYING UP CAN CAUSE PERMANENT AND IRREPAIRABLE MUSCLE DAMAGE.

Practically, both TYING UP and CARBOHYDRATE OVERLOAD are generally caused by feeding too much grain and not giving the horse enough work.

If any ENERGY source, grains and fats in particular, are fed to horses, the horse must be worked to get the energy, supplied in the feed, out of the horses' system. The technique called ENERGY OVERLOADING, sometimes used in performance horses, is very likely to produce TYING UP or related symptoms if not carefully planned as part of the horses' overall preparation.

REMEMBER horses in the wild used energy in the feed for exercise. If in any doubt about the quantity of grain or fat to feed, always underfeed to a little below normal need for the work performed. If this practice of underfeeding is adopted, the chances of the horse getting this condition will be reduced as the horse will need to use all its energy every day in work or performance and therefore will not have any surplus energy left in its body to cause tying up.

The current practices of training thoroughbred racehorses may well be encouraging the possibility of the occurrence of TYING UP. Exercise of the horse for a short period in the early morning, from 45 to 90 minutes for 6 days a week, then rest on Sunday provides a physiological profile which "FITS" the theoretical model causing TYING UP. Whilst it is recognised that the time available for working racehorses can be determined by track availability, employed labour and other factors, changes in training programmes, especially involving some period of long slow work could result in improved fitness and less muscle damage. For those horses in training, which suffer from TYING UP, under the present system of racing stable management, abolition of the rest day and provision of exercise on that day could be of advantage.

The possible causes of TYING UP are still not clarified. What is now known is that the muscle and metabolic condition, now called TYING UP has no relationship to the LACTIC ACID levels in the blood during or immediately after exercise and also has no relationship to any deficiency of VITAMIN E or SELENIUM in the horse. In fact some cases of TYING UP have been observed in horses with high levels of SELENIUM in the body, due no doubt to the overexuberance of people to use SELENIUM when, in fact, it is not generally required.

TYING UP is such a complex problem that researchers are finding it difficult to clarify the causal agents. Suspects include, insufficient supply of oxygen to the muscles, restriction of blood flow, low levels of iodine (I), and electrolyte imbalance, commonly SODIUM (Na), CALCIUM (Ca) and MAGNESIUM (Mg).

The original causative factor of EXCESS ENERGY in the feed in relation to the work requirements of the horse is still prominent as one of the causes of TYING UP and there is a reasonable amount of practical evidence which associates TYING UP with specific electrolyte problems of individual horses.

In New Zealand, in mild cases of TYING UP, low blood levels of MAGNESIUM have been found in the affected horse. These low blood levels were generally found in horses which had a recent change in their exercise programme, or had a period of rest with little ration change before showing the TYING UP symptoms. MAGNESIUM, as an electrolyte, is responsible for the use of energy by the muscle cells and there would appear to be some association between the rations fed to these horses and MAGNESIUM levels.

Lack of sufficient POTASSIUM in the ration and or electrolyte mix has also been suggested as a possible cause of TYING UP. POTASSIUM is responsible for movement of feed components, particularly ELECTROLYTES, between muscle cells,and thus is involved in the control of muscle function.

Insufficient CALCIUM in the ration is also thought to be involved. CALCIUM, as an electrolyte, controls muscle contraction, and any lack of the availability of CALCIUM to the muscles, during work, can affect muscle activity and possibly cause TYING UP.

Data collected on thoroughbreds in training showed that, in that section of the horse population at least, the chances of TYING UP occurring, from measurement of the appropriate enzyme levels in the blood, was greatest in the two year old fillies rather than three year old fillies and colts. Other scientific information also tend to indicate that young female horses are more susceptible to TYING UP than any other category and, in general, females are more susceptible than males.

Some U.S. work has shown that the muscle fibres most involved in TYING UP are those technically known as TYPE 2 or fast twitch muscle fibres. These fast twitch muscle fibres have fewer capillaries, hence less blood supply, than the other muscle fibre types and as a result are more susceptible to blood vessel restriction. As well, these TYPE 2 or fast twitch fibres also have the greatest capacity for storing GLYCOGEN, the muscle fuel, and excess levels of GLYCOGEN have been blamed as a cause of TYING UP.

MILD TYING UP may also be caused as a result of travelling. Two enzymes, the levels of which rise in the presence of the traditional TYING UP, have been shown to also rise in the blood after horses have traveled, due to the amount of exercise and trauma the horse is experiencing during the trip, attempting to stand up and maintain balance in a swaying horse trailer or truck.

The present treatment generally accepted for TYING UP has been to correct the apparent "acidosis" by the use of alkaline salts, especially sodium bi-carbonate. The administration of sodium bi-carbonate (baking soda) is an old remedy, probably due to the fact that baking soda could be purchased at the corner store and did not need a veterinary prescription for use. Sodium bi-carbonate MAY have some value in the treatment of some mild cases of TYING UP. Baking soda may reduce lactic acid build up and buffer the muscle cells. HOWEVER, blood enzyme levels indicated that MUSCLE DAMAGE was still continuing after administration of sodium bicarbonate. The LACTIC ACID is now believed to be released from the muscle cells AS A RESULT of the rapid muscle contraction, and not, as originally thought, causing the rapid muscle cell contraction. The maximum daily dose for sodium bi-carbonate is of the order of 150 grams/day, no toxic symptoms have been noticed up to this level.

Present ideas are that SODIUM BICARBONATE MAY not cure TYING UP as rapidly as previously thought and that the administration of high chloride acid salt preparations may be a better method of approach.

Other methods of possible treatment used separately, or in conjunction with administration of salts may be,

immediate cessation of any exercise, even walking, until the horse has been given electrolytes.
no exercise for at least 6 hours after electrolyte administration.
no general exercise for at least 14 days after TYING UP has occurred.
no grain for at least 14 days after TYING UP has occurred.
increase amount of hay or pasture in the ration
after 14 days less confinement, more exercise, out of the stable into the paddock.
modify training programmes to increase the length of any warm up time,
more work to use up the grain energy inside the horse,
VITAMIN B supplementation, often with brewers' yeast.
Vitamin E supplementation,
magnesium sulphate (epsom salts) supplementation.

BLOOD TEST results can be of value in attempting to clarify why a particular horse has TIED UP. If a blood sample is taken from the horse, when it is showing the symptoms of TYING UP, analysed for ENZYME and ELECTROLYTE levels and then compared with the same readings, already available from previous blood samples taken from the horse when at rest, or from samples taken some days after the horse has TIED UP, again when the horse has suffered no physical exertion, it may be possible to determine that horse's specific needs for electrolyte and other factors which may prevent the condition from occurring again.

Electrolyte supplementation may be of value in the treatment of TYING UP, and is discussed in detail in that section of the book.

Reduction of grain intake on days of reduced work is desirable. This may be difficult, due to the need to change horses' rations slowly as other problems may result. However there are certain feeds, BRAN in particular which can be used to replace grain in rations when work load is reduced, and which will provide the same bulk with approximately the same palatability, but lower the energy intake and hence not predispose the horse to digestive upsets. (Refer to the section on Feed Formulation).

Once a horse has suffered an attack of TYING UP, there appears to be some permanent change which occurs within the muscles as to the method of energy use. Generally horses which have suffered TYING UP once, will be more likely to get the problem again in the future unless changes are made to the feeding and or training programme, after careful evaluation of all pertinent factors.

In horses which are prone to TYING UP, allowing them access to a yard or small paddock as opposed to confinement in a stable all day, enables the horse to get some exercise on a constant basis. This seems to markedly reduce the incidence of tying up and appears to be one of a number of effective management strategies for the problem.

In nearly all instances the problem is MAN MADE and should not occur in most horses. There is always the exception to the rule and some horses may produce typing up symptoms on rations very low in grain. These horses will have specific digestion problems and if the approaches detailed above do not cure the problem, veterinary attention is required.

SYNCHRONOUS DIAPHRAGMATIC FLUTTER

This condition abbreviated to S.D.F. and sometimes called the THUMPS, is a very good indicator of approaching exhaustion and will subsidise and disappear if the horse is sufficiently rested.

SYNCHRONOUS DIAPHRAGMATIC FLUTTER occurs as a result of the lack of certain electrolytes in the horse and the effect that lack has on nerves which affect the diaphragm. This results in the DIAPHRAGM,which separates the thoracic cavity containing the heart and lungs, from the ABDOMINAL CAVITY containing the digestive tract moving or beating, in unison, with the beats of the HEART. Visually, the condition is very obvious when the horses' flanks, on both sides exhibit short sharp co-ordinated movements and at the same time, there may be obvious but not as prominent movement, within the muscle masses, over the hindquarters and down the hind legs, every time there is a heart beat. In severely affected cases, the horse, at rest, may prominently move one hind leg in unison with the heart beat in an uncontrollable action.

The condition is caused by a depletion of the availability of CHLORIDE, POTASSIUM, MAGNESIUM and CALCIUM as electrolytes, combined with a metabolic alkalosis or accumulation of bi-carbonate in the muscle. Reduced CALCIUM levels affect nerve function and this is further aggravated by low levels of magnesium and potassium. Horses affected with the condition should have the appropriate electrolyte supplementation which will correct the problem.

MUSCLE SPASMS

A specific problem, involving intermittent MUSCLE SPASMS has been diagnosed in a number of horses in the U.S. The MUSCLE SPASMS were of about 10 to 15 minutes duration but only occurred at infrequent intervals, generally in the order of about once per month. Blood sampling of the affected horses showed very high levels of POTASSIUM in the blood, immediately after the attack of muscle spasms.

The problem appears to be restricted to horses with heavy muscular build, predominately Quarter horses and does not show any muscle atrophy or wasting. The muscle spasms, which are short in duration and completely unpredictable as to occurrence, can be caused by exercise and or the feeding of lucerne (alfalfa) hay and can also be induced experimentally by given the horse an appropriate dose of POTASSIUM CHLORIDE.

MUSCLE SPASMS in these heavily muscled horses also appears to have some genetic base and predisposition to the problem may well be inherited.

The problem does not currently appear to be nearly as widespread as, what is now called, TYING UP but may be a problem which could develop in the future.

COLIC

COLIC is a general term used by horse people and veterinary surgeons to describe a condition which produces some form of ABDOMINAL or DIGESTIVE TRACT PAIN. The pain is generally caused by some change to the contents of the digestive tract.

Of over 2300 cases of COLIC which were fully evaluated in the U.S., the following significant trends appeared from the results.

1. no breed is affected any more than any other.
2. COLIC DOES NOT appear to genetically related but rather due to management problems.
3. 41% of affected horses were between the ages of one and six, this may be a indication that horse owners are prepared to spend money treating young horses.
4. 51% were mares, 22% were stallions and 27% geldings.
5. distribution of horses, affected by COLIC was representative of the horse population as a whole.
6. deaths, BEFORE SURGERY, from COLIC amounted to only 7% of all affected cases.
7. deaths after surgery amounted to 50% of those horses submitted to surgery.
8. veterinary attention as soon as possible after the horse showed any signs at all of COLIC gave a 90% survival rate in horses affected with the problem.

COLIC CAN EXIST IN A NUMBER OF FORMS.

1. COLIC DUE TO EXCESSIVE WATER INTAKE.

Horses have been known to get colic when allowed to drink large quantities of water when they have just finished work and are hot and sweaty. This is especially likely to happen in the hotter months of the year when hot horses are allowed to drink, to capacity, out of cold mountain streams etc. Allowing a HOT TIRED HORSE to drink unlimited quantities of cold water is a sure way to give an animal colic.

The problem is man made and the remedy is very simple. Allow the horse to cool down, if at all possible, before letting it have access to water. Preferably allow the horse to graze or eat roughage for at least 45 minutes, before allowing access to water. If the horse must have access to water immediately, only allow the horse the first part of the normal drinking pattern and then to thoroughly cool down before being allowed to drink again. Refer Section on Founder.

2. FLATULENCE COLIC

Caused by the horse eating fresh, young, actively growing pasture, especially clovers and other legumes. Such clover contains a large quantity of water in comparison to cellulose or fibre. As such, the clover passes more quickly through the horse's digestive tract and is also broken down faster by the digestive juices because there is little cellulose to hold the plant cells together.

This leads to rapid production of gas in the stomach and the first part of the small intestine. As horses, normally, CANNOT VOMIT, the gas has no escape route and builds up inside the digestive tract. This build up of gas can increase the pressure inside the stomach sufficiently to cause the horse severe pain. Reasonable care with grazing horses, in particular at the spring growth period, will prevent this type of colic occurring.

The easiest way, for the horse, to get FLATULENCE COLIC, is to change to fresh clover or legume paddocks or allow access for some time during the day to areas which contain fresh ungrazed clover or legumes. If the horse is grazing clover in a paddock all the time from the start of, and throughout, the spring season, the digestive tract seems to get used to the young actively growing plant and FLATULENCE COLIC rarely appears. However change paddocks or allow access to fresh ungrazed clover in a good spring, when the horse has not had access to that clover before and flatulence colic may develop within 4-5 hours.

Flatulence colic can also be produced by feeding fresh, wet, young lucerne or clover to stabled horses. In this instance, allowing the green feed to wilt for 3-4 hours before feeding will generally prevent the problem occurring.

3. IMPACTION COLIC – STOMACH

Impaction colic in the stomach is generally caused by the horse getting too much grain in the diet, or else, when the horse gets into the feed shed and eats much more than his daily ration of either grain, intended for his own future use, or else the fowl feed, the dairy cow feed, the dog feed or something similar.

Impaction colic of the stomach has also been reported, in horses which have eaten, in reasonably significant amounts, straw bedding, (barley straw is palatable to some horses), or had a sudden and complete change of roughage from good quality to very poor quality.

Small quantities of wheat, in particular, can cause impaction colic in the stomach. The excessive intake of grain is not able to be satisfactorily attached by the digestive enzymes. and lodges as a "ball" in the stomach and will not move further down the digestive tract. Secondly, and especially with wheat, the ENDOSPERM or "flour" component of the grain rapidly absorb water and swells. Generally the swelling is such that the wet swollen mass cannot pass into the small intestine for further digestion. The swollen wet food then becomes lodged in the stomach and causes impaction colic. EXCESSIVE levels of WHEAT and or POLLARD in the average horse's diet are among the main reasons for IMPACTION COLIC.

Again the remedy for this problem is simple. Make sure the feed shed is not accessible to horses. It will be a lot cheaper to "horse proof" the feed shed than it will be to treat the horse. In addition, you could be without the use your horse for many months whilst he recovers from an attack of IMPACTION COLIC.

Once the feed shed is "horse proof", be careful with the grain content of the ration. Do not overfeed in relation to work load and exercise requirements necessary, do not feed wheat. Wheaten flour is excellent for our daily bread. It is of little value in horse feeding.

4. IMPACTION COLIC OF THE LARGE INTESTINE

Included in this category are the impaction colics of the caecum and the small and large colon. These are parts of the large intestine and the colics are similar.

Impaction colic of the large intestine is generally caused by physical obstruction of the digestive tract by undigested cellulose and fibre. The main causes are poor quality hay, i.e. with a lot of stems and little leaf, mouldy or damp hay or hay containing weeds etc., or ingestion of bedding straw etc. due to insufficient supply of roughage to the horse.

This type of hay or bedding may not be readily broken down by the digestive juices as it passes down the tract and ends up an an undigested mass at the caecum and the colon. The food is normally not in the correct consistency to continue to pass down the gut and hence impaction colic occurs.

Bad molar teeth can also cause this problem. The molars are the grinding teeth, and, if allowed to develop sharp edges, can cause severe pain to the horse, by cutting into the inside of the lips, the gums and the tongue, when it attempts to chew its feed. Horses in the wild, obtaining all their feed by grazing, very rarely develop sharp edges on the molar teeth because the teeth are being used all the time to masticate the food before it is swallowed for digestion. The problems with sharp edges on molar teeth exists when the horse is fed reasonable quantities of grain and chaff and other concentrates. These feeds are readily swallowed and do not need much chewing by the animal. In these circumstances, the molar teeth get much less use than in a grazing situation, and tend to develop sharp edges.

These sharp edges tend to cut into the soft tissues inside the horses' mouth and the pain produced can be such as to prevent proper mastication and grinding of the feed by the horse. Stabled horses on grain and chaff should have the teeth attended to at least every six months, whereas the horse, continually grazing in the paddock, may never need his teeth filed.

IMPACTION COLIC of the LARGE INTESTINE may take some time to develop, often days and maybe weeks, before signs of pain may occur. Remember continual faeces observation is important in assessing horses health.

This form of colic is often a serious problem in horses over 15 years of age or OLDER. Poor quality feed and sharp molar teeth in these old horses can only aggravate the possible problem.

It is possible to confuse IMPACTION COLIC of the large intestine with GRASS SICKNESS. Veterinary attention could be advisable to diagnose between the two conditions.

5. COLIC CAUSED BY IMMATURE WORMS.

The larvae of the RED WORM (Strongylus Vulgaris) migrate throughout the horses' body. During their travels, these migratory stages of the red worm settles in the walls of the arteries, especially those arteries which supply the blood to the intestines and the hind limbs.

Inflammation of the walls of the blood vessels is caused by the immature worms as they develop a protective fibrous covering to ensure their long term survival, for a period of about 8 months, where the larvae maintain a semi- sleeping state before being released, as adults. Upon release of the immature RED WORM LARVAE as an adult, the fibrous swelling remains, even though it no longer contains any IMMATURE WORM. Eventually the fibrous swellings build one on top of each other, within the internal diameter of the blood vessels, eventually getting to the stage where the diameter of the blood vessels are reduced and the blood vessels may even be closed completely. This restriction of blood flow to the intestine can cause colic.

This form of colic should never occur in horses wormed frequently and with sufficient drench. Once the fibrous swellings occur in the walls of the blood vessels, technically called VERMINOUS ANEURYSMS, they do not regress or disappear. Hence it is most likely that if a horse gets colic from this source, it may well continue to be prone to get colic for the rest of its life.

6. COLIC FROM OBSTRUCTION OF THE DIGESTIVE TRACT.

This form of colic may occur in two ways:

a) Due to the intestine twisting, just like sausages or frankfurts, called TORSION COLIC. Simply, the feed is unable to pass the obstruction and often considerable pain develops in the horse, before death.

b) Due to telescoping of one section of the intestine onto an adjacent section of that same intestine, called INTUSSCEPTION COLIC. This can lead to a reduction in the size of the digestive tract and may even cause a complete blockage of the intestine. This is the condition mostly commonly seen in foals stricken with colic.

These forms of colic can occur at any time and are not a result or consequence of bad management practices. There is little the horse owner can do but seek veterinary attention when the animal is affected by TORSION or INTUSSCEPTION COLIC.

7. COLIC FROM OTHER CAUSES:

Colic may also be caused by or as a result of:
changes in feeds and or feeding schedule.
eating hard feed rations too fast.
ingestion of sand.
strangulation.
foreign bodies, e.g. wire in the digestive tract.
sometimes called "hardware disease".
intestinal rupture.
stomach ulcers.
stress following swimming.
pre foaling in mares, due to the size of the foetus reducing the capacity of the mare's digestive tract.
post foaling in foals due to retained meconium,
scours, and intestinal bleeding.

SYMPTOMS OF COLIC

The symptoms of colic all tend to follow the same pattern with the exception of impaction colic of the stomach, due to poor quality roughage, and impaction colic of the large intestine.

These symptoms will generally develop anytime from one hour to some days after the horse has been affected by the causative agent.

As the horse generally gets intestinal or gut pains, the affected animal generally alternates between three classic symptoms:

1. Kicking at the stomach and intestine with one hind leg. The horse actually twists itself into an arc of a circle and will try to relieve pain by kicking its own abdomen and intestines with one back leg.
2. The horse will adopt a dog like sitting position, with the front legs straight and extended forward in front of the body. This position allows the weight of the painful intestines to fall back onto the hind quarters and relieves the pressure on the stomach

and abdominal body walls. This is not a usual posture or position for the horse and the animal will not maintain this posture for any longer than a few minutes at a time.

3. The horse will roll from side to side on its back, again in an attempt to relieve pain.

Other symptoms of COLIC can include:
sweating, especially on the neck and the flank.
twitching of the tail.
biting at the flank.
pawing the ground with front feet.

IMPACTION COLIC OF THE STOMACH, due to ingestion of poor quality roughage will generally be seen as a slow wasting and loss of weight, possible spilling and dropping of feed from the mouth when eating, restricted faeces output. This form of COLIC, which appears to represent less than 1% of a survey of causes of colic, will develop from four to twenty days after ingestion of the poor quality roughage.

IMPACTION COLIC OF THE LARGE INTESTINE shows different symptoms to those described above for the other colics. Impaction colic in the large intestine takes some time to develop, often slowly over a period of one or two months and, on occasions, even longer. The horse initially appears off colour and tired and depressed. This may take up to 5-6 days and the horse just does not behave as its normal self. Eventually the horse will stop eating and drinking and, at the same time, probably stop producing any faeces at all.

At this stage, the horse will start to show the classical symptoms described above in order to relieve the now intense pain which is occurring due to the inability to pass faeces properly.

TREATMENT OF COLIC

Working on the old premise that prevention is better than cure, COLIC, due to excessive water intake, fresh young clover, grain, bad teeth or poor quality hay, and red worms, should not occur if the horse owner adopts reasonable management standards. The other forms of colic may occur in the best managed stables and hence cannot be blamed on poor standards of husbandry.

If the horse shows signs of colic, catch the animal and administer about 4.5 litres (1 gallon) mineral oil down the throat. Stomach tube is the best method, but if that operation is not possible, a long necked bottle is just as good, hold the horse's tongue out over one side of the lower jaw, horses will NEVER bite their own tongue and then SLOWLY pour the mineral oil down the throat, possibly giving in two or three doses to allow swallowing and avoid choking. Then immediately slowly walk the horse around. This is most important as it stops the horse from rolling to relieve the pain, and, in doing so, reduces the possibility of complicating what may a simple case of colic with twisting of the intestines (Torsion Colic). In some cases of mild colic the horse may recover without any treatment, but as the owner is not aware, at the start, exactly how bad the colic is going to be, it is generally advisable to seek veterinary attention. The horse may become so violent and hard to handle from the pain that sedative drugs may need to be given to ensure the safety of humans before any actual colic treatment is commenced.

If the horse recovers from the administration of the mineral oil and slow walking, do not allow access to feed until a reasonable quantity of oil has been passed in the faeces.

Early recognition, diagnosis and treatment of COLIC is essential. There is a very good chance of the horse recovering by itself, if the condition is recognised early enough. If treatment of the colic requires surgery,there is a 50% chance, based on established figures that the horse will not survive, either the colic and or the surgery.

Colic can be relatively easily controlled by veterinarians if action is taken early enough. Delay in calling for professional help in this type of situation may mean the loss of the animal.

GRASS SICKNESS

Sometimes called GRASS TETANY, GRASS SICKNESS is a reasonably common disease in the horses and ponies grazing pastures, in the summer months, in U.K. and Europe. The exact causes of the condition are not known and the symptoms shown by an affected horse are extremely variable.

The main features are behavourial signs, similar to COLIC. Initial symptoms include dull and listless attitude, increased salivation, the horse appears to be "tucked up" in the abdomen and sweating may appear, in patches, over the body, leading to muscle trembling on quarters, shoulders and neck, with the muscles over the back going hard. Partially digested food may appear at the nostrils, indicating an IMPACTION of the LARGE INTESTINE, blocking digesta passage.

In acute cases, death may be rapid, often associated with rupture of the stomach from the excessive amount of food contained in the digestive tract. In the sub clinical cases, some of the symptoms, detailed above, will be evident, and there will generally be a noticeable loss in body weight. It is possible that this loss of weight will occur, WITHOUT any signs of colic being present.

Few horses, which show the clinical signs of this condition recover, death or humane destruction is the most common result. Any horse which shows any signs of the symptoms of GRASS SICKNESS should have immediate veterinary attention, which will basicely be aimed at relieving the impaction of the large intestine and the gases which may be present in the stomach.

HYPERLIPAEMIA

This is a distressing condition with often dramatic results which appears to be prominent in Shetland ponies and donkeys. The condition is not frequent but can be fatal.

The problem is due to an elevated concentration of fat or energy circulating in the blood which in turn causes liver damage.

The liver is important in that it -

1. stores products of digestion.
2. produces enzymes to aid food digestion.
3. detoxifies and metabolises substances.
4. produces blood clotting factors.
5. makes bile which is essential for proper food digestion.

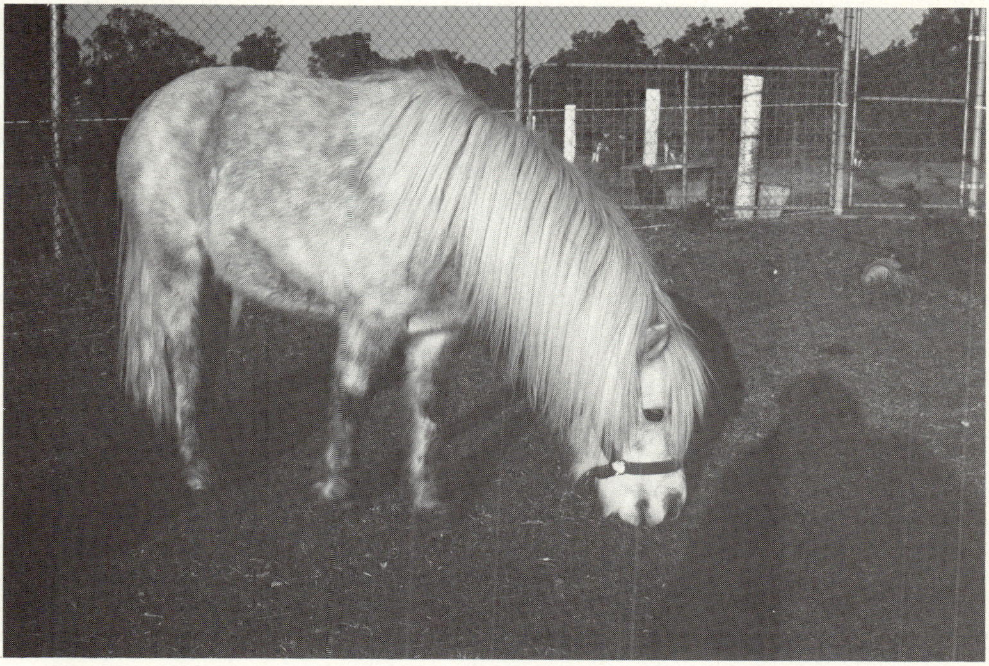

Shetland and miniature ponies are especially prone to HYPERLIPAEMIA.

A horse with a damaged liver can be under considerable stress.

HYPERLIPAEMIA generally occurs in fat ponies or donkeys, particularly mares and jennies in late pregnancy or early lactation, which have suffered a sudden fall in feed intake causing a NEGATIVE ENERGY BALANCE to develop in the horse. Fat deposits in the body are then mobilised to the blood stream and hyperlipaemia develops.

NEGATIVE ENERGY BALANCE can be caused by -

a) internal parasite (worm) infestation.
b) pregnancy.
c) disease.
d) stress, as from transport.
e) insulin deficiency.
f) persistent diarrhoea, often due to a foreign object.

Hormones released into the blood stream, in response to any of the above conditions, stimulate a flow of fats into the blood stream. which creates a NEGATIVE ENERGY BALANCE, more energy being used by the horse than is is either eating and or has stored in the muscles and fat depots in the body.

It would appear that Shetland ponies are more prone to insulin insensitivity than other breeds of horses, and therefore run a higher risk of getting hyperlipaemia. Pregnant and/or lactating Shetland pony mares and donkey jennies are especially prone to the problem.

Clinical signs are depression, inappetance, inco-ordination and muscle twitching, diarrhoea, increased pulse and respiration rate and elevated temperature (above 38.5).

Diagnosis is by blood test with the advice of the veterinary surgeon. Treatment is in two parts -

Firstly, define the cause of the sudden change in energy balance and correct. Immediate correction can be by the administration of calcium borogluconate by mouth, followed by any one of the following – Heparin, insulin, Vitamin B Complex, anabolic steroids, saline drenches and/or electrolytes.

Secondly, and after the immediate problem, attend to regular worm control, make sure the pony or donkey does not get over-fat and if changing the diet do so gradually, being careful to make any energy changes slowly.

STEATITIS

STEATITIS is a problem in foals but only very rarely reported in adult horses. The condition involves widespread inflammatory changes in the adipose fat tissue, that layer of fat immediately under the skin. The condition can sometimes be noted externally by the protrusion and lifting of small sections of skin, due to firm round swellings of subcutaneous fat. On post mortem, changes in the fat in other parts of the horse's body are also obvious.

The exact causes of STEATITIS are unknown but problems with the levels of VITAMIN E and or SELENIUM in the ration have been suggested on preliminary investigations.

RAPID EXCESSIVE OVEREATING

RAPID EXCESSIVE OVEREATING is defined as the horse consuming well in excess of its normal ration in a short period of time, often less than one hour. EXCESSIVE OVEREATING can also occur in the horse which is continually overfed on a daily basis and just ends up getting FAT, managing to avoid any of the nutritional disorders which can affect some horses.

RAPID EXCESSIVE OVEREATING relates to any situation where the horse gets unrestricted access to the feed shed or some other place where it is able to consume much greater amounts of grain and similar feeds than normally allowed. This is always a man-made problem, someone left a stable door open and the horse walked out into a feed shed etc., and unfortunately for the health of the horse and the finances of the horse owner, the problem happens far too often. Horses will very rarely, if ever, overeat on pasture and or hay, they have been eating that type of feed for years and their digestive tract is accustomed to being filled with these roughage type feeds.

Should your horse be suspected of OVEREATING, the following suggestions MAY help:-

1. get the horse away from the offending feed as soon as possible.
2. attempt to make a quick estimate of how much feed, in weight the horse has eaten. Your veterinarian would like to know this when you telephone as his helps his approach to the problem, and while he will understand kilos and bales of hay, he

really will not have any idea of half buckets or coffee tine or ice cream containers or whatever.

3. Always call the vet in these situation, even if it is only a talk on the telephone. Some feeds contain components which can be devastating in a horse. Poultry feeds, contain substances called COCCIDIOSTATS which can cause permanent damage to a horse, even in very small quantities. UREA, inadequately mixed in cattle concentrates can also quickly cause death in a horse.
4. put the horse in a quiet place and call the vet to discuss the problem, describing the symptoms shown by the horse, the estimate of the amount of feed eaten and the approximate time taken for the horse to eat the feed.
5. do not give water until you are sure of the state of the horse. Water will be of no value to a horse with CHOKE or IMPACTION of the STOMACH, in fact it may make either condition worse.
6. if possible take the temperature, pulse and respiration rates, they will be of value to the veterinarian.
7. if there is an increase in pulse rate, due to increased heart activity, the horse may well collapse and, in any case, keep the horse as warm as possible with rugs, blankets etc.
8. having done all this and if the horse still appears reasonable, with no indication of either CHOKE or shock, take the horse for a quiet short walk whilst waiting for the veterinarian to arrive.
9. The veterinarian will be concerned initially with CHOKE, any feed which may be caught in the horses' throat. CHOKE is not common but can occur and affected horses will drop feed and produce white froth from the mouth and nostrils and cough. To check for CHOKE, pull the tongue out to the side of the mouth as far as possible and feel inside with your fingers. The horse will not bite your fingers, as to do so will cause him to bite his own tongue and horses do not do that. Simple CHOKES may be able to be removed by the owner but it is probably a job for the veterinarian.

STOMACH RUPTURE may occur. Remember that horses are unable to vomit relief cannot be obtained in this manner. Fortunately STOMACH RUPTURE is not common, the horse normally has to eat a lot of feed for this to occur and at a rate where the feed going into the stomach is greater, in quantity, than the feed going out. Possible external signs will occur about 30 minutes after ingestion and will include any or all the signs of COLIC, distress, attempting to vomit, and even possibly grinding teeth in pain. If the pain suddenly eases, the stomach has ruptured and any attention will be too late as the horse will be best destroyed.

If stomach rupture does not occur, excess feed will pass through the digestive tract and COLIC will be the next possibility, occurring anytime from 1 to 6 hours after the feed has been ingested.

After 8 hours and no problems then you can then sit back and wait for LAMINITIS or FOUNDER to develop, and this can happen anytime from about 2 days to 14 or more days after the excess feed has been eaten.

THE FAT HORSE

Sometimes the problem has to be faced of a horse which is carrying far too much weight and condition for its size, and has, fortunately, not been affected by any of the many nutritional disorders which can be caused by too much feed and not enough exercise.

For any one of a number of reasons, the horse has to REDUCE weight. Treatment is very simple. Just lock the horse up in a bare yard or stable, allow unlimited access to water, to which salt has been added. The average horse possess enough internal body fat reserves to provide energy for about 5 days of work. This is not an average horse, and is not doing any work. The subject horse has excessive fat reserves and is doing nothing.

Overfat horses fed water and salt for 14 days have had dramatic reductions in body weight with no affect on general horse health. In fact,the health of the horse was probably better after the weight loss than before.

If you feel this treatment a little severe on the horse, still restrict exercise and grazing, delete all grains, concentrates, sweet feeds etc. from the ration and feed the lowest quality hay possible, as long as there is no mould present. Weight will still be lost but not as fast as on the WATER and SALT diet.

CAUTION: DO NOT USE THIS TREATMENT ON HORSES AND OR PONIES AFFECTED WITH HYPERLIPAEMIA.

CONTINUAL AND PERSISTENT OVERFEEDING

In the performance horse industries, especially race horses and pacers, there is an increasing trend to feed young horses much greater quantities of protein and energy in the rations than previously used.

In the period prior to 1950, horses, at 6 months of age, were expected to be about 40% of mature weight, horses as 12 and 18 months of age were expected to be about 60% and 73% respectively.

In the early 1980's, the same horses, at 6, 12 and 18 months were expected to be 44%, 66% and 81% of mature horse weight respectively. This represents an expected increase in growth rate of horses, under 18 months of age, of some 10% over a 30 year period, due no doubt to the increased level of grain and, therefore, energy feeding which is now currently used for young horses. This higher level of grain feeding, in theory at least, is to produce bigger horses and presumably faster horses. In practice the "system" does not quite work like that.

All animals have a normal expected growth pattern and ultimate height, determined by the genetic make-up of the stallion and the mare. As a result of the science of genetics, there is some variation in the ultimate size of offspring from the same parents e.g. the variation in size of suckers in the same litter from each sow.

Nutrition can play a part in determining the ultimate size of all animals but there is a limit beyond which horses growth cannot be increased. In poultry meat production, chickens have been produced which literally outgrew the ability of the rest of the body, especially the heart, lungs, liver and kidneys, to maintain the increased level of growth. This type of work will probably never be undertaken with horses, due to the costs involved but the warning is there.

Normally, the principles of GROWTH in horses is difficult for some people to understand. The principles are simple:

1. Ensure the horse is free of internal parasites, by regular drenching.
2. Ensure adequate levels of protein are available, at all times.
3. Ensure that the Ca/P ratio of the feed is optimum and that the absolute levels of these minerals are also present.
4. Lastly, worry about the energy levels and do not overfeed energy as this will cause problems discussed earlier.
5. Be careful with vitamin/mineral supplements given to growing horses.

If these animals are fed good quality pasture, hay, grain and allied products, they should not need vitamins/mineral supplements, as they should get all they require from the basic feed. There has already been mentioned, in detail, the problems that may occur if some vitamins and minerals are fed, either in insufficient quantities or in excess of normal needs. There is information available which carefully evaluates the effects of the interaction of most vitamins and minerals – the effect of one vitamin upon one mineral when feed intake levels are NOT CORRECT,- There may well be some form of interaction between the various components of vitamin/mineral mixes in the horse which may cause reduced performance or other problems. Humans are able to tell the doctor when a drug has a depressant effect and the medication is generally changed accordingly. If only the horse could talk, they would probably tell us to delete a lot of feed supplements which affect their peak performance, from the ration but which do not show visual or sub clinical signs that can be assessed by man.

As early as 1856, the problem of excess growth of young horses was recognised, " Many thousands of young horses die in consequence of being too well or rather injudiciously fed". In 1898 overfeeding of horses was blamed for a wide variety of problems. In 1912, the problem was again detailed in a very respected text of the time, " in no other way can colts be ruined so surely and so permanently as by liberal feeding and close confinement." Again in 1968, a very respected owner, breeder and trainer of pacers remarked " it is also a fact that mare owners and trainers, despite what their natural inclination might be, seem to prefer slick, stout yearlings that actually have been overfed. Apparently this is an occupational hazard of the yearling selection business and it is doubtful if it will ever change". Again in 1980, "Overnutrition is one of the major feeding problems in the horse industry" and very detailed research by a number of researchers about the same time concluded that "the first step in the treatment of FLEXURAL DEFORMITIES, (leg problems) is the reduction of feed intake.

Many studies with dogs and pigs have shown that numerous bone and skeletal problems do occur from overfeeding. Studies with horses are not as numerous, but those available have produced results consistent with the results in dogs and pigs and reinforce the approach that overfeeding problems do occur in horses. Contracted tendons, especially in young foals 6-12 months of age, have definitely been proved to be a result of overfeeding.

Numerous bone disorders, collectivley termed METABOLIC BONE DISEASE or DEVELOPMENTAL ORTHOPAEDIC DISEASE, and including osteochrondosis, and epiphysitis in particular, have also been diagnosed as resulting from incorrect feeding practices and ration formulation.

Some practical and very experienced race horse trainers are very careful not to accept overgrown and under exercised young horses into their stables. Their own experiences, over the years, have produced a strong feeling the big horses, especially if not exercised as weanlings and yearlings, tend to give more leg problems than a "normal sized horse". These trainers, in some instances, make thorough investigations into the feeding and exercising of the horse up to yearling stage before making any decision about purchase.

THERE IS INCREASING PRACTICAL AND SCIENTIFIC EVIDENCE NOW BECOMING AVAILABLE WHICH SHOWS ADEQUATE EXERCISE OF WEANLING AND YEARLING HORSES IS JUST AS IMPORTANT AS IS CORRECT FEEDING.

Adequate exercise involves allowing the young growing horses to run out in large paddocks, exercising at will, at the same time as making sure the feeding is correct. Adequate exercise DOES NOT MEAN restricting the yearling to a stall or small yard, feeding to the "eyeballs" and taking the horse for a lunge or a walk once in a while.

If all other factors in the preparation of a young racehorse are equal, PADDOCK REARED horses will always stay fitter longer and suffer less breakdown problems than will the same horse reared in a confined space with excess levels of feed available. One of the problems with the thoroughbred industry is that the owner wants the most money for the yearling, the buyer thinks that big shiny yearlings look better, and they probably do on the day of the sale, and should therefore perform better. The racehorse owner, on the other hand, wants a horse which will NOT BREAKDOWN during training. These training breakdowns, often considered "essential" by some trainers, to "toughen up" the horse, will always lead to increased owner costs and possible loss of prize money, as a result of the horse being unfit to race and the additional costs of, hopefully, getting the horse fit again. The problem of OVERFED and UNDEREXERCISED YEARLINGS has been with us since 1856 and will remain with us until yearling horse buyers learn the foolishness and cost of the practice.

Whilst the well grown two year old, with the nice shiny coat may look good in the sale ring, practical experience dictates preference for the horse that may not look as good but has grown up spending by far the greater proportion of its life foraging in large open paddocks. Continual exercise is important for young horses, to condition and strengthen bones, ligaments and muscles. The overfed horse which has spent most of its growing period, locked in a small yard, with little natural exercise will not have the muscle and bone conditioning of the horse, on free range, no matter what the difference in feeding has been.

OSTEOCHRONDOSIS

OSTEOCHRONDOSIS, abbreviated to O.C.D., relates to any condition which involves inflammation of the bone and adjacent areas of cartilage. The condition has been relatively common in growing horses, in the age range of 12-18 months but has now been detected in foals, where the symptoms were observed at about 4 months of age.

Symptoms include swelling or "puffiness" in and around the joints of the lower legs, hocks in particular, especially with foals which are apparently growing faster than normal. The condition seems to appear in a definite order of affected areas, the HOCK being affected first, followed by the STIFLE, then the SHOULDER, the ELBOWS then the FETLOCKS, with often both sides of the horse being affected as well as more than one joint.

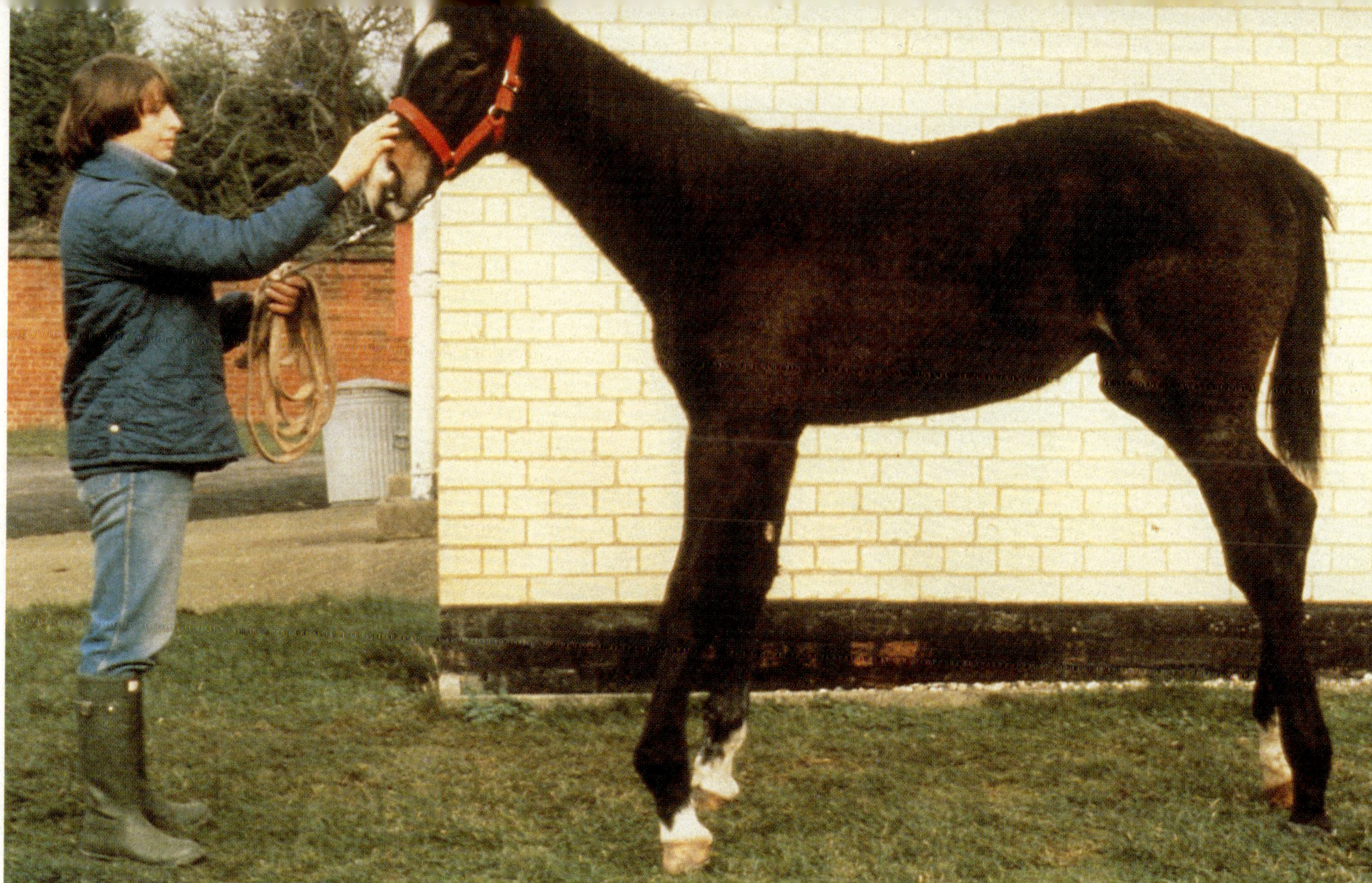

Yearling overfed and underexercised – incurable.

The white tissue is calcium deposited in the aorta – main blood vessel – result of excess Vitamin D in the ration. Refer page 79, same horse.

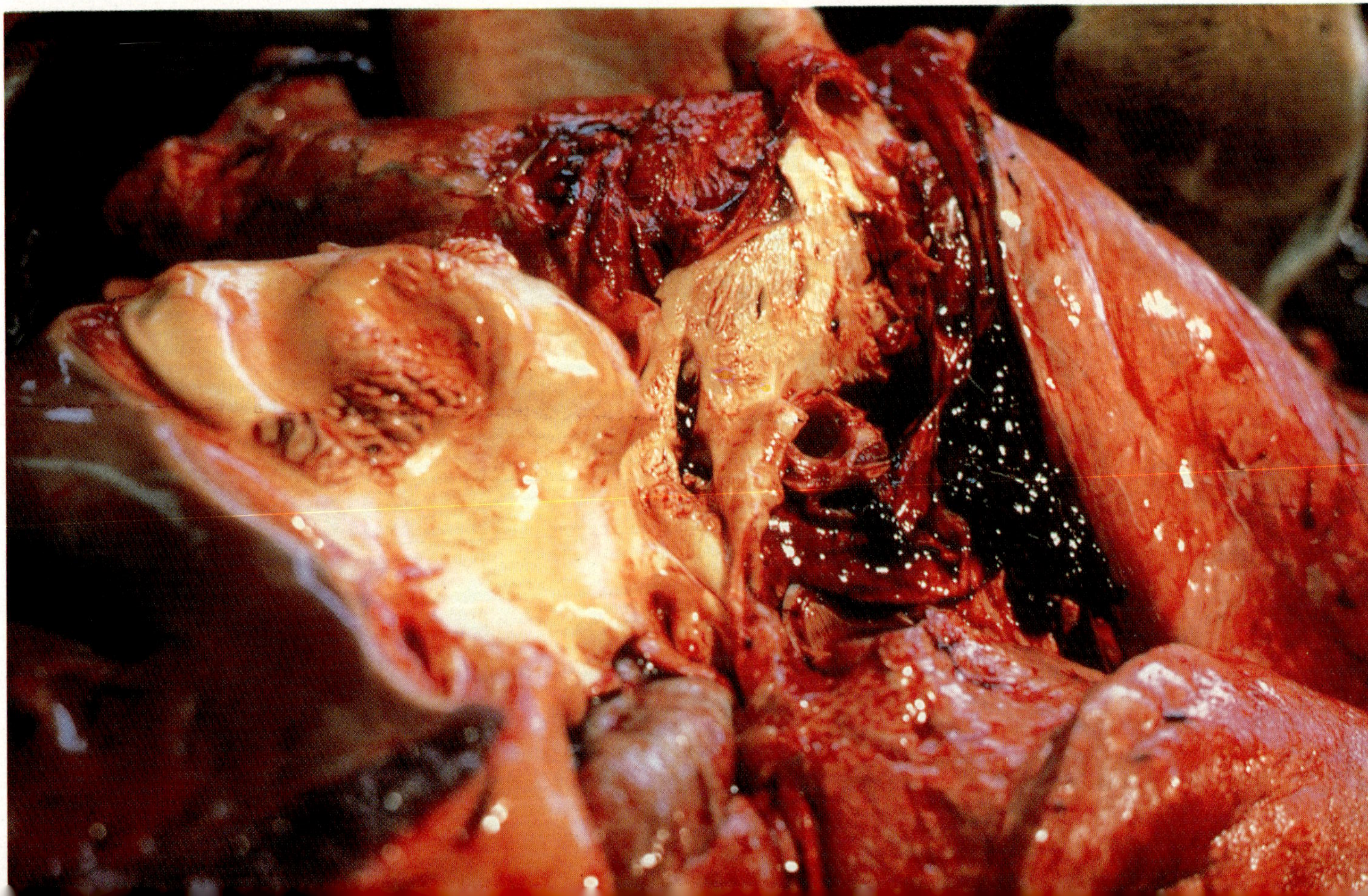

O.C.D. involves separation of the cartilage from the bone and may be caused by a number of factors.

1. O.C.D. is more common in light boned, heavy bodied horses due to the extra weight, of the body, that has to be carried on smaller bones. O.C.D. rarely occurs in either ponies or draught horses, due to the usually larger size of the bones in relation to the total body mass.
2. O.C.D. commonly occurs in a period of fast growth, especially after the horse has been through a period of under nutrition beforehand. This increased rate of growth, immediately after a period of poor growth, appears to cause deficiencies of some of the minerals involved in bone development, CALCIUM, PHOSPHORUS, MAGNESIUM, COPPER and ZINC and also to provide an ideal environment for the development of cartilage disorders.
3. O.C.D. commonly occurs in horses which are overfed either in terms of PROTEIN or ENERGY or both. Excess PROTEIN is able to be converted to energy.
4. Excessive energy in the ration of the young growing horse has been shown to decrease bone density, decrease bone thickness and alter the natural bone growth patterns.
5. High levels of ZINC can lead to O.C.D. High levels of ZINC, in the ration, are similar in effect to high levels of PHOSPHORUS, with the result that, the absorption of CALCIUM is decreased.
6. High levels of grain feeding can reduce PHOSPHORUS availability, due to PHYTATE bonding, and so upsets the CALCIUM/PHOSPHORUS ratio.
7. Genetic make-up or breeding of the horse can also predispose to the problem. There are known strains of thoroughbreds where the genetic problem exists. O.C.D.will generally not appear if the rations are correctly formulated, however if there happens to be a small formulation problem in the ration, O.C.D. can occur.

Treatment of an O.C.D. condition depends on the stage of development.

PREVENTATIVE TREATMENT is the best and the cheapest. This involves monitoring of and adjustments to the feeding programmes of young horses, from birth to mature age of 4 years to ensure correct protein and energy levels, and accurate attention to both AVAILABLE CALCIUM and PHOSPHORUS levels. This can mean reducing the amount of legume hay, specifically alfalfa (lucerne) in the diet, due to the high level of CALCIUM and the low level of PHOSPHORUS, and increasing the amount of grass hay, or mixed pasture hay, usually with lower protein and energy levels but with much better CALCIUM and PHOSPHORUS levels for growth and fitness. This monitoring of the nutritional intake of the young horse MUST ALWAYS be accompanied by the availability of adequate exercise at all times. Correct feeding and adequate exercise go hand in hand, one is of little value without the other in the prevention of O.C.D.

This change of roughage type is desirable as there is no known way of correcting the deficiency of PHOSPHORUS for young growing horses, when grazing alfalfa (lucerne) or being fed a ration based predominately on alfalfa (lucerne) hay.

Whilst the addition of grass and or mixed pasture grazing and or hay to young horses MAY decrease the growth rate slightly, it will generally not affect mature body size to any significant extent and will certainly reduce the possibility of the occurrence of O.C.D. in the young horse.

CURATIVE TREATMENT, that is once the problem has occurred and been diagnosed, will involve complete restriction of exercise, AND CAREFUL ATTENTION TO RATION FORMULATION. Any exercise after diagnosis will ONLY INCREASE the problem on the cartilaginous growth plates and will slow down and sometimes prevent recovery.

EPIPHYSITIS

Also know as PHYSITIS, this condition is one of a number of problems, often loosely termed, METABOLIC BONE DISEASES. EPIPHYSITIS, involves the development of unusual leg shapes, inflamed joints and gait deformities, especially in young actively growing horses, at any time up to about three years of age. It is not unusual for a horse to be born normally but to develop the problem some months after birth.

EPIPHYSITIS can be caused by one one or more of the following:-

BACTERIAL INFECTION
EXERCISE AND TRAUMA
GENETICS
EXCESS PROTEIN
CALCIUM/PHOSPHORUS IMBALANCE

BACTERIAL INFECTION

If a bacterial infection is responsible for the development of EPIPHYSITIS in a horse, there are probably a number of other problems wrong with the horse which should have been detected and diagnosed, BEFORE EPIPHYSITIS EVEN BECAME OBVIOUS. Bacterial infections are commonplace in horses, leading to many conditions which cause the horse to go "OFF COLOUR" or become lethargic, quiet, disinterested in normal surroundings etc. Elevated body temperatures are generally always associated with bacterial infections which in all but the exceptional cases are easily controllable by antibiotic treatment.

EXERCISE AND TRAUMA

Too much work or activity, especially on hard surfaces, in young growing horses has also been blamed as a cause for the presence of EPIPHYSITIS. The continual pounding of the legs of young horses, on surfaces which DO NOT GIVE or do not provide some type of cushioning effect, to each hoof movement, have been blamed for the development of the problem. The horse, after all, developed over time in swamps and marshes and still spends most of its time walking over pasture which has some "GIVE" in it, in all but the driest seasons. Exercise has been particularly blamed for the occurrence of EPIPHYSITIS in two year old pacing horses, who spend considerable amounts of time training on hard surface tracks.

GENETICS

It is well known that inheritance of SKELETAL WEAKNESSES can occur from either or both sire and dam, in exactly the same way as other more obvious inherited genetic problems occur. The potential size and hence possible bone structure and development are all programmed at the meeting of the sperm and the egg, some 11 months before the horse is ever born. This possible ultimate genetic size of the horse can only be obtained if the horse is fed and managed correctly from birth to 4 years of age.

Whilst EPIPHYSITIS, as such, is not is not accepted as being inherited, there are a number of other inherited problems, affecting bone development, which in conjunction with the feeding of imbalanced diets can cause EPIPHYSITIS to occur.

RATION FORMULATION

The main cause of EPIPHYSITIS is a lack of either CALCIUM and or PHOSPHORUS in the ration or insufficient supply of VITAMIN D, from either sunlight and or sun cured hay. The feeding levels of both minerals are discussed, in full, in the chapter on MINERALS and any deviation from levels of CALCIUM and PHOSPHORUS in the ration recommended in that chapter will lead to some type of bone problem, with EPIPHYSITIS being the most common result.

Bone problems can also be compounded by the relationships in the ration, of the following minerals, CALCIUM, PHOSPHORUS and MAGNESIUM in bone development, insufficient MANGANESE in the ration, excess levels of MOLYBDENUM, affecting the utilisation of COPPER and or a deficiency of ZINC.

EPIPHYSITIS can also be caused by making the young horse grow too fast. The ever increasing trend to restrict the exercise of weanling and yearling horses and feed these same horses' rations with higher than normal levels of protein and energy to produce "big horses" which command a higher price at the yearling sales is a practice completely foreign to the horse. Young horses were meant to exercise around the paddocks and the restriction of exercise, by confinement, and the forcing of growth by ration levels of protein and energy, sometimes well above normal accepted limits can cause EPIPHYSITIS, sometimes not occurring until after the horse has been sold and training as a racehorse commenced.

The old saying LET THE BUYER BEWARE is of the utmost importance in this type of situation.

METABOLIC BONE DISEASE

METABOLIC BONE DISEASE, now also known as DEVELOPMENTAL ORTHOPAEDIC DISEASE, is a term currently being used to describe a series of, what till recently were, separate conditions affecting the horse.

The conditions include EPIPHYSITIS, OSTEOCHRONDOSIS, CONTRACTED TENDONS, MALFORMATION OF THE CERVICAL VERTEBRA (WOBBLER), JUVENILE ARTHRITIS and MALFORMATION of the BONES of the FETLOCK AND HOCK.

Previously all these conditions have been accepted as being separate and distinct problems, but recent veterinary cases have shown that some horses are capable of having all the problems at once, based on the failure of CARTILAGE to develop into normal healthy weight bearing bone. In one U.S. study, there was 10% wastage in yearlings, which could not be sold or used due to O.C.D., JUVENILE ARTHRITIS, CONTRACTED TENDONS or WOBBLER SYNDROME, all considered part of M.B.D.

Factors involved in the onset and cause of M.B.D. include, NUTRITION, GENETICS, EXERCISE and CONFORMATION, with NUTRITION and GENETICS being the two main suspects. It is clearly evident that there are a number of nutritionally related problems with young growing horses, to which the answers are not known.

What is known, is that these problems occur in young horses, where the ration has some mineral deficiency and or imbalance, often associated with restricted exercise. What is also known is that M.B.D. and or its apparent many related problems, occur at a nuch reduced rate in young growing horses which are correctly fed and allowed adequate exercise.

NUTRITIONAL SECONDARY HYPERPARATHYROIDISM

NUTRITIONAL SECONDARY HYPERPARATHYROIDISM, often abbreviated to N.S.H. and also called BRAN DISEASE, is a condition in horses which causes more CALCIUM to be removed from the bones, than is being deposited in the bones.

The problem is caused by a reduction in the utilisation of CALCIUM in the digestive tract, causing a reduction in the blood level of calcium which in turn stimulates increased production of the PARATHYROID HORMONE which then acts to release additional supplies from the bone.

Reduction of utilisation of CALCIUM in the body can happen in two ways.

1. HIGH RATION LEVELS OF PHOSPHORUS.

Excessive levels of PHOSPHORUS, in the ration, are known to depress the absorption of CALCIUM, into the small intestine, due to the formation of CALCIUM PHYTIC compounds which are not absorbed in the digestive tract, but which are excreted in the faeces.

2. OXALATES IN HORSE FEEDS.

OXALATES, present in some plant species, when eaten by the horse, bind CALCIUM in the digestive tract and make it unavailable for the the normal functions of BONE formation and maintenance and as an ELECTROLYTE in the horse. Where the grazing intake of the horse is such that the CALCIUM level is ideal but OXALATE is present in the pasture, the OXALATE reduces the availability of the CALCIUM to the horse BEFORE THE CALCIUM IS ABSORBED in the digestive tract. If there is insufficient CALCIUM in the pasture to "satisfy the appetite" of the OXALATE, CALCIUM is then withdrawn from the bones of the horse.

Plants, containing high levels of OXALATE, sufficient to cause NUTRITIONAL SECONDARY HYPERPARATHYROIDISM, include the tropical and sub tropical species, buffel grass, setaria and sometimes on green panic, kikuyu, guinea grass, para grass, pangola grass and signal grass. OXALATE has also been found in grazing lucerne (alfalfa) and lucerne hay (alfalfa hay).

OXALATE problems are now known to occur in horses when the CALCIUM/OXALATE ratio in the grass is 0.5/1.0 or less, and this generally occurs when the total OXALATE concentration, in the DRY MATTER, exceeded 0.5%. The OXALATE content of lucerne, does not, in general, approach this danger level, although there have been isolated instances, where initial symptoms of BIG HEAD have been observed in horses grazing or being fed lucerne and which have been corrected by the feeding of additional CALCIUM to the affected horses.

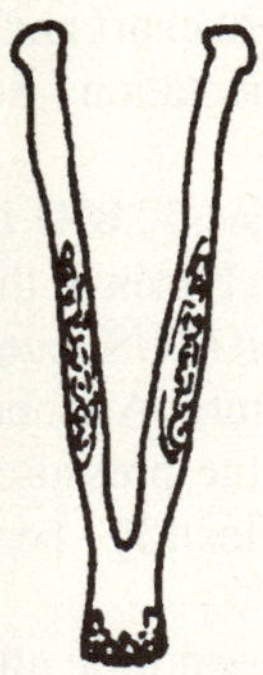

NORMAL JAW

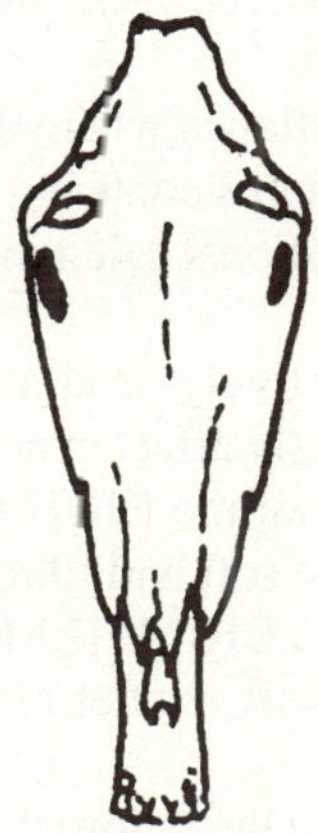

NORMAL WIDTH

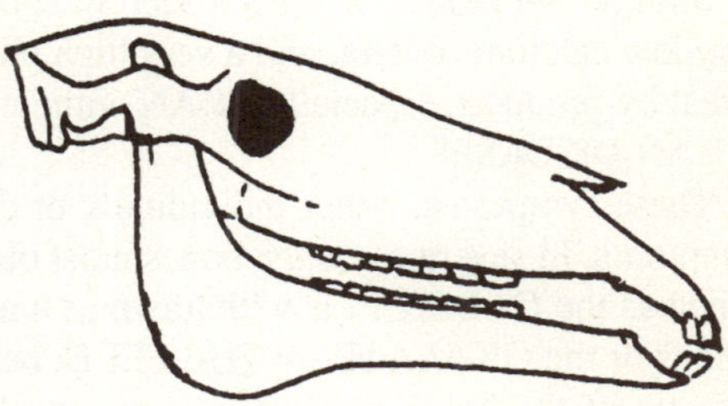

NORMAL SIDE VIEW

INCREASED JAW WIDTH

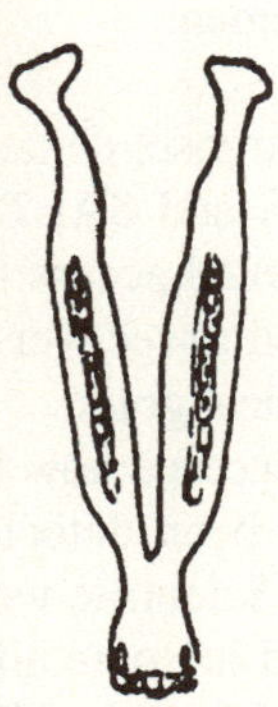

INCREASED HEAD WIDTH

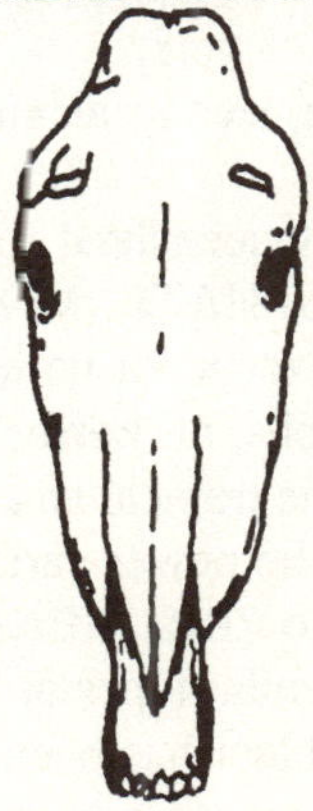

RAISED FRONTAL BONES

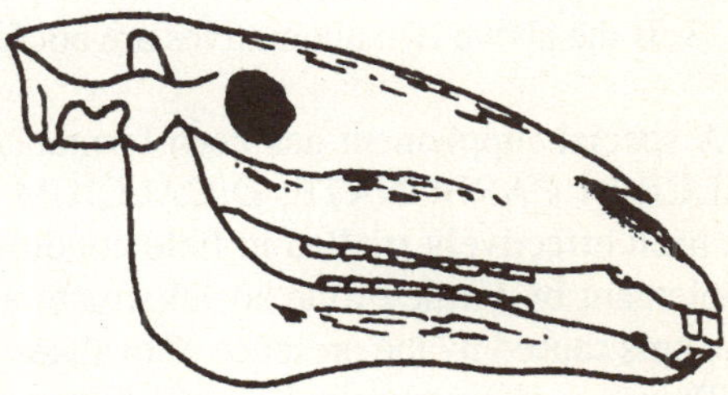

"BIG HEAD"
NUTRITIONAL SECONDARY HYPERPARATHYROIDISM

Cattle and other grazing animals are not affected by the OXALATE component of these pasture species, indicating the vast differences in the way in which the same feeds are utilised differently in the two animals.

Symptoms of N.S.H. include wasting and loss of weight, shifting lameness and general stiffness, shortening of gait, reluctance to move, irritability, loose teeth, especially in adult horses, loss of calcium from the bones, swollen joints and possible bone fractures, and even inability to get up from the ground if the horse is badly affected, all a function of reduced enzyme activity occurring as CALCIUM is removed from the bone to balance the high PHOSPHORUS levels.

Similar symptoms have been seen in earlier studies where horses were fed diets with a very low calcium content, and a very high phosphorus content – e.g. cereal chaff and grains, cereal by-products, especially BRAN without additional calcium supplementation – so called "BRAN DISEASE".

These symptoms, either individually or collectively, lead to the classical "BIG HEAD" symptoms. In severe cases the bones most obviously affected are the thin bones of the head, which as the CALCIUM is withdrawn as a result of the HIGH PHOSPHORUS level in the rations or the OXALATE IN THE FEED, become soft and fibrous in nature. As soon as the strength of the bones are lost, as a result of CALCIUM REMOVAL, the pressure of the fluid under the "bones" causes the face to swell, sometimes significantly, hence the common name "BIG HEAD".

Provided the condition is detected at an early stage before there has been little alteration to the bones of the face, the problem can be cured by correcting the CALCIUM intake of the horse. However once the horse is mature, over four years of age, and the condition is in a reasonably advanced stage, facial bone changes MAY be permanent.

Where any of the above pasture species are to be used for horse feeding then corrective measures must be taken to avoid oxalate problems. These are:

1. Graze horses on other species where possible.
2. Maintain a mixed sward of plants and sow clovers and other grasses with kikuyu. Haifa white clover is valuable in this regard as it appears to be the only clover that will persist in kikuyu stands for any length of time.
3. If the above two alternatives are not feasible, feed a calcium supplement.

A special supplement has been formulated in Queensland for this purpose, containing CALCIUM CARBONATE, DICALCIUM PHOSPHATE, MOLASSES and SALT, and has been effectively trialled in field conditions. Except for horses prevented access to the supplement by virtue of the social structure in mobs, all horses appeared to recover from problems caused by the presence of oxalates in some tropical and sub-tropical grass.

There are also recent indications that some of the newer varieties of lucerne now being sown may contain oxalates. Symptoms similar to "BIG HEAD" have been detected in horses being grazed or fed on hay made from particular types of lucerne. Scientific work in the United States has shown that the oxalate problem has been detected in some alfalfas (lucernes) in that country. The present level of scientific knowledge of OXALATES in alfalfa (lucerne) shows CALCIUM/OXALATE ratios of between 1.7/1 and 3.9/1 or about 3 times greater than the ratio which is currently accepted as being in the dangerous category.

ANAEMIA

Anaemia is the term for the condition which features a decrease or reduction in the numbers of RED BLOOD CELLS, in a given volume of blood. As soon as a horse has an "off day", an unexplainable lack of energy or just does not perform as expected, a perceived reduction in the level of RED BLOOD CELLS is blamed, by many people, as the cause of the problem.

ANAEMIA, resulting from a lack of IRON in the diet of the horse VERY RARELY IF EVER OCCURS.

Nearly all the common horse feeds contain more than adequate IRON for the horse's daily needs. In addition, the horse possesses the ability to self regulate the amount of IRON it uses and stores within its body, any excess being stored in the mucosal lining of the digestive tract from where it is transferred, by a protein bonding, sometimes called "BIOAVAILABILITY" to the bone marrow for the production of additional RED BLOOD CELLS. The rate at which these additional red blood cells are produced depends on two things, firstly the normal loss, the average RED BLOOD CELL lives for about 150 days and secondly any abnormal loss, generally as a result of either loss of blood from an injury or loss of blood as a result of an internal parasite infestation.

Apart from ANAEMIA caused by massive blood loss, due to injury and to internal parasite infestation, the other recognised causes of ANAEMIA are:

1. a lack of HAEMOGLOBIN building material in the horse, very rare, genetically related and incurable.
2. an absorption imbalance, within the horse, which results in the production of RED BLOOD CELLS which function with a reduced level of activity.
3. a disease problem which actually dissolves RED BLOOD CELLS and is incurable.
4. a dietary deficiency of FOLIC ACID, a member of the VITAMIN B COMPLEX.
5. a possible VITAMIN E deficiency in the diet.
6. drug induced, especially from the use of some anthelmintics and tranquilisers.

The symptoms of ANAEMIA include very pale mucous membranes, lips, gums, eyelids etc., due to lack of blood, lethargy, loss of condition and a tendency to become tired and lazy earlier than normal, exactly the symptoms of a wormy horse.

Contrary to common belief, ANAEMIA IS NOT CAUSED by any of the following:- growth, hard work, pregnancy and lactation or "off days".

Should your horse appear ANAEMIC, the problem is either very simple, massive loss of blood from an injury or internal parasite infestation, both of which you should be able to recognise and control. If these causes can be discounted, then the services of a veterinarian are required as the problem is one which requires professional attention, NOT THE ADDITION OF MORE IRON TO THE HORSE.

HEAVES

HEAVES also known as BROKEN WIND, CHRONIC OBSTRUCTIVE PULMONARY DISEASE and EMPHYSEMA is characterised by prolonged and persistent dry coughs, often not very loud, accompanied with double movements of the flanks on expiration or when breathing out, sometimes called "double expiratory lift". HEAVES is the outward sign of problems in the horses' lungs.

The condition is a SECONDARY DISEASE, caused by and associated with changes in the LUNG tissue, consisting of allergic lung tissue reactions etc, which can be caused by:-

1 – the presence of dust in the feed, stable bedding etc.

2 – inadequate stable ventilation.

3 – infection, which in turn can be caused by bacteria and or viruses.

4 – Neutrophils, the white blood cells which increase in number to fight a bacterial and or viral infection, are themselves able to cause lung damage, leading to a horse, so affected, producing the symptoms of HEAVES.

5 – parasite infestation, primarily resulting from larval forms of worms, migrating through and damaging the lung tissue.

6 – allergy.

7 – infection from other horses.

8 – oedema

HEAVES decreases the tidal volume of the lungs, and or reduces the amount of air which can effectively be handled with each breath and therefore reduces the overall oxygen intake of the horse and can also causes increased heart rates.

HEAVES OR C.O.P.D. IS IRREVERSIBLE.

The condition is often blamed upon dusty feeds and some horse trainers go to great lengths to reduce the possible dust level in feeds, without paying any attention, at all to any one of the additional seven possible causes detailed above. In fact some trainers develop a paranoia about dusty feeds, that has to be experienced to be believed, yet one has only to walk into their stables to realise that air circulation could also do with some improvement.

English research work has shown that there are some 65 individual and specific organisms which can be carried in dust and can cause HEAVES. Of these 65, some 53 or 82% were found in hay, some 29 or 45% were found in straw whilst 28 or 43% were found in both hay and straw.

It is therefore logical that dusty hay and or straw can be incriminated as ONE of the possible causes of HEAVES. It is also possible, as these organisms are microscopic and only visible under a microscope, that HAY and STRAW did not contain any of these infective organism and in fact the HEAVES was a result or one or more of the other seven causes detailed above.

Practical solutions for horses, affected with HEAVES, include:-

1. if possible, put out on pasture away from the stabled environment. It has been proven that horses affected with HEAVES, recover from the condition when removed from the stabled surroundings and put out to pasture, yet again develop the symptoms of HEAVES when returned to the stable. The response is due to the increased air movement outside as opposed to restricted ventilation, within the stables.
2. if the horse MUST be kept indoors, the aim should be to reduce the exposure of the horse to dust at all times.

a) improve air ventilation in the stalls, this is probably the most important aspect of HEAVES control. Physical modifications to the stables to increase air flow, without causing obvious air draughts may be necessary. Installation of overhead fans, new ventilation openings at normal horse nose height, and above, and other modifications, dependant on the structure of the stables, should be considered.

b) ensure the horse is thoroughly drenched. Any tissue damage already in the lungs, from past worm infestations is permanent, but you should stop any more such damage, from larval worm migration, occurring.

c) any feed bins should be lifted off the floor to chest height.

d) any hay fed should be spread out or teased out for about 10 minutes before feeding and then placed in a hay net, in the stable. This practice will have a dramatic effect on lowering the micro-organism count of the hay. Similar treatment of straw bedding will also markedly reduce the level of micro-organism content. The problem with teasing or separating the straw is that it MUST BE DONE OUTSIDE the stable and the teased straw then placed inside, after at least 10 minutes. TEASING of straw bedding, within a stable, will only increase the possibility of the horse getting infected as the micro-organisms will be released at the bottom of the stable where there is little air circulation, no matter what the stable design.

e) any hay fed should be thoroughly soaked in water for at least five minutes, preferably with a little bentonite added to the water.

f) hay cubes or wafers can be subsituted for hay, without additional treatment, if the hay cubes contain bentonite as a binder.

g) reduce hay level and increase pellet level in the ration

h) changing from lucerne chaff to oaten or wheaten chaff is of no value, all chaffs are as dusty as each other.

i) change from straw to wood shavings as bedding.

The occurrence of HEAVES and or allied breathing problems can also be associated with the problem of clean stalls. URINE and FAECES, to-gether or individually, are able to produce large amounts of AMMONIA gas which can not only be offensive to smell but which may affect the lungs of the horse.

Recent research work with young foals clearly shows that, up to age 6 months, the continual presence of URINE and FAECES in stables can predispose the foal to attacks from FOAL PNEUMONIA. It is known that AMMONIA gas, in horse stables stays near the floor, the exact area where young foals spend most of their time resting, meaning that the foal will breath much more ammonia gas than its mother, who, rarely lies down and, for the greater part of the day has her nose much higher above ground level.

AMMONIA levels are determined by ventilation and air movement, the more the air movement the less the chance of AMMONIA affecting the foal. One of the obvious practical solutions to a reduction in the problem is to increase the amount of air movement through the stable.

The effect of the AMMONIA level in the stable is generally compounded by some type of stress suffered by the foal, new stables, new feed, changed feeding times or any other small item which may not be obvious to the feeder but which is noticeable to the foal.

HIVES

HIVES, also called PROTEIN BUMPS, NETTLE RASH, HEAT BUMPS, SWEET FEED BUMPS and URTICARIA is a condition where a number of small swellings, welts or pimples appear on the skin of the horse. The problem can be due to any one of a number of causes, including, insect bites, allergies to drugs and or feed additives, insecticides and INCREASED PROTEIN LEVELS IN THE RATION.

When HIVES are caused by increased protein levels in the ration, it is, generally, due to the production of AMMONIA, from the excess protein which cannot be excreted from the horse in the normal manner and shows as HIVES. If increased protein level in the ration is the cause, reduction of the protein content of the diet will cure the problem.

EXHAUSTION

EXHAUSTION occurs when the horse shows a total loss of strength and an inability to continue to work at an acceptable level.

FATIGUE, on the other hand is a state of weakness or tiredness after exertion but the horse will still have the ability to continue, even if only for a short period of either time and or distance before it becomes exhausted.

EXHAUSTION can be caused by:-

1. depletion of GLYCOGEN availability to the muscles. This can even happen where the horse still has left considerable levels of FAT reserves, as the FAT reserves are not being mobilised as quickly as the muscles are using the GLYCOGEN.
2. ACCUMULATION OF LACTIC ACID
3. ELECTROLYTE IMBALANCES and or REDUCED AVAILABILITY OF SUPPLY. The most severe ELECTROLYTE decreases will be measured from 30 minutes to 4 hours after the completion of a ride or race.

Factors which can affect each or all of the above three primary causes of EXHAUSTION include increased environmental temperature and oxygen consumption of the body cells, which increases 10% for every 1 degree CENTIGRADE increase in body temperature. This increase in body temperature, in turn, decreases the horse's AEROBIC working capacity, increase the probability of respiratory alkalosis and decreases the amount of blood available to the working muscles as blood is sent to the skin to assist in heat loss.

The time taken for EXHAUSTION to occur depends on the horse's AEROBIC working capacity, properly trained and conditioned horses having much better AEROBIC working capacity than untrained and unfit horses and on the availability of FREE FATTY ACIDS (FATS) with the amount of OXYGEN being transported in the RED BLOOD CELLS, the key to the whole problem.

When the total of the humidity reading and temperature exceeds 150, with temperature being measured in FAHRENHEIT, the horse is able to lose sweat in critical amounts and may not be able to dissipate or lose heat adequately. Exhaustion then sets in.

(For those who measure temperature in CENTIGRADE, degrees C can be converted to degrees F by the formula 5F=9C+32.)

Symptoms of EXHAUSTION include:

1. horse unwilling to move
2. disorientated, lethargic
3. delay in reduction of pulse rate, which should be back to 70 beats/minute after 20 minutes with drop in these levels levels commencing to occur immediately upon the completion of exercise. Low pulse pressure can be indicative of possible shock occurring whilst high pulse pressure can be indicative of the possible occurrence of LAMINITIS.
4. get shallow increased respiratory rate, combined with an elevated body temperature. Above 41 degrees C (105.8 degrees F), oxygen use exceeds supply and tissue damage will result. If RECTAL TEMPERATURE DOES NOT FALL to 38 degrees CENTIGRADE (100 degrees FAHRENHEIT) within 10 minutes of ceasing hard exercise or performance. RECTAL TEMPERATURES may not be very accurate, in this situation, due to possible dilation of the ANUS, due to exhaustion.
5. the horse will probably be dehydrated. The SKIN PINCH REBOUND TEST MAY BE OF SOME USE. The horse has to be extremely dehydrated for this test to work but pinch a bit of skin, generally around the shoulder, if it does not return to the normal flat position within 5 seconds, the horse has a SEVERE dehydration problem. PARTIAL DEHYDRATION CANNOT BE DETECTED BY ANY SIMPLE TEST.
6. PACKED CELL VOLUME (P.C.V.) will rise from normal levels of 35% to as high as 55%.
7. decreased intestinal sounds
8. in male horses, complete lack of penile tone.

Treatment for EXHAUSTION should be aimed at replacing the lost body fluids and electrolytes. The severely exhausted horse can lose up to 50 litres of fluid, and treatment with fluids should continue until the horse shows some type of visual response by urinating, having a decreased heart rate, increased gut sounds etc. This fluid treatment will consist of INTRAVENOUS administration of a solution containing the appropriate electrolytes plus oral administration of the same solution. The use of straight drinking water will be of little value to an exhausted horse, the primary cause being mainly massive electrolyte loss, with water loss being associated with electrolyte loss and being the secondary cause.

If treatment for EXHAUSTION, at the time of occurrence, was inadequate, it is possible for POST EXHAUSTION SYNDROME to occur up to three days after the problem occurred. Symptoms of POST EXHAUSTION SYNDROME include digestive tract, kidney and liver malfunctions, synchronous diaphragmatic syndrome, laminitis and tying up.

In order not to have a horse suffer EXHAUSTION, the following tips are provided:-

1. increase the ability of the horse's muscles to use oxygen for energy use, by a training programme of long slow work, increase AEROBIC working capacity and provides conditions in the muscle which allow the horse to handle increasing LACTATE levels better.
2. attempt to obtain a decreased level of ELECTROLYTE concentration in the sweat.
3. get the horse to be able to use fats as a source of energy better, related to increased oxygen utilisation by the muscles as a result of long slow work.

4. need a reduced resting PACKED CELL VOLUME, conditioned ARABIANS seem to have this feature better than any other breed.

WHITE MUSCLE DISEASE

SELENIUM DEFICIENCY, in the horse, has been diagnosed as WHITE MUSCLE DISEASE, abbreviated to W.M.D. and also known as NUTRITIONAL MYODEGENERATION.

Considerable difference of opinion exists as to the SELENIUM requirements of horses. Levels of from 0.1 to 2.5mg SELENIUM/day

For a 450kg horse have been mentioned in the scientific literature. A daily SELENIUM intake of 45-50mg for the same 450kg horse would be considered toxic.

Fortunately most of the feeds analysed for selenium, contained in excess of the horses' daily needs, and research work has also shown that horses can tolerate up to ten times the acceptable selenium level in their food, without showing toxic effects. U.K. information provide SELENIUM levels in oats and hay at 0.03 mg/kg D.M. which means that a 450kg horse eating about 9 kg of DRY MATTER/ day would have a SELENIUM intake of 0.45mg/day.

Selenium deficiency associated with WHITE MUSCLE DISEASE, in foals, has been diagnosed in parts of the U.S.A, Victoria, Western Australia and New Zealand. The disease appeared in specific conditions, where the mares were grazing in are certain soils were known to be selenium deficient, with a SELENIUM content of 0.5 UG(MILLIGRAMS)/GRAM of soil. WHITE MUSCLE DISEASE had a marked seasonal occurrence occurring much more frequently in Spring when it was felt the accelerated growth of the pasture, may have reduced the total selenium intake of the horses. Spring also happens to be the foaling time in the SELENIUM DEFICIENT regions and newly born foals show the symptoms of WHITE MUSCLE DISEASE, better than any other class or type of horse.

The pastures, which were being grazed before and at the time of occurrence of the WHITE MUSCLE DISEASE did not contain lucerne, which is recognised as containing adequate levels of selenium for horse needs. WHITE MUSCLE DISEASE, in foals, can be corrected if early diagnosis is made, particularly or the horses are bred on soils known to have a SELENIUM deficiency problem.

SYMPTOMS of WHITE MUSCLE DISEASE, in foals, can occur from birth up till about 12 months of age and include muscle dysfunction, especially inability to stand for any length of time, leaking of milk from the nose or mouth after suckling, elevated breathing and heart rates. On occasions, the actions of a foal, suffering from WHITE MUSCLE DISEASE has been confused with COLIC, due to similar leg actions of the affected horses.

WHITE MUSCLE DISEASE is very difficult, if not impossible to cure, if NOT DETECTED IN THE VERY EARLY STAGES. Veterinarians now have available a number of tests which can be carried out on likely affected foals to correctly diagnose the problem. Complete recovery of a foal diagnosed as having WHITE MUSCLE DISEASE is not good, evidently once muscle damage has occurred, it is very difficult, if not impossible, to correct.

BROOD MARES and progeny, grazing on pasture in localities and or soil types known to be low in SELENIUM should be treated with SELENIUM on a preventative basis,

BEFORE WHITE MUSCLE DISEASE occurs. The feed is generally supplemented at the rate of 0.1 to 0.2 P.P.M. SELENIUM, equal to about 0.9 grams. Alternately, the mare can be fed at the rate of 1 gram of SELENIUM/day or given a 10 ml SELENIUM injection once a week. SELENIUM supplementation of pregnant mares should start at least 6 weeks before the expected birth of the foal as the passage of SELENIUM across the placenta to the unborn foetus is not very efficient.

At birth, a blood sample should be taken from the foal and immediately analysed for SELENIUM level. Any foal at risk from low levels of SELENIUM should be treated by intra-muscular injection at birth, two weeks and six weeks of age as SELENIUM is NOT transferred from mare to foal in the milk to any degree.

WHITE MUSCLE DISEASE, occurring in stabled horses on mixed rations, is generally NOT related to the stable feed as most concentrate or hard feeds fed to stabled horses have adequate SELENIUM levels. Any such problem generally occurs in horses past weaning age and will probably be as a result of a period of grazing on pasture with borderline SELENIUM levels, prior to entry into the stables.

SELENINOSIS

SELENIUM EXCESS in the diet, produces a condition known as SELENINOSIS, ALKALI DISEASE, BOBTAIL DISEASE or BLIND STAGGERS and can be caused by the horses eating plants which accumulate large amounts of SELENIUM, as in the U.S.A., or by the administration to the horse of SELENIUM overdoses, either by injection or in the feed. SELENIUM can accumulate in the body and its excretion rate is EXTREMELY SLOW, SELENIUM accumulation producing symptoms which include loss of appetite, loss of hair, with the mane and tail falling out first, disintegration of the hoof wall, blindness and paralysis.

SELENIUM is one of those minerals which does not allow any mistakes. Once the effects of SELENIUM LEVELS, either TOO HIGH or TOO LOW, take effect, the damage is virtually permanent.

Cases of SELENIUM toxicity have been reported in horses, feed SELENIUM, additional to that already present in the feed and at the same time grazing pasture which had adequate levels of SELENIUM in the pasture. The additive effect of SELENIUM in the feed and SELENIUM in the feed supplement have been sufficient to cause SELENINOSIS

ALWAYS SEEK PROFESSIONAL ADVICE IF ADOPTING ANY FEEDING TECHNIQUE WHICH MAY PRODUCE ADVERSE RESULTS IN THE HORSE. THERE IS OFTEN A NUMBER OF INTERRELATED MATTERS TO CONSIDER WHICH REQUIRES PROFESSIONAL ASSISTANCE.

VITAMIN D EXCESS.

The effects, on the horse, of administration of VITAMIN D, in levels in excess of the horses' daily needs have been carefully documented in a number of cases.

VITAMIN D, when fed in excess of the horses' continuing daily needs, can have some dramatic effects on the health of the horse. The excessive Vitamin D will initially cause wasting and loss of condition and weight, dry faeces, and markedly decreased ability to exercise. More advanced stages of EXCESSIVE VITAMIN D administration can cause CALCIUM to be deposited in soft tissues such as blood vessels, heart, lungs and kidneys. This irregular deposition of CALCIUM can occur in horses, of any age, and can cause irregular bone development which will be permanent.

The toxic level of VITAMIN D has not been established in the horse, but in other animal species, it is 10 times normal requirements. There are several reported cases of these sorts of problems occurring, in practical situations, from the USE and or OVERUSE of mineral vitamin supplements containing what appear to be reasonably high levels of VITAMIN D.

Research studies have also shown that mares, fed about ten times the accepted level of Vitamin D during pregnancy, have produced foals which have died shortly after birth, due to deposition of calcium in the blood vessels. Rupture of the large blood vessels coming from the heart has then occurred, due to build up in pressure from the heart, attempting to pump the same amount of blood through a much smaller CALCIUM restricted artery. Growing horses, fed excess levels of Vitamin D, develop ossification of the bone joints – too much calcium is laid down the joints become stiff and the animal becomes permanently lame.

Any changes in the horse, such as CALCIUM deposit in the blood vessels, irregular bone development, lameness etc. are PERMANENT and IRREVERSIBLE, and recorded case history indicate that any horse so affected has never recovered from treatment, so extreme care should be taken when feeding VITAMIN D supplements to a horse.

BIOTIN AND HOOF GROWTH

Hoof growth, in horses, is determined by nutrition as well as by genetic make-up or heredity. There is little one can do about the genetic reasons for the hoof problems, but there are methods that can be taken to assist the possible nutritional problems.

1. Ensure the horse has adequate levels of protein and energy in the ration. Poor hoof growth in the form of weak walls, sand and quarter cracks, weak frogs etc. will be more prevalent when the protein and energy levels of the diet are not adequate.
2. Ensure that in all periods, except very wet seasons, that the hooves are "dressed" with an appropriate hoof dressing. Hoof tissue contains on average about 35% moisture and hoof moisture content should be maintained at that level,for optimum hoof growth.

   Hoof dressings should be able to supply moisture to the tissues, allow moisture to enter into the hoof tissues and at the same time stop the moisture, already present, from drying out. The cheapest and best practical hoof dressing is boiled down beef or mutton fat. Other dressings which can be used include horse oil boiled down horse fat – but this product is not often readily available as horses do not get very fat and the recovery of horse oil from horses is very low.

   Other proprietary hoof dressings are available which are generally based on horse beef or mutton fat, often with lanolin (wool grease) added. Other commonly accepted hoof dressings, such as neatsfoot oil and stockholm tar, are not recommended as they generally dry out the hoof, and this is contrary to the aims of hoof dressing.
3. If the above steps are followed and the horse still has hoof problems, it may well be that that there is a need for supplements of methionine and/or biotin. METHIONINE is an amino acid and would be available in lucerne hay, soybean meal and pasture.

Hence horses with hoof problems on a diet principally of grain and cereal hay may need supplement of this specific amino acid. BIOTIN is a member of the Vitamin B Complex. Very recent research work has shown that a daily dose of 15 mg of biotin over approximately 5 to 6 months will assist horses with chronic hoof problems, sand cracks, quarter cracks, etc and that once the problem has been corrected, the continual addition to the feed of 1-2 mgs of BIOTIN/horse/day will ensure better continual hoof growth.

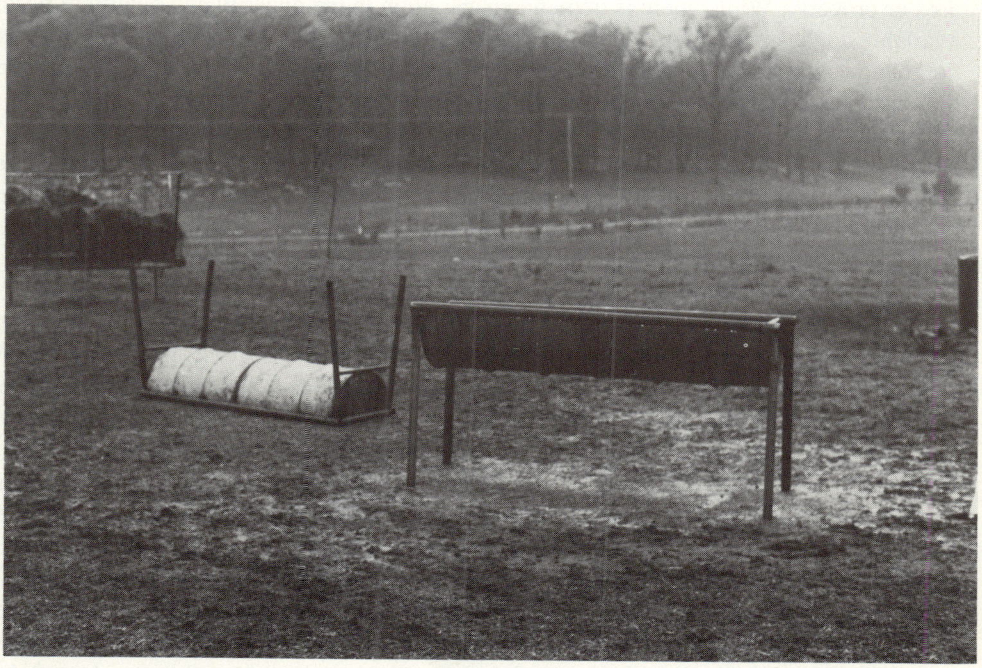

Supplementary feeders on pasture – beware of possible injuries from the legs on the feeder which is upside down. – bad management.

19. PASTURE FEEDING

Feeding on pasture is the natural way of maintaining horses. Horses evolved and developed over millions of years as animals whose sole diet was obtained from growing plants and horses have specifically developed a digestive and metabolic system which allows them to transform growing plants into energy in a digestive tract vastly different from other grass eating animals. The horse is the ONLY SINGLE STOMACHED animal which exits on grass alone and for this reason has a specifically developed large intestine which has the ability to allow breakdown of fibre or cellulose to occur and absorption of the products from that process to take place into the bloodstream.

Grazing of horses occurs in many different parts of the world and on many different pasture species, all of which produce reasonable horses under grazing conditions. It is not the intention of this chapter to detail names and or mixtures of pasture species applicable to all those areas of the world where horses are grazed, that would be an impossible task.

It is however the intention to detail the important points, with reference to grazing horses on pasture, which will apply no matter what part of the world the horses are grazing pastures. It will be up to the individual reader to seek further information, on a local district and or property basis, as to the best way to grow satisfactory pasture for horses in his or her area or property. Whilst there is tremendous variation in the quantity and quality of pasture available to horses, dependent largely on soil type, pasture species present, fertiliser programme, seasonal circumstances and rainfall and stocking rate, there are large areas where horses can breed, grow and maintain condition satisfactorily on pasture alone.

Pasture consists of growing plants whose composition of PROTEIN, ENERGY, MINERALS and VITAMINS will in fact be changing daily as the plant grows and matures. The growth habit of all plants is determined by the four seasons of the year but all plants must at some stage within the 12 month period produce seed. Seed is vital for the natural survival of the plant because, without seed production, the plant would not be able to commence a further generation in the next growing season.

Annual plants are so called because they have a growing period of less than 12 months and at some stage, during that 12 month period, that plant will not exist in the pasture. The ANNUAL plant will, at the end of its growing season, produce seed which normally drops onto the ground, where the seed waits for some stimulation to germination to produce the next years growth. Dependent on the species of plant, this stimulation can depend on one or more of the following, rainfall, air temperature, soil temperature, humidity and day length.

PERENNIAL plants are plants which remain in the vegetative state throughout the year and do not have any period where the vegetative form of the plant is not present and visible in the pasture. Despite the continual vegetative growth, PERENNIAL plants still seed, even if seeding is secondary to the survival of the plant. Kikuyu, a grass species which is very common in sub tropical and tropical areas and, which produces large amounts of vegetative growth, will produce seed in the form of very fine thread which is visible for about 2 days only. If you do not know what to look for and the particular time of the year when kikuyu seeding takes place, you would completely miss the kikuyu seeding.

PASTURE FEEDING

The digestive and metabolic functions of the horse have adapted over time and are quite capable of handling the variation of the individual feed nutrient content which occurs in pasture.

Excess PROTEIN can be stored as energy and it is possible for the horse to lose up to 50% of its total body PROTEIN content before it starts to get near death. The horse will certainly lose body condition and weight but it will still stay alive as far as protein is concerned.

Excess ENERGY can be stored in both internal fat depots, within the abdominal cavity, in particular, and also within the muscle tissue for re-use.

The important VITAMINS A, and E, are both contained in green actively growing plants, in the case of A and E and from sunlight in the case of D and, all three being fat soluble, any excess can be stored inside the fat depots for use at some later time. The other VITAMINS of the B COMPLEX and C are made within the horse, B COMPLEX in the large intestine from fibre or cellulose breakdown and C from GLYCOGEN which is part of the energy system.

Mineral storage in the horse is excellent. The horse has the ability to store any excess levels of any mineral present in the pasture within its body for later use, subject to natural self limiting processes which allow the horse to excrete any excess levels of minerals, derived from pasture species.

Average to good quality pasture should be able to provide all the feed nutrients required for any horse which is either resting, breeding, growing, spelling or doing light work. The problems of pasture feeding of horses start when we ask performance horses, horses doing medium levels of work or above. to be able to satisfy all their nutrients requirements from pasture. The work load requirements, and hence the nutrient requirements, of the horse are then starting to exceed what can be obtained from most pastures.

The best example of this is the SALT requirement of the horse. One thing the horse cannot store in its body is SALT. Any salt not used virtually immediately will not be stored for future use but will be excreted from the horse. In the natural situation, the horse does not tear around at a fast pace and sweat on a hot day. Horses on free range will rest in the heat of the day and any exercise will be at the cooler parts of the day or at night. when sweat production and hence salt loss will be considerably reduced and the salt requirements can be met from that contained in natural feed. Man, however, decides for any one of a number of reasons, to make horses sweat excessively, often in temperatures where the horse in the paddock would be resting under the shade of a tree and due to this action immediately increases the sweating horses need for salt to be added to the ration.

The availability of all the important feed components from pasture will be discussed in the following sections in this chapter.

The problems in PASTURE FEEDING of horses requires an understanding of the interrelationship of the many factors which affect pasture growth and the intake of pasture by horses. These problems can be divided into the following sections:

1. SOIL FERTILITY AND PASTURE PRODUCTION
2. PASTURE GROWTH
3. STOCKING RATE
4. GRAZING PREFERENCE
5. PASTURE GROWTH AND NUTRIENT CHANGES
6. PASTURE CONSUMPTION AND WATER INTAKE
7. PROTEIN AND ENERGY IN PASTURE
8. VITAMIN AND MINERAL CONTENT ON PASTURE
9. LABELS FOR PASTURE
10. WEEDS
11. SUPPLEMENTARY FEEDING ON PASTURE.
12. COSTS OF KEEPING A HORSE AT PASTURE.

SOIL FERTILITY AND PASTURE PRODUCTION

SOIL FERTILITY is a term used to describe in a collective manner the mineral content of a particular soil. This mineral content, consisting of PHOSPHORUS, SULPHUR, NITROGEN, MOLYBDENUM, CALCIUM, COPPER, ZINC, etc. combined with water and sunlight is what plants use to produce vegetative tissue and hence horse feed. A soil of HIGH FERTILITY will have adequate levels of all these minerals, essential for plant growth present in the soil and in a form which can be used by the growing plants. A soil of LOW FERTILITY will either have all these minerals present but in levels less than desired or may have one or more minerals present in inadequate amounts whereas all the other minerals levels may be satisfactory,

Very few soils can be termed of HIGH FERTILITY, with all minerals present in the correct amounts for optimum plant growth. Even if the soil could be classified as HIGH FERTILITY, in its natural state, after some years of farming and or grazing, the fertility level of that soil will be reduced, in comparison, to its original fertility or mineral content as minerals will go from soil to plant, from plant to horse and then sold off the property in terms of live horses. The reduction in soil mineral level will, on a yearly basis, will be so small as to be invisible but over a period of years, reductions in soil mineral levels can be detected on soil analysis and plant growth studies.

Any form of grazing is a MINING operation, minerals are mined from the soil, as growing pasture, or grains and oilseeds harvested from plants which are then transferred to horses as feed to allow horses to grow and perform.

The mineral content in the soil will be reflected by the mineral content in the pasture and subsequent horse feed, produced on that soil. If the soil is deficient in adequate NITROGEN for optimum plant growth, any pasture growing on that soil will be deficient in PROTEIN. The exact same situation will apply with SULPHUR, SULPHUR deficiency will lead to reduced PROTEIN levels in the feed. REDUCED PROTEIN levels in horse feed does many things, including restricting growth rate and affecting performance.

Reduced PHOSPHORUS levels in the soil will affect overall water utilisation, by the growing plant, which in turn will affect the uptake of most of the TRACE or MICRO-MINERALS form the soil, by the pasture. And so the list can go on but this is a book on feeding horses, not soil chemistry and plant growth.

PASTURE FEEDING

The problem of the mineral content of soils and therefore of feed growing on those soils is further compounded by the tremendous variation which can exists in the types of soils. Within the HUNTER VALLEY area of N.S.W., recognised as one of the premier horse breeding areas of the world, there are 34 different soil types on about 1.8 million hectares, some of high natural fertility and excellent for horse activities and other soils of such low fertility and with other problems, that there are best left covered with timber and never used for grazing. It is not unusual to have 5 and 6 different soil types on the one property. No where is this more evident than in some parts of NEW ZEALAND, where a property can have an area of SELENIUM DEFICIENT soil in one part of the farm and the balance of the property can be of a soil type with no SELENIUM problems at all. As the the margin of error for SELENIUM INTAKE by the horse is very small, too much can be as dangerous as too little, the need for horse owners, on properties of this type, to understand a little about soils is very evident.

Some particular areas of the world have had long standing reputations as being excellent for breeding horses because of the calcium or lime in the soil in the water. Personal observation over a long period of time, tend to indicate, that in fact these areas do not possess a special calcium level, but rather the soils have high natural phosphorus levels. Remembering the necessary relationship, between calcium and phosphorus, in the formation and maintenance of bone, it is probably not surprising some people may have confused a supposedly high natural calcium level with a high actual phosphorus level in the soil. The end result as far as the horse is concerned would be very similar.

It is possible, with most soils, to be able to correct a plant growth problem by the use of fertiliser. However, as there are well over 50 or so different fertilisers available for use in promoting and encouraging plant growth, it is important that the correct fertiliser be applied and this requires a knowledge of soils, fertilisers, plant growth and horse nutrition to produce the best results.

Phosphorus deficiency, in the soil, is one of the main problems affecting plant growth, both in terms of total production and in plant mineral composition. Phosphorus deficiency is easily corrected by the application of super-phosphate to the soil. Methods of application and rates to be used depend on many factors, including the natural soil phosphate level and it is suggested that concerned horse owners should seek local expert advice on their individual problem. Nitrogen is responsible in plants for growth and protein level. The less nitrogen available in the soil to growing plants, the lower will be the total quantity of green feed produced. As well, the feed that is produced will be lower in protein than normal. As protein is an important component of horse feeds, judicious and careful use of nitrogen fertilisers on the correct pasture species will ensure production of better quality horse feed.

Artificial Nitrogen, as a bagged fertiliser, is expensive and if not applied under the correct conditions, may be completely wasted.

Natural Nitrogen produced from legumes such as clovers, lucerne and allied species, when established properly, using inoculated seed, is then utilised by the other plants, especially grasses. Clovers however, need super-phosphate for adequate growth but, where practical, the use of super-phosphate on clovers will not only produce more total feed, but will also produce nitrogen at a much less cost than nitrogen fertiliser applied from a bag.

Correct pasture management including fertiliser application, will in present knowledge, increase carrying capacity often two fold and, at the same time, produce better quality feed.

PASTURE GROWTH

The old saying "the eye of the master fattens his stock", as applicable to the cattle business, is directly applicable to horse feeding. Whilst the objective of cattle feeding is to fatten as quickly as possible in order to make as much money as possible, the objective of horse feeding is to maintain the horse in an acceptable condition, at the same time allowing the horse to perform at a required level, without nutritional problems occurring.

Astute and experienced horse feeders are able to tell whether a horse is "doing", that is, maintaining condition as required. The inexperienced horse owner may find this a little difficult, and often overfeeds concentrates and grain when in fact the horse has plenty of feed in the paddock to eat. The application of the principles of BODY CONDITION SCORING, as described earlier in this book, provides an ideal system which allows anyone, after only nominal training to be able to assess the condition of the horse and following on from that, the amount of feed the horse should need.

PASTURE GROWTH is going to vary tremendously, dependant on:-

1. SEASON OF THE YEAR – SUMMER GROWING SPECIES.

SPRING GROWTH is always the best feed, although often on some pastures for a short period of time, it could be described as too good in that the combination of high water content and low cellulose or fibre levels can lower considerably feed utilisation. Sometimes it is necessary to provide the horses with hay, AD LIB or free choice so that they can adjust their fibre needs between the high water content pasture and the low water content hay.

SUMMER GROWTH in average seasons is always reasonable horse feed and suitable for most horse needs.

In AUTUMN, the quality of the pasture will decrease as the summer growing species will be seeding and some level of feed supplementation MAY be desirable, dependant on pasture species, soil type, rainfall and temperature.

In winter, the grazing value of SUMMER growing plant species is not very high as this is the time of the year when these plants have their "holiday".

SEASON OF THE YEAR – WINTER GROWING SPECIES.

AUTUMN -this is the time of germination and or commencement of growth of all winter growing species. The ANNUALS will germinate and the PERENNIALS, despite having remained in the vegetative state over the summer, will suddenly "green up" and start to grow, due to a drop in temperature accompanied by rainfall. Generally there is no problem with high water content at this time of the year as in freshly growing plants as in SPRING.

WINTER, dependant on temperature, plant growth will be reasonable as long as natural nitrogen can be produced in the soil. If soil temperatures drop to a low level, natural soil nitrogen production will cease and winter growth of grasses, but not legumes, will reduce considerably, unless applications of nitrogen fertiliser are made. Any such applications of artificial NITROGEN fertiliser should be carried out with care on pastures to be grazed with horses, as NITRATE poisoning problems can occur. In some parts of the northern hemisphere, temperatures are so low in winter as to completely stop plant and pasture growth and hand feeding then becomes necessary.

SPRING, as with summer growing species, SPRING growth of winter species increase dramatically as soon as the air temperatures start to warm up but as the plants are at the end and not the start of their growing season, the problem of high water, low fibre content of spring growth is generally not present.

SUMMER Winter growing species generally seed at the end of Spring or in early summer, indicating that the SUMMER season is the period of low production.

Ideally, in a grazing situation, it would be desirable to be able to produce the same amount of feed, of the same desirable quality from each hectare or acre of land on each day of the year.

Unfortunately, nature does not allow us to do that.

The best we can do is to endeavour to sow a mixed pasture which contains both grasses and legumes of both Summer and Winter growing habit. That may be possible in some areas but may not be so in others, due to soil type, rainfall or some other agronomic reason. Even if it is possible to get a pasture of mixed summer and winter growing species established, at some stage in the future, the pasture will change composition to become either winter or summer dominant. This change could occur within one year and is largely dependant on two things. Firstly the effect of rainfall after establishment. If this rainfall happens to be summer dominant, then the species change will be to summer species and vice versa. Secondly in a pasture of mixed species, grazing will be occurring throughout the year, meaning that some plants will not get their "holiday". This will cause some plants to disappear from the pasture mix.

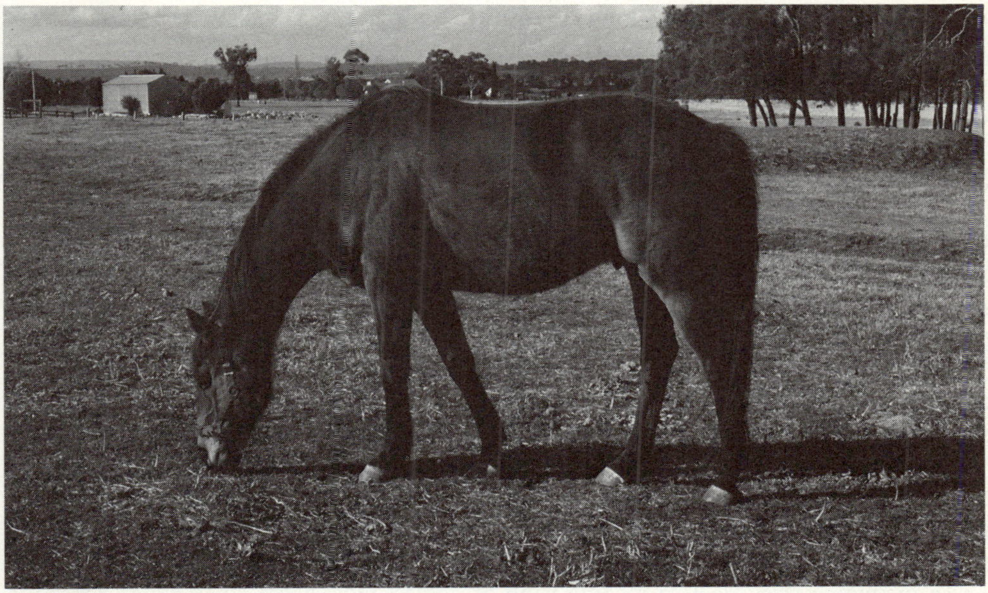

Short but adequate pasture, horse still in good condition but may need some supplementary feeding.

If a mixed pasture is either not possible or desirable, then separate plantings of summer growing species and winter growing species should take place. These separate plantings in, different paddocks, do allow for better pasture management and better long term pasture productivity, as the differing grazing practices, for summer and winter growers, can be applied to the separate paddocks.

STOCKING RATE

Horses on pasture are stocked for convenience, not to fatten as quickly as possible as in the case of cattle. In a cattle situation, stocking rate is normally assessed to ensure that the animals will grow as fast as is possible on the feed available, subject to the variations of normal seasonal plant growth.

Different types of pasture in different areas have a nominally assessed carrying capacity, i.e. 2 cows and calves to one hectare (common on good irrigation pasture) to a possible extreme of one cow and calf to 15 hectares or more generally in the very dry areas of Australia.

This tremendous range of carrying capacities is based on the ability of the pasture, IN NORMAL SEASONS, to keep both the cow and calf in good to fat condition.

The stocking rate of horses is determined by a number of other considerations beside keeping the horse in reasonable condition from the grazing available on an area of pasture.

There are two extreme grazing situations with a multitude of in-between variations.

1. PASTURE AS THE ONLY SOURCE OF FEED.

Horses are renowned fussy pasture feeders. Horses do not graze a pasture evenly, as will cattle. Cattle will generally eat all the feed growing in a pasture and leave very little, except that growing in dung patches, or around weeds, e.g. thistles etc.

Horses on the other hand will tend to graze some areas of pasture to the ground whilst an adjacent area of apparently the same species composition will not be touched. All the reasons for this selective grazing are known only to the horse itself but some of the problems are bound up with the FAECAL EXCRETION HABITS.

Horses are known to pass or excrete faeces in particular areas in a paddock, sometimes know as "ROUGHS". Before defecaeting most horses will smell the faeces, currently on the ground. The mare will smell the faeces and, if produced by herself or another female, will stand in the same spot and defecaete one horse length away. If the old faeces has been produced by a gelding or stallion, the mare will move on until she finds female smelling faeces. This mares' habit, of deciding where to defecaete means that the total area covered by the FAECES, or ROUGHS is slowly increased in size. Geldings will defecaete anywhere, not being very fussy at all whilst stallions, in the paddock situation, will always defecaete on top of another stallion or mare faeces, unless using FAECES to delineate or mark out their territory in which they will defecaete in a large circle, sometimes covering acres or hectares of ground. Horses will NOT generally eat pasture contaminated by faeces, partially explaining the apparently ungrazed areas in a horse paddock.

To overcome this selective grazing habit of horses, most horse studs which run large numbers of horses on pasture generally put a mob of cattle in the paddock after the horses have been removed. Generally called "followers", these cattle will clean up the areas of pasture which the horses have not eaten. If this practice is then followed by pasture harrowing, especially in the colder months of the year, the new pasture regrowth will be the best obtainable in the seasonal conditions prevailing at the time.

Due to their fastidious grazing habits, the generally accepted stocking rate for horses is normally 40-50% above that of cattle. Two cows and calves to one hectare then, in practice, becomes one brood mare to 0.75 hectares, and one cow and calf to 15 hectares becomes one mare and foal to 23 hectares. These types of stocking rates are based on the horses growing satisfactorily on a complete pasture diet and not receiving any supplementary feed of any type.

The stocking rate can be increased above these suggested limits, i.e. more horses on the same area of grazing, but some form of feed supplementation will be required by the animal to maintain normal growth and maintenance.

In practical terms, geldings are considered to need about 60% of the amount of pasture as one lactating brood mare and foal, whilst weanlings and yearlings are generally classed as geldings for most purposes. The lower body weights of weanlings and yearlings, and hence their lesser needs per day of total feed intake, means that when stocked at the same level as geldings, they are able to grow to the optimum ability.

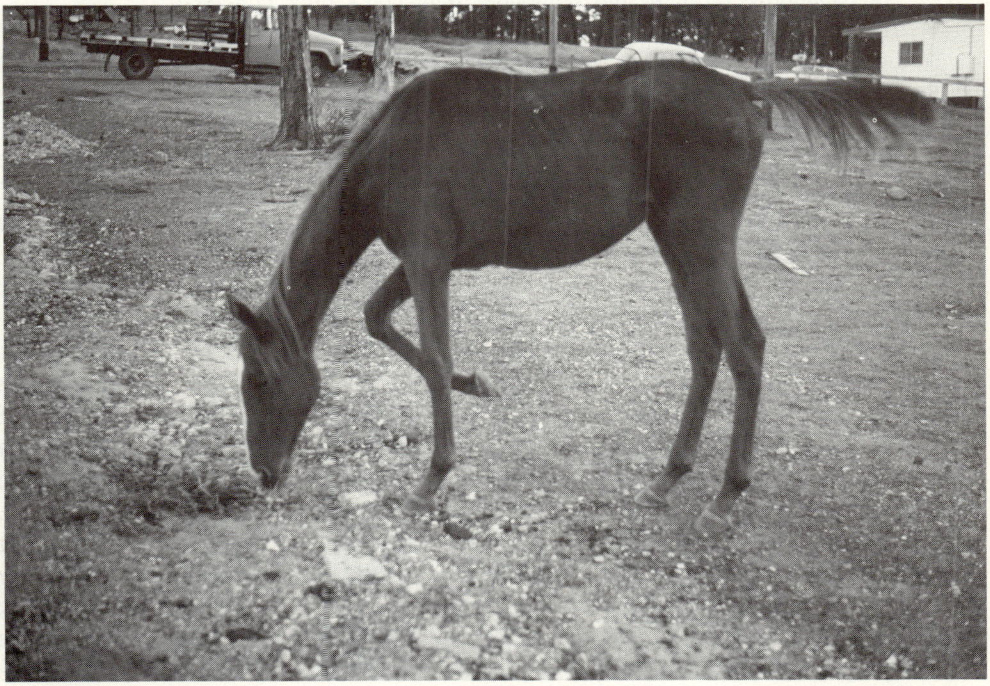

Lack of paddock feed – needs some level of hand feeding depending on the work load of the horse.

2. PASTURE AS A PARKING LOT.

The other extreme of pasture grazing for horses is where the pasture is virtually used as a "parking lot" on which to place the horse whilst most of its feed requirements are supplied from grain, concentrate and roughages and what the horse gets from grazing is a bonus. This "PARKING LOT" approach is often a common situation, especially in areas within, adjacent to or close by cities and towns where the value of the land is such as to restrict, in many instances, the grazing of horses at "normal" stocking rates. The one major problem with this type of concentrated grazing operation is that the horses generally end up eating the ROUGHS and so quickly become re-infected with internal parasites, requiring continual attention to the drenching programme.

3. PASTURE AS PART SOURCE OF DAILY FEED INTAKE.

The problem, in this situation, is to try and estimate how much feed the horse is actually getting from the pasture and how much concentrate and or grain and or hay needs tc be provided to supplement the pasture intake and provide a satisfactory ration for the particular horse.

The level of feed supplementation for pasture fed horses can vary tremendously, and is dependent on:

1. The ability of the feeder to assess the level of pasture production, especially re seasonal variances.
2. the ability to use BODY CONDITION SCORING effectively to control weight and condition of the horse.
3. The palatability of the pasture compared to the concentrate type feed.
4. The cost of supplementary feed.

To those where the expense of feeding the horse is on no concern, then there is probably no need to worry about the pasture growth and production, just use the paddock as a bigger PARKING LOT.

To those who are concerned about feeding costs, and as will be shown later, pasture feeding costs are inevitably cheaper than purchased horse feeds, the use of the BODY SCORING SYSTEMS are an ideal way of working out what your horse needs. Once you become proficient in using either one of the BODY SCORING SYSTEMS, you will be able to adjust, within reason, the HARD FEED intake so that the horse is getting the most out of the pasture and the rest is coming from the bag or the bale.

Remember the seasonal variations in pasture growth which will occur. As an example, and this probably applies in many cases, take a situation where the cow and calf stocking rate is accepted at 1 to 2 hectares. This would be a stocking rate applicable to a large area of Australia. Converted to brood mares gives a stocking rate of 1 to 3 hectares, in geldings at a rate of gelding to 1.5 hectares. At a stocking rate of three geldings to 1.5 hectares the area would be considered to be overstocked by 300%.

In terms of feed supply the area of 1.5 hectares would probably support the three geldings on good condition for about 3-4 months of the year, assuming normal seasons. For the rest of the year some form of feed supplementation would be necessary as it would be most unlikely that the paddock could produce the quantity of feed required to keep the horses in a desired physical condition.

If you want to get some idea of the DRY MATTER production of the pasture and you do not feel competent to visually assess the physical quantity of pasture production, fence of a small area generally in the corner of the paddock. Make sure the enclosed area contains pasture represented of the whole area. Get a wooden or metal square either 1/2 square metre in area or 1 square metre in area and periodically cut the pasture inside the square at ground level and weigh the pasture cut. This will give you a wet weight, so to get a DRY MATTER, leave in the sun for two days, identical to making hay and then weigh when dry. This "HAY" will contain about 12% moisture so divide that weight by 11 to get the DRY MATTER weight for the area cut and then multiply that by the necessary factor to get to production/hectare or /acre.

LOW PASTURE STOCKING RATES

This problem is the reverse of the overstocked problem but can produce some problems in some horses. Understocked pastures, especially on "fertile" soils (soils with high levels of natural phosphorus) may cause problems with inactive brood mares and ponies. Founder has been diagnosed in these types of horses at low stocking rates, particularly on 'hayed-off' or mature feed. The seed content of the dry pasture on the fertile soil has been sufficient to produce the problem. Overfat mares, at the start of the breeding season are also commonly recognised as being much more difficult to get in foal than mares carrying less weight and or increasing in weight during the mating period.

GRAZING PREFERENCE

The preference, for eating particular types and or species of plants, can vary greatly amongst horses.

The grazing horse is able to determine which growing plants to eat, initially, by the SMELL, TOUCH secondly and then once in the mouth by TASTE. SIGHT has nothing to do with what a horse eats, due to the position of the eyes on the horse's skull, it is unable to see, when grazing, anything within about 1.2 metres of its mouth.

SMELL is a very powerful sense in the horse and is undoubtedly the reason why horses will not, unless very short of feed, eat grass growing around their own excreta or faeces.

TOUCH is also a vital sense. The TACTILE hairs which grow on the lips of the horse have been developed, by nature, to allow the horse to sort out the good feed from the bad. The show ring practice of cutting the TACTILE HAIRS from the horses' nose, whilst cosmetically desirable, removes one of the two vital senses which the horse possesses in selecting what to eat. Whilst this may be satisfactory when the horse is in a fully hand fed situation, where what the horse eats is controlled by the feeder, any horse, which derives part or all of its feed intake from grazing, should have the TACTILE HAIRS present on the nose, otherwise there is always the possibility of the horse eating some plant which can cause problems and even death.

TASTE in a horse is acute, they are able to distinguish many different tastes, but it is very much an individual thing. Some horses have been seen discarding or spitting out, from the mouth, pasture plants which they have just eaten, while other horses have not done so. TASTE is the last line of feed acceptance or feed rejection before the feed enters the digestive tract.

There have been some studies done on the palatabilities or grazing preferences of SOME grazing pasture species. The problems with using the results of these trials are as follows:-

1. pasture selection preference is generally based on studying a specific select number of plant species and generally has not covered a very wide range of species.
2. the trials have been restricted to certain areas.
3. most of the trials have been on green, actively growing pasture, yet in some parts, dried, hayed off pasture is equally as good as a horse feed.
4. no consideration has been taken of soil fertility and or fertiliser application. It is well known with cattle, that from a practical viewpoint, they have a decided preference to graze pasture on soils with a high level of PHOSPHORUS, and certainly do much better on that type of pasture than any other. No such information is available for the horse.
5. Not only is palatability of the pasture species important but it is also essential to ensure that it will not affect the horse. In some parts of Australia, a grass species, called SETARIA,is extremely palatable to horses, is recommended, by some people, to be the main grass in horse pastures, yet it is also proven and well known, by other people, to contain high levels of OXALATE and to produce BIG HEAD.

The summary of all is is that if you live in an area where grazing preference trials with horses have taken place and you have the same pasture species, on the same soil type, with the same fertiliser treatment, then the result are applicable to your property, individual horse differences considered. However if you do not live in that area or do not use those species in pasture, for any one of a number of agronomic reasons, the results are of little value to you.

Horses are very adaptable animals, especially in the grazing situation and you can learn a lot more about their grazing preferences, on you property, eating your pastures, by closely observing what they will and will not eat. The occasional walk over the paddock will reveal those pasture species which they like, as they will be short and close to the ground and those pasture species they do not like, all of whom will be much taller and bigger in growth habit.

PASTURE GROWTH AND NUTRIENT CHANGES

As a pasture grows the level of FIBRE or CELLULOSE, PROTEIN, ENERGY and WATER in the pasture changes. Horses will do best on pasture which is:

actively growing.
about mid-season.
about 10-15 cms (4-6 inches) in height.

This type of feed will have the best balance of fibre or cellulose, protein, energy and water for most horses. The practical problem is that it is impossible to get pastures to grow like this every day of the year.

The phases of pasture growth can be simplified as follows:

1. YOUNG ACTIVELY GROWING

The early stages of growth at the start of the season, corresponding to Spring growth for summer growing species and Autumn growth for winter growing species. Pasture is young, fresh and, in Spring, literally growing in front of your eyes. This type of pasture is generally reasonable in protein and energy but low in fibre or cellulose and high in water. Pasture, at this stage,is not an optimum diet for most horses as the digestible nutrient level is low and the horse cannot eat enough per day to get sufficient protein and energy to satisfy its daily needs. In the paddock horses, generally, have a mixed intake of pasture consisting of fresh new seasons' feed and the old mature feed remaining from the previous season's growth.

The balance of the old, dry, mature feed and the fresh, actively growing feed in the pasture mix overcomes any excessive water intake problem. In the situation where only this fresh young actively growing green pasture is available, supplementary feeding of hay will be of considerable benefit. The hay will balance out the nutrient levels and also slow down ingesta flow due to the high water level of the fresh pasture.

In most grazing situations involving fresh young growth, horses will eat hay, fed to them, provided the hay is of reasonable quality. Horses seem to be able to adjust their requirements for DRY MATTER in this regard provided the hay is fed on a regular basis, i.e. available all the time in a hay rack or fed at the same time each day.

2. MID SEASON ACTIVELY GROWING PASTURE

This is the ideal horse feed, corresponding to Summer growth in summer growing species and some, but not, all winter growth in some winter growing species. The protein, energy and other nutrient levels are as high as the individual pasture species can produce, dependent of course on the seasonal conditions. The fibre or cellulose level is ideal for adequate breakdown in the large intestine and the water content is not too high to cause nutrient absorption problems in the gut. The length of this period in each pasture growth depends very much on the species concerned as well as the seasonal conditions during the period of growth. The period normally continues until the first flower or signs of seeding appear in most plants.

3. FLOWERING STAGE

As soon as the pasture species start to flower, changes take place within the plant, which reduces the nutrient level, and also the overall digestibility of the plant, to the horse. The process of flowering is the start of the period when the plant decides to ensure enough seed is produced to continue the next generation in the next season. Up to this stage all the protein and energy in the plant have been directed towards stem and leaf production, both parts of the plant which the horse will eat.

Flowering, however, starts the process where the nutrients leave the leaves, in particular, to form the flower. The end result of this is a gradual lowering of the protein and energy levels of the total plant.

A further change in the FIBRE or CELLULOSE, within the plant at flowering, also reduces the availability of the reduced level of protein, energy and other nutrients to the horse. Up to the pre-flowering stage, the plant cells were held together, initially with hemi-cellulose, readily digestible by the horse and as the plant grows, this hemi-cellulose was gradually replaced by cellulose, which is also digestible in the horse's stomach and intestines.

The act of flowering causes all the remaining hemi-cellulose to change to cellulose, and then causes some cellulose to change to lignin. Lignin is not nearly as digestible in the horses' digestive tract as is cellulose, and hence, with a reduction in protein and energy levels, due to development of the flowers and further reduced availability of these nutrients, due to the development of lignin in the plant tissues, these types of pastures are not nearly as complete for some forms of horse feeding.

4. SEEDING STAGES – MATURE DRY PASTURE

Once seed is produced, there is a further reduction in the protein and energy levels of the stems and leaves, by far the greater amount of the protein and energy now being concentrated in the seeds or grain, and a lesser availability of those nutrients to the horse, due to an increase in the lignin levels, especially in the stem. This increase in lignin levels is necessary so that the stem can support the maturing seed. If the plant cells did not have increasing lignin levels, the weight of the seed heads would cause the stem to bend and break. If this were to happen the seed would not mature and hence the plant could not properly prepare itself for the next generation.

PASTURE CONSUMPTION AND WATER INTAKE

Young actively growing pasture can have a water content of up to 90% in the early stages of growth, generally leveling out at about 80% water in the growth stages prior to flowering. Some native pasture species and some tropical and sub-tropical species may well have lesser water content than this, at corresponding stages of growth. The horse body weight determines the weight of food which can be held in the gut and the problem which may exist with horses at medium or hard levels of work, is that they may not be able to absorb enough nutrients from the total daily feed intake from pasture, to satisfy their needs.

A 450 kg. horse at rest needs about 7.0 kgs. of dry matter per day. With pasture at 80% water content, the horse would have to eat at least 35 kgs. of green actively growing pasture to get this 7.0 kgs. of dry matter.

The same horse in hard work could need up to double that amount or 14kgs of dry matter per day which, when converted to pasture containing 80% water, would mean an approximate daily consumption of 70 kgs. of growing pasture.

Under these conditions horses with reasonable work demands may not be able to eat enough material to extract all the food nutrients that they need for their expected level of work.

Basically, these horses will spend a lot of time getting rid of the excess water in their body, principally by urinating, and hence the feeding of hay, in particular and possibly other feeds, is of value in this situation.

In order to compete at expected levels, performance horses, with medium to heavy work loads, will need supplementary feed even if they are obtaining some of their nutrient requirements from pasture.

PROTEIN AND ENERGY IN PASTURE

CRUDE PROTEIN

The level of CRUDE PROTEIN in green feed varies greatly with the stage of growth of the pasture. The following will give an indication of the AVERAGE RANGE of protein values that can be expected in reasonable pasture.

All these values are presented on a dry matter basis so that comparisons can be made with the more concentrated feedstuffs to be discussed later.

AVERAGE VALUES CRUDE PROTEIN

1. Actively growing mixed pasture Spring	18-20%
2. Mid-season mixed pasture	14-18%
3. Mixed pasture flowering	8-12%
4. Mixed pasture dry and hayed off	6-12%
5. Actively growing lucerne	18-26%
6. Lucerne in flower	14-18%
7. Kikuyu well fertilised	14-16%
8. Kikuyu not fertilised	6-10%
9. Tropical pastures improved and mixed actively growing	10-14%
10. Tropical pasture improved seeding or hayed off	6-10%
11. Native pasture-Spring	6-10%
12. Native pasture-later in the season	4-8%

This list is by no means comprehensive and there are other situations and pasture types which will not be listed here.

Local inquiry of your veterinary surgeon, agronomist, livestock officer, or similarly qualified person should provide you with the data, appropriate to the individual situation.

Provided the stocking rate of horses is reasonable, and the pasture is not being used as a PARKING LOT, most horses should be able to obtain their complete protein needs from pasture.

The exceptions to the general rule may be lactating brood mares. These may need some form of protein and or supplementation, especially if the pasture has hayed off or dried up due to seasonal weather patterns.

Native pasture is generally not high enough in protein to adequately support brood mares in all but the short Spring period and protein supplementation is generally desirable to these animals on this type of feed.

Native pasture, in the temperate areas and most tropical pasture of native origin, are only capable of adequately supporting mature dry horses, as far as protein is concerned. Horses which require reasonable levels of protein for growth and/or performance will need some form of protein supplementation when grazing this type of feed.

An important point to remember is that the CRUDE PROTEIN present in growing pasture is completely balanced, i.e. it contains the 10 essential AMINO ACIDS, necessary for optimum horse performance and growth.

ENERGY

All pasture contains energy in the form CARBOHYDRATE, contained within the plant cells and in the form of hemi- cellulose, cellulose and the indigestible lignin which are components of the outer plant cell walls. The more readily available forms of CARBOHYDRATE energy are generally not present, in any quantity in the leaves or stems of mature plants, but are in fact found in much larger quantities in the seeds and grains produced by most plants.

On a dry matter basis, which allows comparison of the pasture types with grains and other feeds, pasture can have an energy content of between 15% and 65% dependent on the pasture species and the stage of growth.

Energy requirements of horses vary considerably, dependent on the amount of exercise required, but a reasonable practical rule of thumb which has survived the test of time by producing results over many horses without producing many problems, provides the following values:

a) Horses at rest or with little energy and work requirements.
Ration energy level no higher than 45% and in fact can be lower.

b) Hacks and led-in type horses which need to look attractive and pleasant, but need to be calm and obedient in the show ring.
Ration energy level no higher than 45%.

c) Horses with medium work loads such as stock horses actually working, active pony club horses and performance horses in the early stages of training. Ration energy level no higher than 50%.

d) Horses with heavy work loads, performance horses in full training, show jumpers and eventers, race horses and pacers, endurance horses and similar animals. Ration energy level from 50 to 65% energy, dependent on the size of the horse, the work load and the stage of preparation.

Most actively growing young pasture of mixed composition such as rye grass and clover, or most pasture for a period in Spring, will have an energy level of around 60 to 75% on a dry matter basis. In theory, this type of feed should be able to support and supply the energy levels for any performance horse, and in fact, over supply the energy level for horses with low work requirements, and hence low energy needs.

In practice, problems exist when grazing horses on this type of fresh young actively growing pasture.

Pasture contains up to 80% water and the problem with performance horses, on this young actively growing feed, is that they need up to 50 kgs. of green pasture per day to retain 10 kgs. of dry matter. Some 40 kgs. of the total intake, or 80% can in fact be water. The DRY MATTER intake of performance horses can DOUBLE in weight, from the period of no training to the period of peak physical activity, meaning that some 100 kgs of pasture may have to be eaten by a performance horse, in order to obtain sufficient nutrients for the physical exercise. Performance horses can suffer digestive problems on this type of feed, due to this high water intake, and in this situation it is often necessary to feed some form of hay to the animal to increase the dry matter intake as a proportion of the total ration and to decrease the actual water intake of the animal to allow a slowing down of ingesta flow in the digestive tract. Slowing down the rate of passage of ingesta flow will lead to better nutrient absorption by the digestive tract, and generally less likelihood of the horse suffering nutritional disorders.

As pasture matures, the energy level decreases as the hemi-cellulose changes to the less digestible cellulose to support the larger quantity of stem and leaf being produced by the plant.

Most mixed pastures in mid-season growth would have an energy level on a dry matter basis, of 30-55%. This type of feed should therefore be able to supply the energy needs of most types of animals with the exception of horses with heavy work loads, and performance horses in full training.

As the energy level has decreased and the cellulose level increased, there has also been a reduction in the water content of this type of feed, and generally horses can obtain all their dry matter needs with adequate energy levels, without any likelihood of nutritional disorders appearing.

Pasture which is flowering or seeding, immediately has a reduction in the available energy levels as the reasonably digestible cellulose is changing to lignin to allow the plant to support the seed head, so that the plant survives for the next generation.

This type of pasture generally has an energy level of less than 30% and, in fact, the energy level is below the desired value for virtually all animals. In practice the horse will utilise stored energy in the body, in the form of fat laid down between the muscles in periods of grazing younger pasture. In the early stages the feeder will not notice any changes in the horses conformation, but after a period of time the horse will start to lose condition.

No exact figures can be stated for this period of time before the horse will start to lose condition, as it will depend on:

1. The pasture mixture previously fed.
2. The fertiliser history of the paddock.
3. The size of the horse.
4. The workload of the animal.
5. The amount of supplementary feeding that the horse has received prior to the pasture drying off.

Generally most horses on dry mature pasture will require some form of energy supplementation, dependent on the workload.

The one possible exception is on some soils, which contain high natural phosphorus levels, the native pasture species tend to retain the seed on the plant rather than the seed fall off onto the ground. These pastures will have a higher energy level than that quoted above for dry mature pasture. In practice the energy levels may rise up to 40-45% on this type of feed.

VITAMIN CONTENT OF PASTURE

VITAMIN A

All green feed contains carotene, the factor required for the production of Vitamin A inside the horse. In addition, Vitamin A can be stored inside the liver so there is no need to feed a Vitamin A supplement to horses on pasture.

VITAMIN B COMPLEX

With the possible exception of Vitamin B1, (thiamine), needs of performance horses, all the other B Group Vitamins are present in more than adequate levels in green feed. B1 deficiency generally only occurs when the horses have access to poor quality hay and grains, and even if some form of supplementation of this type of feed is taking place to horses on pasture, the animal will generally get sufficient thiamine (B1) from the pasture to provide for its usual requirements.

VITAMIN C

In terms of present knowledge, horses do not need Vitamin C in their rations, either on pasture or when completely hand fed. VITAMIN C is made inside the digestive tract from GLUCOSE which is the main source or energy supply for the horse.

VITAMIN D

Not present in green feed but comes from sunlight or sun cured hay. Reasonable access to either will provide the horse with all its needs.

VITAMIN E

Readily available in all forms of green feed.

VITAMIN K

The horse has a positive Vitamin K balance, that is, it excretes more Vitamin K in the faeces than it takes in by mouth. Hence Vitamin K supplementation is not necessary to any horse.

MINERAL CONTENT OF PASTURE

COMMON SALT

Most growing plants contain relatively low amounts of SODIUM and CHLORINE, the two elements which make up common salt.

COMMON SALT is essential for horse nutrition as it is easily removed from the body by the sweating mechanism and the horse does not have any ability to store common salt in the body. Horses, which sweat excessively, can lose considerable quantities of common salt, from their bodies, and this has to be replaced to allow the body cells to function properly.

Grazing horses, either resting or spelling or having very low work loads are able to obtain sufficient SODIUM and CHLORINE from the growing plants for their daily needs. Any horse however which is grazing and performing at a work load which causes a reasonable degree of sweating, will require daily supplementation with common salt.

CALCIUM AND PHOSPHORUS.

Pasture species vary considerably in their actual content of CALCIUM and PHOSPHORUS as previously shown.

In practical terms, the situation can be summarised as follows. Most improved pastures contain sufficient CALCIUM and PHOSPHORUS, both in absolute amounts and within the desired ratios, to provide the average horse with the required quantities of both minerals. This is assisted by the ability of the horse to be able to store any excess of both minerals in the bone tissue, provided there is no interference from other minerals in the ration. This ability to store both CALCIUM and PHOSPHORUS allows the animal to accumulate the two minerals in times of plenty and to draw on those body mineral reserves in times when the pasture may not contain the desired levels of either or both.

Exceptions to the above statement are as follows.

1. GREEN GRAZING OATS and similar grazing winter cereal crops, BARLEY and WHEAT, are surprisingly low in CALCIUM and high in PHOSPHORUS and some form of supplementation is required to horses, where most or all of the feed requirements are obtained from grazing green winter cereals.

2. With a number of sub-tropical and tropical grasses, including kikuyu and kikuyu based pastures, there is always the problem of the presence of OXALATE in the plants which renders the CALCIUM unavailable to the horse.
3. LUCERNE has a high level of CALCIUM, both in terms of absolute amounts and in the ratio with PHOSPHORUS, and the feeding of pure lucerne, or straight lucerne hay to horses under three years of age MAY cause a possible PHOSPHORUS deficiency.

IRON

All pasture species contain more than adequate levels of IRON to support the requirements of any type of normal healthy horse and there is no technical need for any type of iron supplementation for grazing horses.

Similarly, the same comments apply to the availability of MAGNESIUM, SULPHUR, ZINC, COPPER, COBALT, MANGANESE, MOLYBDENUM, SELENIUM, IODINE and FLUORINE. With very few and individually specific exceptions, which are detailed in full in the chapter on minerals, grazing horses will be able to obtain all their needs of these minerals from pasture.

HORSE GROWTH ON PASTURE

Despite the fact that horses have grazed, bred, survived and performed on a pasture diet for years, very little is actually known about the absolute, or physiological or mathematical details of how horses grow and perform on pasture, when compared to commonly accepted roughages and "hard feeds".

This lack of technical data is undoubtedly a factor of the tremendous variation in pasture types which horses graze, as well as the lack of facilities and possibly finance to do the experiments. Some horse people have just accepted that horses survive on pasture.

One particular experiment carried out in the U.S. measuring the growth rates of yearlings, under controlled conditions of grazing ALFALFA (LUCERNE). At controlled stocking rates of 1 yearling to 0.7 hectares (1.71 acres), these horses showed daily LIVE WEIGHT GAINS in the range of 0.22-0.59 kgs (0.5-1.3 lbs)/horse/day. Allowing for the natural variation, between horses, in genetic ability to grow, these growth rates were very similar to those recommended by the N.R.C. The conclusion from this experiment was that grazing lucerne was the complete horse feed for yearling horses.

Practical problems in interpreting these results include that of stocking rate and rainfall. The researchers clearly adopted a stocking rate which allowed the horse population to be equated to the lucerne growth. Had the stocking rate been increased or the rainfall less than normal, then these results may not have occurred.

All this goes to show is that PASTURE, of most types and species composition, is ideal horse feed but STOCKING RATE or CARRYING CAPACITY needs to be adjusted to make allowance for variations in pasture growth which in turn will be affected by soil fertility, fertilizer application and rainfall.

LABELS FOR PASTURES

LABELS, indicating the names of the feed components and the concentration of those components are generally required, by law, to be placed on any horse feed WHICH HAS BEEN PHYSICALLY ALTERED, CONTAINS AN ARTIFICIALLY PRODUCED COMPONENT OR IS AN ARTIFICIAL MIXTURE OF A NUMBER OF COMPONENTS.

LABELS are NOT REQUIRED, BY LAW, to be placed on pasture.

The problem with the use of labels, is that people start to think that all the necessary feed components are in the labeled products, generally supplements and or pre-mixed ready to use feeds, and that none of these feed components are present in normal grazing pasture.

NOTHING COULD BE FURTHER FROM THE TRUTH

Before the advent of all these various feed supplements, prior to about the early 1900's and which are now available to "feed" to horses, they bred, grew, raced and survived on pastures. They did this simply because good quality pasture CONTAINS ALL the feed components which the horse needs.

Very simply, if that had not been the case, the horse would not have become adapted to use the feeds it does, to survive, or alternately, the horse population would have died out due to a nutritional problem.

The main problem from the average horse feeders' angle, is that it has never been explained to them just what pasture contains compared to other feeds and feed supplements. At times, the various labels, on feed supplements and pre mixed feeds, are completely bewildering and confusing, and the additional advertising material, provided with most of these products, tend to indicate that each product is absolutely essential for the survival of the horse.

The preceding sections of this chapter should be sufficient to show that pasture contains all the feed nutrients required by the horse. The main problem with pasture feeding comes with performance horses. Any horse, expected to work at medium or higher levels of activity, is not able to get sufficient energy, in particular, from pastures. Hence the need for the feeding of an additional energy source, commonly grain, which is itself deficient in some other horse feed nutrients, principally VITAMINS, MINERALS and AMINO-ACIDS, and so some type of feed supplementation may be required at this level of activity.

WEEDS

A WEED is a plant with no economic use, or a WEED is a plant growing where it is not wanted. Man is unable, for a number of reasons, to use the vegetative parts or the seeds of plants commonly called weeds.

This book is not going to provide a list of the various weeds which may affect horses. With the many different climates, soil types and pasture species that are used for horse production, any such list would never be complete. This book will detail the various categories into which weeds can be grouped and it is up to each individual, to determine at a local level, whether any plant is a weed and the method of control and or eradication.

1. INDICATORS OF LOW SOIL FERTILITY

There are a number of plants (weeds) which will appear in a pasture as the soil fertility declines. The decline in soil fertility will occur, as a result of the slow but gradual removal of plant nutrients, basically minerals, from the soil,without replacement. This mineral removal occurs because the plants need minerals from the soil to grow, the horses eat the plants and so take out most of the minerals for their own use, returning only very small quantities back to the soil in the form of urine and faeces.

If these minerals are not returned to the soil, commonly by fertiliser application of some specific type, there will be a gradual decline in soil fertility as the natural soil making processes from the bed rock beneath the soil are not able to make soil minerals as fast as they are being removed.

With this decline in soil fertility, there will be changes in the plant population some weeds will appear in the pasture, happy to survive and, in fact, encouraged to develop by the declining mineral level of the soil. These weeds are generally NOT PALATABLE to horses but as they increase in number and cover a greater area of the pasture, their presence will reduce the overall carrying capacity and production from the paddock.

The common cure for these types of weeds is to apply some type of selective spray. Application of the correct fertiliser, to restore soil fertility, may well do the same thing as sprays PLUS increase the content of desirable plant species and hence produce better horses.

2. INDICATORS OF HIGH SOIL FERTILITY

Some weed species are often an indicator of high soil fertility. They will be very profuse growers, often attaining considerable size but are always unpalatable to horses and, in most instances, to other livestock. These weeds cannot be reduced in number or in size by the application of fertiliser, as they only grow on the good soil anyway. They can only be controlled by either establishing a more vigorous pasture, which literally grows faster than the weeds and crowds them out or alternately by chemical methods. Some of these high fertility weeds may require a combination of the two methods to achieve some degree of control.

3. RESTRICT PASTURE PRODUCTION

There are many weeds which affect pasture production, simply by competing with the pasture species, no matter what the level of soil fertility. These weeds generally have a flat or prostrate form and cover the ground, preventing any productive plant species from growing on the covered area. These weeds always possess the ability to grow slightly faster than the productive pasture plants, especially early in the season or growth cycle. All these weeds are unpalatable to horses and definitely reduce the productive capacity of the pasture.

The methods of control consist of establishing plants which can grow faster than these types of weeds, early in the growing period and so dominate the weed as the weed is currently dominating the existing pasture and or the use of chemical methods of weed control.

4. AFFECT HORSE HEALTH.

WEEDS which affect horse health can be divided into two groups.

A. PHYSICAL INJURY

There are a number of weeds which have thorns, spikes and other projections on the stems and leaves. It is not unusual for a horse to have some of these thorns or spikes penetrate the lower legs, in particular, causing infections, pain, lameness etc.

B. CAUSING ILLNESS AND OR DEATH.

These are the weeds to be wary of, they are often palatable to the horse, not all the time but generally at specific times of the year or when there is nothing left to eat in the paddock. They will either act suddenly as in the case of CYANIDE POISONING, possibly leading to death within minutes of being ingested or they slowly accumulate in the horse over a number of months until the excess levels get to the stage where the horse shows external signs of a problem. The best example of this is BOBTAIL DISEASE in the U.S. where SELENIUM accumulates within the horse, due to the ingestion of certain plant species which accumulate SELENIUM from the soil.

These types of plants need to be identified and the way in which they MAY KILL or permanently affect a horse understood. Some species of these types of plants need to be eradicated and destroyed, others such as the SELENIUM accumulating plants, in the U.S. are too widespread to economically eradicate and are only eaten when other and better horse grazing gets short, so in this instance a changed grazing strategy and or supplementary hand feeding has to take place.

LEVEL OF HAND FEEDING ON PASTURE

The amount of hand feeding that each individual horse may require, when grazing pasture, is dependent on the following factors:

1. Stocking rate on the pasture
2. Drenching programme for the horses
3. Stage of maturity of the pasture
4. Work programme or use for the horse

Even though it is desirable to consider all these points, it is important to remember that the average horse is a "lazy" feeder and will prefer to eat concentrate, hay, chaff and other foods, provided by the owner, rather than forage around the paddock and eat the pasture on the ground. This feature of horse's eating habits is generally a function of the better palatability of the prepared feeds and the animals preference to wait for the "convenience" foods, rather than forage around the paddock.

If the horses are continually waiting at the gate to be fed, then it is most likely that one of two alternatives are happening. The first is that the grazing area is completely eaten out and the horses are only able to obtain their fodder needs from hand feeding. The second reason would generally be that, whilst the grazing area will provide sufficient pasture to adequately maintain most horses, the level of hand feeding allows the horse to substitute the more expensive purchased feeds for the cheaper pasture.

Many instances have been observed where the horses will not move, at any time during a twenty four period, from the general hand feeding area despite the fact that there is more than sufficient grazing pasture available in the paddock.

Horses are worse than spoilt children as far as eating habits are concerned. Horses are also very lazy eaters and can often put it over, or fool, the person feeding the horse.

Grains and other concentrates always appear to be more palatable to the horse than pasture, even if the pasture is the best available in the peak of the spring season.

No matter what quantity of concentrate or grains the horse is given, it will always eat those feeds in preference to any pasture growing at the time. Horses will always substitute grain and allied feeds, for pasture in their diet.

The situation has been seen many times where up to 5 kgs of grain or pellets have been fed to horses with access to pasture and the pasture at the time is growing faster than the horse can eat it. The horses are simply substituting the more palatable, more easily digested, less difficult to obtain and generally more expensive feed for the cheaper and generally equally good quality pasture available on the ground.

In this type of feeding situation, the horse is probably doing just as well on the prepared feeds as they would do on pasture, but at increased expense to the owner.

Reduction in the level of grain feeding, in most of these instances, has had no effect on the condition of the horse as it has only caused the horse to spend more time grazing and receive a greater proportion of its daily fodder needs from the pasture.

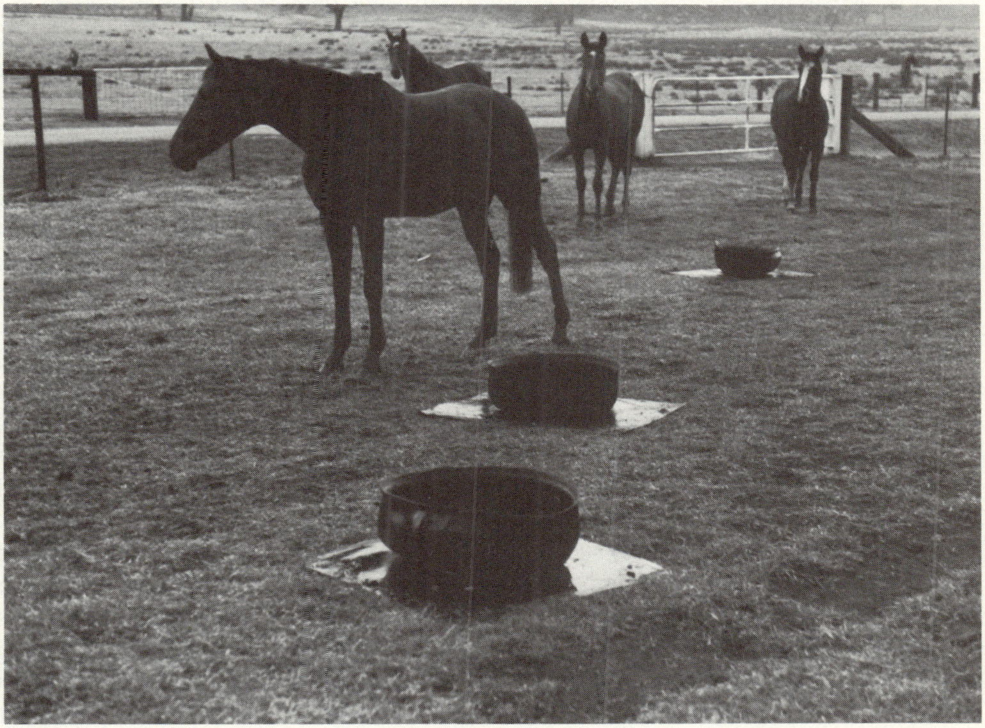

Thoroughbred yearlings being supplementary fed in ideal feeders.

The main problem in reducing grain feeding in these situations is not a horse problem but a HUMAN PROBLEM. The horse has to learn that the grass is as good as the grain and the human has to realise that the horse will stand at the gate, or feed shed, or whatever, waiting for its feed. Provided the human resists the temptation to provide some hard feed, the horse will eventually realise that grazing is the answer to the problem of an empty stomach.

Generally most horse properties are overstocked relative to the normal carrying capacity of the same properties when looked upon as a cattle operation.

Factors to consider when trying to assess a reasonable stocking rate are:

1. Season of the year. Carrying capacity will always be best in Spring compared to other seasons.
2. Natural soil fertility. Pastures on soil with high levels of natural phosphorus will always have a higher carrying capacity than pastures on soils with low natural phosphorus levels.
3. Pasture composition. Native pasture species are generally notable to support as great an overall stocking rate as pastures which contain improved pasture species. These improved pasture species will vary tremendously, due to the many climatic zones and soil types.
4. Normal carrying capacity. Each area generally has a normal carrying capacity which the established landowners have determined, over a period of years,andisthe generally accepted stocking rate that will allow them to satisfactorily grow and fatten cattle and stay in business.

These figures, if available, should be used as a guide by the horse feeder as to the number of animals that can be satisfactorily run on an area without the need for hand feeding. Remember that any cattle carrying figures supplied must be increased by about 50% to allow for the selected grazing habits of horses.

For horses on pasture, supplementary feeding is often the same as giving lollies or candies and chocolates to children. Children will always eat the lollies and chocolates first even though they may not be of much value. Horses will always eat grain and other supplements first, even though they may be able to get the same quantities of food nutrients from the pasture.

Preference will always be shown, by horses, to feeds which are chaffed, ground, pelleted or prepared in some manner. Even if the palatability of the feed is the same as pasture, or even less palatable, practical tests have shown that horses always prefer convenience foods. The mere fact that the horse ate all his rations of grain and concentrate, when grazing actively growing pasture is only an indication that he has substituted that grain and concentrate for actively growing pasture, and is having an easy time in obtaining his feed.

The problem can also exist with horses, fed large amounts of grain and/or concentrate in pasture situations, of an interruption in constant ingesta flow through the gut. This can cause any number of nutritional disorders which are dealt with in this book. This intermittent gut flow is simply due to the fact that the horse may wait around the feeding area, for hours, for the normal time of feeding grain and or concentrate. The animal, then generally, consumes the concentrate ration as quickly as possible and then usually does not graze again for sometime as the digestive tract is full. Dependent on all the circumstances the horse will commence grazing when it again feels hungry, causing, at times, considerable variation in gut fill.

The horse continually on pasture and deriving all its feed from that source, will generally maintain a reasonably consistent gut fill and ingesta flow and should not suffer the potential problems of horses being fed excessive levels of concentrate and substituting that concentrate for growing pasture. Horses can be educated to graze during most of the day and night, provided the level of supplementary feeding is carefully adjusted by the horse feeder. As the use of horses vary considerably, and each owner has separate aims and wishes as to the horses' ultimate achievements, the extent of supplementary feeding to horses on pasture is an individual decision. The details outlined above should help those people to assess their actual feeding programmes, hopefully at a lesser cost than at present.

COSTS OF KEEPING A HORSE AT PASTURE

Provided the horse can maintain itself and perform on pasture alone, this is normally the cheapest way of feeding horses.

Most people generally feel that the cost to feed a horse on grass is very small. It is if you do your calculations on the estimated cost to reduce 1KG of DRY MATTER but it is necessary to look at the alternate uses for that DRY MATTER, the most common, of which, is feeding the same pasture to cattle and selling beef.

The correct way to assess the cost of feeding horses on grass is to assess the alternative income that may be generated from that same area of grass by some other use, in this example beef production.

Let us take an area where it is possible to carry say, one cow to 2 hectares, and to produce from that cow one vealer type calf per year. At say, a net return on farm, after sale costs, of $300, the gross income per hectare will amount to $150.

Horses are accepted as notorious finicky or selective graziers, and, generally, to allow a horse to maintain itself in good condition on pastures alone, requires at least 50% more area than to graze a cow and calf and to produce a satisfactory vealer.

Our comparative horse would then need 3 hectares to graze satisfactorily for an income, foregone from the inability to run cattle on the same area of $450. This horse at pasture is then costing $8.65/week. (1989 values).

No consideration has been taken of the cost of drenches etc., in fact it would be more expensive for one horse, on a yearly basis, than the cost of drenching etc. would be for one cow and one calf.

Dependent on your own area, the carrying capacity and cattle returns may vary, but the principles of the calculation remain the same.

The average horse, grazing pasture at reasonable stocking rates should be able to obtain all its nutrient needs from the mixed green feed, with the exception of salt and calcium, and/or phosphorus when grazing particular pasture species. Pastures do not come with labels on them similar to prepared feed supplements, but despite this fact average quality mixed pasture will contain virtually all the feed needs of most horses.

Problems start to occur in feeding horses on pasture when:

1. Carrying capacity or stocking rate is higher than normally accepted, the PARKING LOT approach. In this situation the problem will largely be one of reduced total dry matter intake with a resultant decrease in the total amounts of the individual feed nutrients that the horse is able to consume and the possible need for some level of supplementary feeding.

2. When pastures dry off and mature and decreased nutrient availability, (generally protein and/or energy), takes place in the plants due to seeding process.
3. When horses are performing at medium or higher levels of work and generally are not able to satisfy their energy needs from pasture.

The combination of factors affecting the final decision about the desirable level of supplementary feeding on pasture, e.g. stocking rate, season of the year, size of horse, work load, pasture composition, pasture maturity, and the horses' previous feeding history are many. It is hoped that the explanation of the principles involved will enable people to understand the feed nutrients that are available in most pastures and allow informed decisions to be made as to the type of supplement, if any, that the horse may need.

SPECIFIC PASTURE PROBLEMS

LOCO WEED POISONING

LOCO WEED (ASTRAGALUS and OXYTROPIS species) poisoning frequently occurs in the same areas as the problems of SELENIUM TOXICITY and the two are sometimes incorrectly diagnosed. LOCO WEED poisoning is caused by organic substances and is not related to SELENIUM TOXICITIES. The LOCO WEED needs to be grazed for some period of time before the symptoms become obvious. These include abortions, birth defects, and loss of weight. There is generally always some permanent destruction of parts of the nervous system.

SWEET CLOVER POISONING

This will occur as a result of what could be called spoiled sweet clover hay and or silage being fed to horses. Spoiling involves any reduction in hay quality, due to the presence of moisture at the time of hay making, leading to the development of mouldy hay. In silage production, quality can be markedly reduced, due to inadequate sealing of the silage pit or stack, allowing the entry of oxygen and the resultant change in the silage, from feed to a type of compost.

These changes cause the coumarins in the clover to change to dicoumeral which in turn causes internal and external bleeding in the horse, stiffness and lameness, etc. The condition can only be avoided by not feeding such damaged hay and or silage to horses.

CYANIDE POISONING

Fodder species of the summer growing SORGHUM family, including Johnson grass, Sudan grass, and the various hybrid Sorghum fodders all contain compounds called cyanogenetic glycosides which are changed inside the horse to hydocyanic acid which produces CYANIDE poisoning. A similar problem can also occur with other plants, namely Arrow grass, wild black cherry, chokecherry, pincherry and flax, which also contain the same dangerous factor.

The level of the cyanide producing products are highest in these plants during rapid growth, immediately following cold weather, in periods when soil moisture is lacking, causing wilting, and whenever the leaves change to a bluish green colour instead of maintaining a green colour.

The condition of cyanide poisoning in horses is called ENZOOTIC EQUINE CYSTITIS and symptoms include urinary incontinence, hind leg inco-ordination and muscle twitching over the hindquarter. The condition can be FATAL, death can occur within one hour of eating sorghum plants if the level of the cyanogenetics glycosides in the plants is high enough. Very few horses ever recover and then not completely. Sorghum hay, if made correctly from actively growing plants will be free of the problem. However sorghum hay made from wilted plants will probably still contain the dangerous factor. IF AT ALL POSSIBLE, DO NOT GRAZE HORSES ON SORGHUM OR ALLIED SPECIES. There is also the possibility that grain harvested from SORGHUM crops, grown under conditions of moisture stress may also contain the toxic factor.

FESCUE TOXICITY

FESCUE (FESCUE ARUNDINACEA) is a cool seasonal perennial grass, well known for its ability to tolerate heavy grazing and changing weather conditions. Grazing pregnant mares on FESCUE can produce problems, some of which will include unusually thick placentas, extended pregnancies, abortions and AGALACTIA or no milk production in the mare. In a survey of pregnant mares, 27% of mares grazing Fescue during their pregnancy had foaling difficulties whilst of mares grazing non fescue pasture, only 8% had foaling difficulties.

There appears to be some relationship between these problems and the low Selenium content of the fescue pasture, but this matter still has to be clarified.

Pregnant mares should not be grazed on fescue pasture, if at all possible, secondly encourage clover and legumes to grow amongst the fescue but if the pasture mix on the property is such that the grazing of fescue dominant pastures cannot be avoided try and get the mares off fescue for the three months prior to foaling. If this is not possible, allow the mares unrestricted access to lucerne hay whenever grazing fescue.

RYEGRASS STAGGERS

Occurs when horses eat RYEGRASS which is infested with certain fungi and moulds. The damaged ryegrass can cause considerable metabolic changes within the horse, leading to the development of muscle tremors, gait inco-ordination and tetany.

PHOTOSENSITIZATION

PHOTOSENSITIZATION occurs when the horse eats plants which contain chemicals which affect the composition of the skin and allow sunlight to produce changes in skin tissue. The problem can also occur as a result of liver damage. PHOTOSENSITIZATION can be caused, in horses, by the intake of pastures containing ALSIKE CLOVER and ST JOHN'S WORT and some other plant species. The PHOTOSENSITIZATION is generally accompanied by liver damage.

LEGUME PASTURE

Any pasture containing legumes which are affected with the mould RHIZOCTONIA LEGUMINICOLA, causing the production in the legume of a toxic factor called SLAFRAMINE, may cause excessive salivation in horses after ingestion. This problem can develop into diarrhoea and loss of weight. The mould will develop in conditions of high humidity and or rainfall, and apart from removing the horses from the affected pasture, there is no known treatment. The mould will disappear when the period of high rainfall and or humidity ceases and the weather returns to a drier phase.

HIGH OXALATE PASTURES

refer NUTRITIONAL SECONDARY HYPERPARATHYROIDISM

in the chapter on NUTRITIONAL DISORDERS.

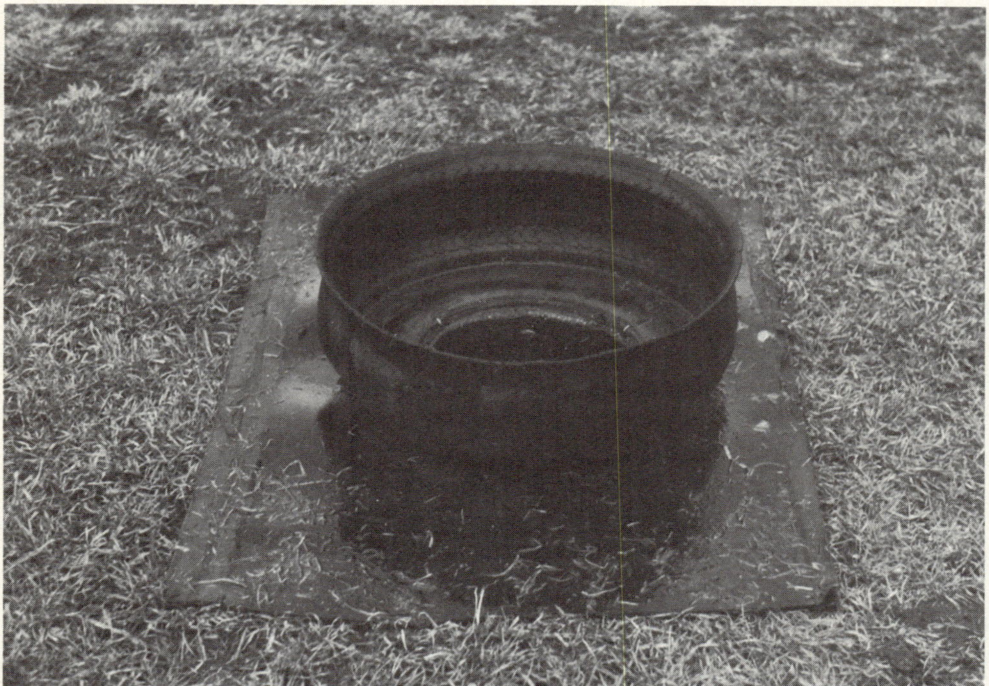

Close up of an ideal paddock feeder, old car tyres and belting, little chance of injury to horses.

20. COMMON HORSE FEEDS

The most common horse feeds are classified into a series of groups based on PROTEIN and ENERGY content, on a DRY MATTER BASIS, not AS FED. The figures provided are based on averages and there will often be considerable variation in actual PROTEIN and ENERGY content of various feeds, due to SOIL FERTILITY and seasonal circumstances during the growing period. The various details of PROTEIN, ENERGY and T.D.N. content are summarised in table form within the chapter.

LOW PROTEIN, LOW ENERGY FEEDS

CEREAL HAY - CEREAL CHAFF - CHOPPED CEREAL HAY

C.P. about 8.0%. D.E. about 1.90 MCal/kg.
T.D.N. about 45% 7.90 MJ/kg.

Included in this category is both OATEN and WHEATEN HAY and the CHAFF made by chopping such hay into small lengths. Chaffing hay does not alter the feed nutrient values in any way, the process only allows more rapid attack by the enzymes, within the digestive tract of the horse.

These feeds contain enough protein to maintain dry adult horses in reasonable condition for short periods of time, but have an energy level which is insufficient for any activity but survival. CEREAL HAYS and CHAFFS also contain low levels of CALCIUM, very high levels of PHOSPHORUS, very low VITAMIN A activity and a high LIGNIN content. When used as the major proportion of the roughage intake of dry adult horses, these feeds require supplementation with CALCIUM and VITAMIN A and will have a poor digestibility due to high LIGNIN or FIBRE content.

Due to the above technical deficiencies with these feeds, they are NOT RECOMMENDED to be fed to any of the following types of horses:-

LACTATING MARES, ANY GROWING HORSE,(foals, weanlings and yearlings), and ANY PERFORMANCE HORSE.

The use of oaten or wheaten chaff, as a horse feed, is a legacy of the days in the cereal growing areas when large teams of draught horses were used for farming. In those times,it was logical for the farmers to cut their hay from the paddocks and use that hay or chaff to feed their horses. However, it must be remembered that the horses in those areas would, in most seasons, only be on the cereal chaff and hay for a period for about four months per year. For the rest of the year, the horses generally had access to green pasture which, in adult horses, would allow excess protein, energy, calcium and VITAMIN A, to be stored in the body, for use during the period of the year when CEREAL HAY and or CHAFF, provided the bulk of the diet.

When CEREAL CHAFF and or CEREAL HAY provides the bulk of the roughage portion of the ration, as in fully hand fed stabled horses, there is no opportunity for the stabled horse to build up body reserves of CALCIUM, PHOSPHORUS and VITAMIN A from any green feeds so there are no body reserves from which the horse can draw upon to satisfy the deficiencies in the cereal roughages.

In most areas, chaffs made from lucerne and pasture hay are cheaper to feed than the cereal chaffs when consideration is taken of the protein, energy, mineral and vitamin contents and hence there is little reason on technical or economic grounds to feed cereal chaff, unless it is produced on the property at minimal cost and fed to the horses on that property.

LOW PROTEIN, HIGH ENERGY FEEDS

MOLASSES

C.P. varies 2-9%. D.E. about 3.40 MCal/kg.
T.D.N. about 60%. 14.00 MJ/kg.

MOLASSES is commonly made from sugar cane or sugar beet but may also be made from citrus and maize (corn). The protein present in MOLASSES varies considerably, dependent on the the soil fertility in which the original crop grew, from which the MOLASSES was extracted. The PROTEIN is also mostly NON PROTEIN NITROGEN and therefore of little value in horse nutrition. For practical purposes, the PROTEIN content of MOLASSES is ignored when calculating horse rations.

Every 1 kg of molasses contains 500 gram's or 50% of sugars. This energy level is sufficient to provide enough energy to most horses, performance horses excepted. However the energy will not be effectively utilised unless the molasses is supplemented with a protein source that raises the total protein of the ration above the 8% level.

Molasses is often used in many pre-mixed feeds, pellets etc. as a "binder" at levels of 2-3% of the total ration and some of the SWEET FEEDS contain levels of MOLASSES as high as 10%. Molasses is a handy feed component, especially from the palatability angle. Molasses to horses is like lollies to children, although there are some horses which find molasses unpalatable. Molasses should never be used in horse feeding to disguise the taste of bad feeds. Horses will eat mouldy grain or hay, wet hay, weevil infested grain etc. if the taste is sufficiently disguised with molasses. The feeding of cheap feeds to horses in this fashion is definitely not recommended as the molasses does not decrease the main problem of mould, moisture, weevils etc. and the horse may suffer a digestive upset from these types of feeds. It is false economy to use molasses in horse feeding in this manner.

CORN AND COB MEAL

C.P. about 6.0%. D.E. about 3.00 MCal/kg.
T.D.N. about 73%. 12.30 MJ/kg.

Common in maize growing areas where husk is removed from the cob of corn and the whole cob, plus grain, is generally hammer-milled to produce a meal. There is a reduction in levels of PROTEIN and ENERGY compared to maize (corn) grain as the cob is low in all nutrients and the inclusion of the cob with the grain will dilute these levels and markedly increase fibre content.

Feeding corn and cob meal is really only recommended to horses with low work loads and even then the animal would need to have access to high protein feed as 6% protein is probably the bare minimum level of protein needed to keep a horse alive.

FATS AND OILS

ANIMAL FAT

C.P. 0% D.E. about 8.00 MCal/kg.
32.80 MJ/kg.

ANIMAL FATS, used in horse feeding, consist of any fat derived principally from cattle and sheep.

VEGETABLE FATS

C.P. 0% D.E. about 9.00 MCal/kg.
36.90 MJ/kg.

VEGETABLE FATS are the oils which are derived from oilseeds, normally by the solvent extraction process and commonly called, polyunsaturated oils used for household and industrial cooking. Included in this category are SUNFLOWER OIL, SAFFLOWER OIL, SOYBEAN OIL, COTTONSEED OIL, CANOLA OIL etc.

These fats or oils, whether of animal or plant origin are used in horse feeding at low levels (1-3%) of the ration as a binder to hold the feed components to-gether or in larger quantities as a source of energy.

MEDIUM PROTEIN, MEDIUM ENERGY FEEDS

HAY

HAY quality, the term used so frequently by horse people, can be defined as being dependent on:-

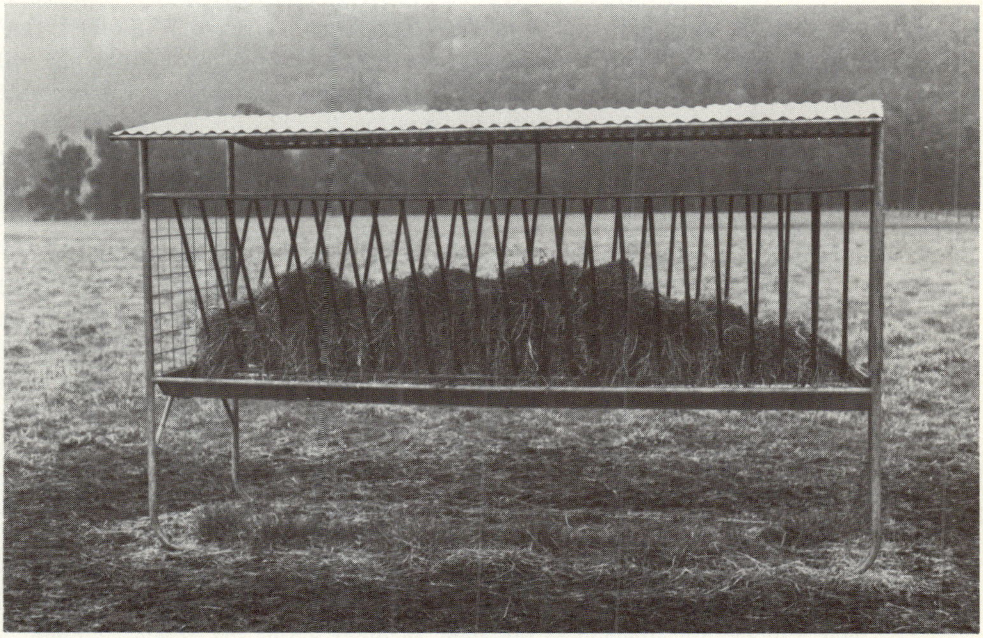

Close up of covered hay rack.

1. STAGE OF MATURITY when the crop is cut.

In order to achieve the maximum amount of retained nutrients in HAY, is should be cut at the stage when the first flowers appear. At this time, the plants will contain the maximum levels of PROTEIN and ENERGY, the content of the various MINERALS and VITAMINS, remaining fairly constant, no matter what the stage of cutting. The exception to this rule will be the CAROTENE level, the pre-cursor of VITAMIN A. Green colour AT CUTTING is indicative of CAROTENE level, so the less the green colour of the material, being cut, the less the CAROTENE level.

The stage of flowering is relatively easily seen with plants of the LEGUME family, these plants produce prominent visible flowers. With members of the GRASS family, flowering is not so obvious, so to obtain the greatest concentration of nutrients in the hay, cutting is done at the "BOOT STAGE", when the seed head just starts to appear from the top of the stem.

As flowering and seeding progresses, the nutrient concentrations in the pasture will decrease BUT the FIBRE level will increase in turn leading to the production of greater weight of hay/hectare but with reduced feeding value.

2. PRESENCE OF WEEDS BEFORE CUTTING

The crop should be weed free, especially containing no noxious or undesirable weeds. WEEDS with large fleshy leaves such as thistles, docks etc. take longer to dry than the grass and or legume being used for hay, with the result that when the desired species are dry enough to bale, the large leafed weds are still moist, leading to the development of mould, within any bales containing such weeds.

3. PROBLEMS AT HAYMAKING TIME.

HAY MAKING is entirely dependent on the weather which occurs AFTER THE HAY has been cut. Provided ideal weather conditions follow cutting, top quality hay will probably be made. However, is is possible for the best quality hay at mowing to become a second or third grade product at baling, dependent on:-

1. any rain which falls on the crop after cutting and before being placed in the shed. Rain can occur at various stages during hay making and the effect of rain on hay can be considered from the following:-

   A – rain after baling, hay still in the paddock. Dependent on the amount of rain, will only affect the outside of the bale, and will probably not penetrate inside the bale, to any extent. Provided the bales are turned to get the wet bottoms dried out before shedding, little damage will be done to baled hay in all but heavy rainfall.

   B – rain on hay after mowing and before raking. Can affect quality, will probably get some leaf loss but if the weather conditions, immediately following the rain are ideal for drying, reasonable hay can be made.

   C – rain on hay after raking but before baling. This is the worst time to get rain on hay, the compact windrows are unable to be teased out completely to dry and quality will always suffer if rain falls at this time.

2. Air temperature at time of baling. Baling should always take place when the hay is 12% moisture, this is the level at which mould will not develop and where the leaf will remain attached to the stem, in other words the greatest amount of nutritious feed will be harvested. Even if the hay is tested with a moisture meter,

the decision as when to bale is a human one and even 30 minutes delay in the start of baling can lead to hay being produced which is drier than normal resulting in much less leaf than normal, particularly if there is a rapid increase in temperature during the hay baling operation. It is for this reason that most professional hay producers tend to bale during the night.

4. HANDLING OF THE HAY AFTER MAKING.

After baling, the hay has to picked up off the paddock and transported to a shed. This involves the use of elevators, machines which pick the hay up from the ground and moved to a level where the bales can be stacked on truck etc. for transport to the shed. If the hay is baled at a moisture level which is considered too dry, any leaf, which was on the hay in the windrow, will not be present on the outside of the bale having shaken or fallen off during baling and or transport. This especially applies to any hay made from leguminous species of plants. such as ALFALFA (LUCERNE) and the CLOVERS. The presence of leaf on the outside of a bale of hay should indicate baling at the correct moisture level. Up to 10% of the nutrients present in the pasture can be lost from the hay, due to incorrect handling procedures after baling.

5. BUYING HAY

A – smell the bale for a pleasant aroma, any unusual smell should be followed by a check for dampness, mould, or similar conditions. Ask can you open a bale to have a look inside - any reasonable hay supplier should always oblige to this request.

B – check to make sure that the leaf stays attached to the stem when you open the bale up. If hay has been baled too dry, the leaf will tend to fall off the stem, when a bale is opened up. As most of the food nutrients are in the leaf, this is the part of the plant that the horse should get. It is of little value, if the leaf is so dry as to fall onto the ground and be trodden upon by the animals as they eat the coarser, and not so valuable, stems.

C – the more flowers and or seed present in the hay, the more mature the hay was at cutting and the greater the amount of fibre and a reduction in the levels of the necessary feed nutrients.

D – colour is the last item to consider when buying hay. Many people consider that the greener the lucerne hay, the more the potential Vitamin A content. A number of studies have shown that the loss of carotene, the Vitamin A precursor, occurs more rapidly than loss of colour. Refer to the section on vitamins for a more detailed analysis on this topic.

HAY can be made from any one of three types of pasture.

A. All legume B. All grass C. Mixed grass and legume.

The preferred horse feeding hays are generally those made from plants of the legume family, the most favoured being ALFALFA or LUCERNE HAY, although similar hays can be made form many of the plants in the clover family. In the production of LEGUME HAY, the horse feeder should be more interested in the leaf content of the bale than the stems, the reason being that the leaves contain 66% of the energy and 75% of the protein in the total mix of leaves and stems.

Also, on average LEGUME HAY, compared to GRASS HAY, contains higher energy, twice the amount of protein, 3 or 4 times the amount of CALCIUM, equivalent levels of PHOSPHORUS and 5 times the amount of CAROTENE, the precursor of VITAMIN A.

ALFALFA HAY-LUCERNE HAY

C.P. about 16-20%. D.E. about 2.30 MCal/kg
T.D.N. about 54% 9.40 MJ/kg.

Good to excellent quality LUCERNE (ALFALFA) HAY contains a protein level sufficient to provide the needs for all types of horses. The protein, present in lucerne hay, also provides the ten essential amino acids that ALL horses require for optimum feed utilisation. The ENERGY level of LUCERNE (ALFALFA) HAY is sufficient for any horse which is doing nothing - AT REST -, or which has a LIGHT WORK LOAD. Lucerne hay also provides more than adequate levels of Vitamin A, Vitamin D, Vitamin E and reasonable levels of Vitamin B. All the necessary minerals are present in adequate levels with the EXCEPTION of PHOSPHORUS for growing horses. The CALCIUM to PHOSPHORUS ratio is about 4.1, but can extend to 6.1, which means that there can be a problem with a lack of PHOSPHORUS, in the ration, if lucerne hay is the only feed supply to young growing horses, possibly leading to some form of METABOLIC BONE DISEASE or DEVELOPMENTAL ORTHOPAEDIC DISEASE.

Any mature horse, over 4 years of age, including the week-end horse, the pony, most horses at rest or spelling, and even horses doing up to one hours work per day can perform and maintain good body condition on a diet of lucerne (alfalfa) hay alone.

When the specifications of a good average horse feed, for MATURE HORSES, is analysed, lucerne (alfalfa) hay fits the details better than any other feed.

ALFALFA CHAFF-LUCERNE CHAFF

LUCERNE or ALFALFA CHAFF, sometimes known as CHOPPED HAY, is simply lucerne hay cut up into small pieces and as such there is no change at all in the protein, energy or other nutrient levels in the chaff, as opposed to the hay. CHAFF or CHOPPED HAY is only as good as the hay from which it is made.

The comments applying to lucerne hay are therefore directly applicable to lucerne (alfalfa) chaff.

Some manufacturers of LUCERNE (ALFALFA) CHAFF or CHOPPED HAY, however, use techniques to "enhance" the apparent value of inferior quality hay when used to make chaff. The hay is often steamed before passage into the chaff cutter. The application of a fine jet of steam allows the leaf to "come back" and means that the dry leaf does not fall off to the bottom of the chaff cutter but ends up in the bag. After a few days in the bag, the leaf tends to revert back to its original moisture level and may "powder" on feeding. As leaf contains the most food nutrients as opposed to the stem, powdered leaves are of little value to the horse. A second technique sometimes practiced is to apply a fine spray of green dye to the hay just prior to entry into the chaff cutter. Whilst this green dye gives the impression that the chaff is made from top quality fresh hay, such in fact may not be the case. DYED CHAFF can be readily detected by placing some of the CHAFF in a glass of water for a couple of hours, any green dye present will colour the water green.

PREPARED ALFALFA-LUCERNE SUPPLEMENTS

These are available in three forms - dehydrated lucerne meal, lucerne cubes and lucerne pellets. As with LUCERNE CHAFF, the quality of these products will depend on the quality of the lucerne used in the process. These processes DO NOT increase the value of the lucerne, they only make the feeds, easier to handle, store or for the horse to digest.

DEHYDRATED LUCERNE (ALFALFA) MEAL

Involves the collection of fresh lucerne (alfalfa) from the paddock by means of forage harvesting, conveyance of the freshly cut material to a dehydration plant, generally close to the source of supply, and the preparation of a lucerne (alfalfa) meal. Technically, the meal has food nutrient values similar to the lucerne (alfalfa) hay, although there may be a reduction in the availability of protein, due to the use of artificial heat in the drying process. The energy costs in terms of oil, gas, or electricity for drying is generally too high in relation to the possible sale price of the lucerne (alfalfa) meal to make the production of this type of feed an economic operation, when compared to other horse feeds. Presently there is little dehydrated lucerne (alfalfa) meal used, due to very restricted availability.

LUCERNE (ALFALFA) CUBES

LUCERNE (ALFALFA) CUBES and LUCERNE (ALFALFA) WAFERS, which are shortened lucerne (alfalfa) cubes, are made by exactly the same process. The production of either product is an-in field process in that the large self propelled machines move directly into the standing crop in the paddock and produce cubes or wafers.

LUCERNE (ALFALFA) CUBES or LUCERNE (ALFALFA) WAFERS are generally preferred over LUCERNE (ALFALFA) MEAL, for feeding horses, as the lucerne (alfalfa) content in the cube is generally not ground as finely as in the dehydrated lucerne (alfalfa) meal, and hence, in horse feeding, there is likelihood of less digestive tract disturbances occurring. Secondly, horses fed cubes will spend more time on eating and digesting, and may not suffer any possible problems of wood chewing, windsucking etc., which arise in horses which tend to consume the feed rapidly.

LUCERNE (ALFALFA) PELLETS

Lucerne (alfalfa) pellets are generally made in a stationary plant, similar to as is dehydrated lucerne (alfalfa) meal. In fact, in some plants either lucerne pellets or dehydrated meal can be produced, dependent on the market demand.

As with lucerne (alfalfa) cubes, the protein and energy content of the pellets will depend of the quality of the lucerne (alfalfa). which is used as the base material. The protein and energy levels undergo little change in the pelleting process, hence, from a horse feeding angle, pellets can be regarded as a direct substitute for hay and/or lucerne chaff.

Lucerne (alfalfa) pellets are generally more expensive than lucerne (alfalfa) hay, and as the market will vary with the seasons and supply of hay, it would be necessary for cost comparisons to be made at the time of possible purchase.

LUCERNE (ALFALFA) SUPPLEMENT COMPARISONS

In a comparative trial where LUCERNE (ALFALFA) was fed in four physical forms, CUBES, PELLETS, CHOPPED HAY and LOOSE HAY, no differences in digestibility of either DRY MATTER, PROTEIN or GROSS ENERGY were detected between the four methods of physical feeding.

When the horses were allowed to eat as much of the feeds as they wished, AD LIB or VOLUNTARY INTAKE, the greatest consumption was in lucerne cubes, some 16.5 kgs/day, about 18% increase, as opposed to the other three forms of lucerne which were all about the same at 13-14kg/day. The mares fed on the lucerne cubes gained more weight than when fed on the same amount of lucerne hay, possibly due to less waste. The cubes were eaten at a faster rate than hay but provided the horse was able to satisfy its appetite with lucerne cubes, no vices such as wood chewing etc. developed.

ADVANTAGES OF LUCERNE (ALFALFA) CUBES AND PELLETS.

1. less wastage, often up to 10% on a DRY MATTER basis.
2. less storage space required, about one fifth of that needed for the same weight of lucerne.
3. less dust, provided that the cubes and or pellets are made correctly.
4. less manure
5. particularly good for old horses or others with teeth problems, pellets tend to have no trouble eating cubes or pellets when compared to the problems with hay.
6. if MINERALS and or VITAMINS are incorporated, can get better distribution than simply adding to the feed.

DISADVANTAGES OF CUBES AND PELLETS

1. Any added VITAMINS may be destroyed in the production process.
2. unable to tell the quality of the original feeds, once in the pellet or cube form.
3. reduced digestive tract fill, wood chewing etc. may increase dramatically, compared to the feeding of hay.
4. poorly made cubes and pellets will easily break apart and may make a greater dust problem than hay. This breakage can be caused by manufacturing problems and also by adding too much fat to the cubes and or pellets.
5. pellets are expensive to produce when compared to other types of feed.

GRASS HAY

HAY made from grass species can be divided into two types:-

a – hay made from what are known as IMPROVED GRASS species.

b – hay made from what are known as NATIVE GRASS species.

IMPROVED GRASS HAY

C.P. about 6-14%	D.E. about 1.77-2.10 MCal/kg.
T.D.N. about 45-50%	7.25-8.60 MJ/kg.

IMPROVED GRASS species included in this category include the many types of RYE GRASS, PHALARIS, (Canary grass), PASPALUM, FESCUE, BERMUDA GRASS, (Cynodon spp.), BLUE GRASS, TIMOTHY, ORCHARD GRASS, COCKSFOOT etc. These grass species are generally introduced or planted species and not native to the area concerned. In some instances, the native species is of such quality that it can be considered an improved grass, as far as hay making for horse feeding is concerned,

The range of values indicated above are typical of those which would apply to a grass hay, made when the plant is in the "BOOT STAGE" and do not apply to mature grass hay. This book does not allow sufficient space for each type of grass hay to be separately evaluated and it is doubted if such an evaluation would serve any useful purpose, due to the wide range of areas, soil types, growing conditions and hay making under which these hays can be produced.

In comparison to legume hay, principally ALFALFA or LUCERNE, any grass hay will contain about half the PROTEIN content, and about 75%-90% of the ENERGY content. As with legume hay, the protein in grass hay will contain the 10 essential AMINO ACIDS, required by the horse.

Top quality grass hay will be suitable for feeding to all types of horses, except young growing horses, where a PROTEIN supplement of some type will be required to raise the protein level to about 18%. The advantage of grass hay over legume hay, for the feeding of young growing horses, is the levels of CALCIUM and PHOSPHORUS in the hay. In all species, except ORCHARD GRASS, the CALCIUM content is at least equal to and sometimes up to double the PHOSPHORUS level, making grass hay much more preferable, in this regard, for feeding to growing horses. With ORCHARD GRASS, the PHOSPHORUS level exceeds the CALCIUM level by about 25%, requiring some CALCIUM supplementation if ORCHARD GRASS is the only hay being fed to young growing horses.

HAY, made from mature plants of these species, will have nutrient values approaching and possible less than the lower levels indicated above, indicating their value as a source of roughage for mature horses with very restricted work loads.

HAY made from native grass species will vary considerably in nutrient content but rarely will the protein and energy levels exceed the minimum levels stated above. Most hays, made from native grass species, will provide maintenance rations only for mature horses.

MIXED GRASS-LEGUME HAY

C.P. about 11-17% D.E. about 2.00-2.20 MCal/kg
T.D.N. about 50-52% 8.20-9.00 MJ/kg.

Often termed PASTURE HAY, these hays are generally made from a pasture which contains varying proportions of grass and legume. The ideal balance is 50% of each but the pasture composition will depend considerably on soil fertility, seasonal conditions and age of pasture, as these combined factors will generally encourage the predominance of one or other of the pastures species.

By far the most common pasture hay, especially in Australia and New Zealand, is hay made from a mixed pasture of rye grass and subterraneum clover. Rye grass, white clover hay is common as is phalaris, subterraneum clover mix. In the U.K., mixed pasture is based on rye grass/white and red clover and in the U.S.A., orchard grass/white clover, timothy/white clover, fescue/white clover and bluegrass/white clover are the general pasture mixes for hay making.

The actual nutrient values of these hays will vary, dependent on the proportions of grass and legume present in the mix and the stage of the maturity of the pasture at cutting. If the mix is 50/50 grass and legume and is cut at the correct stage, for maximum nutrient yield, good quality pasture hay is as good as average quality LUCERNE or ALFALFA hay for all horses, and specifically for young growing horses, as the CALCIUM level will generally always exceed the PHOSPHORUS level, avoiding the potential problems which may occur in bone development with young growing horses, fed predominately lucerne or alfalfa hay.

HAYLAGE

HAYLAGE is made by cutting pasture, as for hay production, allowing the pasture to wilt in the field, for varying lengths of time, up to 24 hours and then baling in very compressed tight bales, attempting to maintain a moisture content of about 50%. A similar and second method of making a commercial product, similar to HAYLAGE, is to collect the pasture from the paddock and transport to a factory where corrections are made to the pasture for water contents, molasses is generally added and sometimes a micro-organism culture. The product is then sealed in plastic bags of about 22 kg (50lb.) capacity and, when fed, has a brown or brown-gold colour with a sugar smelling odour. There may be some problems in getting some horses to eat HAYLAGE and similar products. Both farm produced HAYLAGE and the the commercial product are promoted as a cure for HEAVES.

Practically, the HEAVES problem requires attention to seven separate possible causes, feeding of wet feed is only one of these causes. Secondly, HAYLAGE type products contain about 50% water and when the cost of the actual DRY MATTER, contained in the HAYLAGE and HAYLAGE type products is considered, they appear to be a very expensive way to buy water.

BLISTER BEETLE

The BLISTER BEETLE is a deadly insect, distributed throughout the U.S.A. and Canada, living primarily on legumes and soybean. When ALFALFA (LUCERNE) HAY is made, the BLISTER BEETLE can be baled in with the hay and when ingested by the horses, produces a very toxic substance, called CANTHARIDIN. There is no known treatment for the effects of CANTHARIDIN, in the horse.

Affected horses produce symptoms including severe irritation and inflammation of the lining of the oesophagus, stomach and intestines, colic and death normally follows within 6 to 48 hours after ingestion of the BLISTER BEETLE.

The only cure for the problem is to examine all hay before purchase to ensure that it is free of BLISTER BEETLE.

MEDIUM PROTEIN MEDIUM ENERGY FEEDS

RICE

C.P. about 7-13%.	D.E. about 3.20 MCal/kg.
T.D.N. about 76%.	12.00 MJ/kg.

RICE, with the HULLS removed, is used as a grain, for horse feeding, in tropical areas where it is freely available, and cost effective when compared to the price of other horse feed grains. The RICE grain is readily eaten by horses, with an energy level slightly below that of maize. RICE contains reasonable levels of LYSINE, in comparison to other grains which are generally very deficient in LYSINE content.

As with OATS, RICE has the same CALCIUM and PHOSPHORUS problems, detailed for that grain.

OATS

C.P. about 8-12%. D.E. about 3.20 MCal/kg.
T.D.N. about 70%. 13.10 MJ/kg.

Oats is the most commonly accepted horse grain and is used by many people as the basis for energy rations. Oats contains the least amount of ENERGY of any of the grains, and the greatest amount of FIBRE, and is the safest of grains to feed any horse. Most performance horse trainers always start their feeding programmes on oats, build up the level of grain intake to the desired weight/day, and then replace oats with grains, of higher energy contents, initially BARLEY and then MAIZE. This practice, of grain substitution, allows a higher energy intake into the horse, within the same weight of feed and is an important part of the correct approach to conditioning performance horses.

Slowly increasing the physical level of oats to the maximum intake, and then replacing oats with grains of higher energy content, will allow the horses' digestive tract to gradually change to the increasing levels of energy and should reduce the likelihood, if not eliminate, the possibility of digestive tract upsets arising from rapid changes in diet.

OATS can vary dramatically in quality. Studies have shown that the weight of oat grain samples can vary by as much as 30% for the same volume of grain. Plump well filled oats are the desired type to feed horses. Pinched grain, generally grown under less than favourable climatic conditions, will always be lighter in volume weight than plump well filled grain. This difference in weight, of the same volume is a function of ENDOSPERM or ENERGY content, LOW volume weights are indicative of low endosperm content, and this re-enforces the need to measure horses feed on weight not volume.

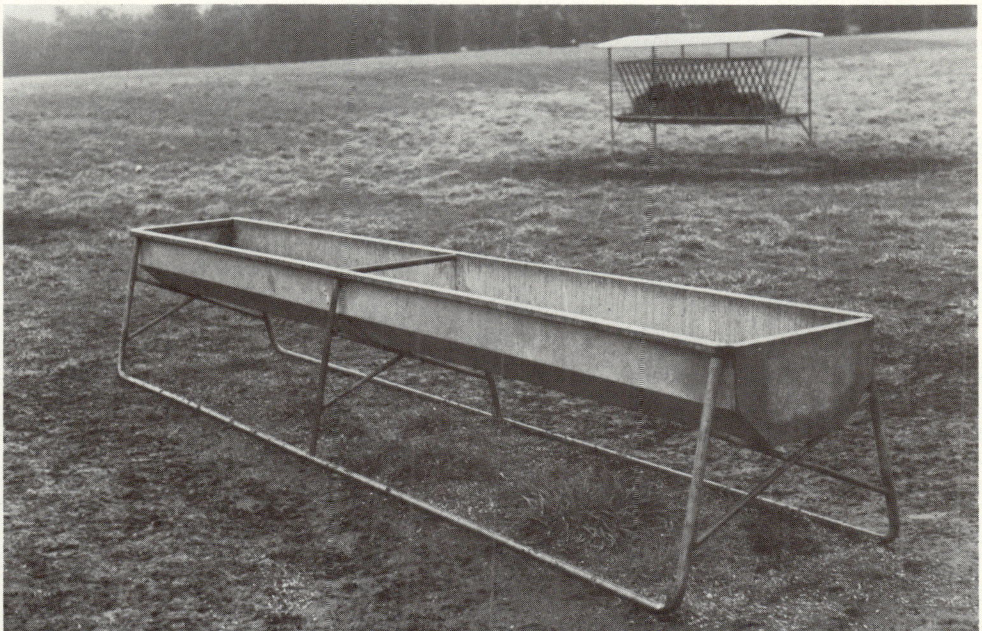

Excellent paddock feeding facilities

In common with all grains, OATS contain low levels of CALCIUM and high levels of PHOSPHORUS, and CALCIUM supplements MAY need to be added, dependent on the amount of OATS being fed in the total daily ration.

GROATS or OATEN GROATS are simply oats with the hulls, or outer covering, mechanically removed befores sale. HULL removal reduces fibre level by about 75% and increases energy level by about 8%. and in doing so considerably reduces the "safety factor" or margin of error in oat feeding, compared to other grains.

BARLEY

C.P. about 8-14%. D.E. about 3.50 MCal/kg.
T.D.N. about 77% 14.30 MJ/kg.

For practical purposes, BARLEY contains the same protein levels as oats, but has a higher energy content. This higher energy content is a result of a decrease in the fibre level of barley compared to oats. Barley is an excellent horse feed and can be readily used in horse rations. Volume weight of barley may well vary as for oats because both crops are generally grown in dry land situations and soil fertility and rainfall during the growing period can affect the development of the grain.

BARLEY has the same CALCIUM and PHOSPHORUS problems as OATS.

SORGHUM

C.P. about 10-12%. D.E. about 3.60 MCal/kg.
T.D.N. about 77% 14.70 KJ/kg.

SORGHUM, also known as MILO and or KAFIR, is a reasonable feed but there are some problems with the grain, that detract from its general use as a common horse feed. The hard outer seed coat, on the sorghum grain, can slow down digestion and it is not uncommon when feeding sorghum to horses, to observe whole sorghum grains in the faeces, even after sorghum has been fed for some period of time. For adequate digestion, by horses, SORGHUM grain needs to be mechanically treated in some way, cracked, rolled, ground etc.

The brown coloured SORGHUM grain may contain varying levels of tannic acid which can cause palatability problems and, at times, complete rejection of the grain by horses. The level of tannic acid appears to be related to the variety of sorghum, WHITE coloured sorghum grain having very low TANNIC ACID levels, but the average horse feeder is not going to be in the position to be able to state the variety required when purchasing his feed.

There is also the problem that the sorghum grain may in fact contain prussic acid - a poison which can cause death. All members of the sorghum family produce prussic acid during the growing period, and if the plant grows continually without any set back, especially due to reduction in moisture supply, then there is generally no need to be concerned about prussic acid levels in the grain. If however the grain is harvested from plants which have suffered moisture stress, especially in the late stages of grain development, then there is a possible chance that the grain may contain prussic acid. The horse feeder is not going to know this until he gets a very sick horse or maybe one which is dead.

The same CALCIUM and PHOSPHORUS problems exist with SORGHUM as described with OATS.

MILLET SEED

C.P. about 11% D.E. about 3.60 MCal/kg.
T.D.N. about 75% 14.80 MJ/kg.

The seeds of various types of MILLETS are sometimes fed to horses. The seeds are small, with a tough outer hull which is not removed at harvesting. The grain generally requires coarse grinding, to assist digestion, before feeding to horses. MILLET is extremely low in LYSINE content and LYSINE supplementation is definitely required, if millet is being fed to growing horses.

CEREAL RYE

C.P. about 12% D.E. about 3.84 MCal/kg.
T.D.N. about 76% 15.70 MJ/kg.

As with OATS and BARLEY, there will often be considerable variation with the nutrient levels of CEREAL RYE, as the grain is generally grown under dryland conditions and soil fertility and rainfall can affect these components. The main problem with CEREAL RYE, for horse feed is one of PALATABILITY, very few horses will eat CEREAL RYE as a grain.

The problems of CALCIUM and PHOSPHORUS levels as detailed for OATS also apply to CEREAL RYE.

WHEAT

C.P. about 8-15%. D.E. about 3.85 MCal/kg
T.D.N. about 80%. 15.80 MJ/kg.

Despite the protein and energy levels, WHEAT is not a recommended feed for horses. The problem with wheat is the low FIBRE level, compared to other grains, and the nature of the ENDOSPERM which is milled to produce flour. Bread is made by mixing yeast with flour and applying heat. This causes the moistened flour to swell. The digestive tract of the horse contains bacteria similar in action to the yeast bacteria that are used in bread making. When a horse eats wheat, these bacteria cause the flour portion of the grain to swell. This in turn will slow down the rate of the food through the intestinal tract, and if the rate of passage is slowed down, combined with large quantities of wheat, complete blockage of the digestive tract may occur. In practical terms, the end result of all this is some form of colic or similar problem. If WHEAT must be fed to horses, it should not make up any more than 25% of the grain portion of the ration and the horse should be slowly introduced to the wheat over a period of 4-5 weeks.

The same CALCIUM and PHOSPHORUS problems exist with WHEAT as with described with OATS.

MAIZE

C.P. about 10-13%. D.E. about 3.90 MCal/kg.
T.D.N. about 84% 16.00 MJ/kg.

MAIZE, also known as CORN, is an excellent horse feed. It is the preferred energy supplement for performance horses because it contains the least amount of FIBRE of any grain and the greatest amount of energy, per unit weight. There is less variation in the weight, of any volume, of maize, compared to oats or barley, as most maize is grown under high rainfall or irrigation conditions.

MAIZE is sometimes called a "hot feed". This undoubtedly refers to the low fibre and high energy levels of the grain, in comparison to the other grains. Corn is really only a feed for horses which have consistent and continual need for large quantities of energy. Race horses and pacers in training, polo and polo-crosse horses in the season, endurance horses, eventers and show jumpers in full competition, are the type of horses that benefit from the use of corn as an energy supplement.

The most common mistake made with the feeding of corn is when a change is made from say oats to corn on a volume basis. A 4 litre ice cream container of oats contains about 3.1 kgs of grain at an energy level of 3.20 MCal/kg, or 9.90 MCals of energy. The same container holds 4.3 kgs of corn at an energy level of 3.90 MCals/kg or 16.77 MCals of energy. Hence the same volume of corn has 70% more energy than the same volume of oats.

When a change in the type of grain being fed takes place, allowance must be made differing ENERGY DENSITY levels, affected by the different volume weights and the different energy contents.

The same CALCIUM and PHOSPHORUS problems exist with MAIZE as described with OATS.

BRAN

C.P. about 14%. D.E. about 3.30 MCal/kg.
T.D.N about 67%. 13.50 MJ/kg.

BRAN is a by-product of the flour milling industry and is part of the outer coating of the wheat grain. BRAN can be sold as GIANT BRAN, BROAD BRAN or FINE BRAN, dependent on the size of the product or often a mix of the three and called "straight run" BRAN. Bran is generally recognised as a laxative, i.e. it causes the digesta in the intestinal tract to flow faster than normal and it is capable of absorbing many times its own weight in water. The protein level in bran is sufficient to maintain adult horses, but is not enough to allow mares to lactate to the best of their ability, or to allow young horses to grow to their potential. The energy level of bran is adequate to provide sufficient energy to adult horses at rest, but is insufficient for more energy demanding purposes, e.g. lactation, growth and performance. BRAN contains low levels of CALCIUM 0.15% and high levels of PHOSPHORUS 1.40%, most of which is in the PHYTATE form, virtually rendering what little CALCIUM is present unavailable to the horse. Unless CALCIUM supplements are used when BRAN forms any part of the ration, a CALCIUM deficiency will occur, commonly called BRAN DISEASE, or NUTRITIONAL SECONDARY HYPER-PARATHYROIDISM.

Bran can be used as a special purpose feed as follows:-

a) As a means of getting the horse to eat various supplements. The obvious situations are the administration of worm drenches in the feed, to spread the intake of vitamin and mineral supplements, and to help the intake of fats being fed to top performance horses, no more than 0.5 kg of bran would be necessary for this purpose.

b) As a means of preventing fast eating horses from gulping or "woofing" their feed. Some horses are fast eaters and there is always the fear that they may get digestive upsets if they eat their grain and concentrate ration too quickly. Some people try to get around this problem by increasing the bulk in the ration by the addition of bran. This can, however, lower the energy level of the ration and needs to be considered for performance horses.

c) As a means of reducing the horses' energy intake on days of restricted work, and hence, possibly, overcoming any TYING UP problems Most racing and training stables do not exercise their horses on the track on Sundays. If grain were fed on Sunday at the same volume as feeding on week days, and the horse not worked on that day, there is a good chance that the horse will suffer from the tying up - azoturia syndrome when the animal is worked again on Monday. Bran is used to replace all or most of the grain component in the ration on the days of restricted work. ON an energy density basis, BRAN contains one third or less the energy of grains so the reduced total energy intake of the same volume of BRAN means that the horse is much less likely to get tying up - azoturia symptoms when work is again commenced.

d) When letting horses down after training, when they go for spelling. It is not unusual for horses to race on Saturday and be on a float to the spelling paddocks on Sunday. In this situation, it is not desirable to transfer the horse immediately from a predominately grain ration to pasture overnight. It is much better to let the horse adjust to the spelling situation by slowly reducing the grain intake, over say a two or three week period. This is simply done by slowly reducing the content of grain in the ration, and replacing that grain with bran. The next step is to slowly reduce the bran content of the ration to nil, and the horse should then have a digestive tract properly adapted to the utilisation of pasture.

The bacteria and enzymes in the horse's digestive tract are specific to the type of feed being used. These valuable and essential aids to digestion can increase or decrease their respective levels over a period of days, and sometimes weeks. They cannot, however, adjust overnight, and complete removal of heavy levels of grain feeding and straight onto pasture in a 24 or 48 hour period can not be of benefit to any horse.

e) As a laxative for horses which are hard in the faeces, often called "bound-up". Increasing the amount of bran in the ration and decreasing the amount of grain, will often help animals in this situation to return to normal faecal output and consistency.

f) As a "filler" for hacks and led in horses. These animals are required to show not only their best conformation, but also their best manners in the show ring. Many of the problems of "fizzy" hacks and mis-behaving led-in horses is due to too much energy in the ration. The overfeeding of energy to these horses, such as from grains or the meals derived from oilseeds, is undesirable and will only tend to produce an animal which may not behave itself in the show ring. If feeding bran to these types of horses. it is necessary to ensure the quantity being fed does not act as a laxative and increase the rate of ingesta flow.

POLLARD - WHEAT MIDDLINGS

C.P. about 16%. D.E. about 3.42 MCal/KC.
T.D.N. about 78%. 14.00 MJ/kg.

As with Bran, this feed is a by product of the flour milling industry, and is best described as flour unfit for human consumption. POLLARD is a very fine feed and its use is not advocated in horse feeding as it can absorb water, become compacted in the stomach and cause digestive upsets and possibly colic. There is also information available from slaughtered horses which indicate that the feeding of reasonable levels of POLLARD to a horse can lead to increased deposition of fat around the heart. POLLARD has exactly the same CALCIUM deficiency and PHOSPHORUS excess problems as outlined above for BRAN, except the level of PHOSPHORUS is generally much higher than in BRAN.

CEREAL MILLING BY-PRODUCTS

There are a number of other products available for horse feeding, which consist of various mixtures of broken grain, bran, wheat middlings, pollard and other by products of cereal milling. These products are marketed under various names, the most common of which is MILL RUN. The nutrient composition of MILL RUN will vary, dependent on its actual physical make-up but will approximate the details supplied for BRAN and POLLARD. HOMINY FEED is a BY-PRODUCT of CORN STARCH manufacture and is a mixture of corn bran, corn germ and part of the starchy portion or endosperm of the grain. Generally contains about 4% fat. PROCESSED GRAIN BY-PRODUCT consists of various grain portions left over from the processing of grain for flour and beer. Can include wheat bran, brewer's dried grains, wheat middlings, and other grain fractions.

WHEY POWDER

C.P. about 17.0% D.E. about 3.61 MCal/kg.
T.D.N. about 78.0% 14.80 MJ/kg.

As a horse feed, WHEY powder is used as a carrier or base for feed supplements, in which the various vitamins and minerals are mixed. Most of the energy component in WHEY powder is in the form of the milk sugar, LACTOSE, which is broken down inside the horses' digestive tract by the enzyme LACTASE. This enzyme disappears from the digestive tract between two and three years of age and the feeding of large amounts of WHEY POWDER after LACTASE disappearance can lead to problems with diarrhoea. The price of WHEY POWDER is such that its use is restricted to being a carrier for vitamin and mineral supplements.

RICE MILL BY-PRODUCT

Various by products are obtained from the milling and preparation of rice for human consumption. Various names are given to individual fractions, dependent on the country involved. In Australia, RICE POLLARD is accepted as the total mill run, consisting of RICE BRAN, RICE GERM, RICE POLLARD and sometimes, broken RICE GRAINS. RICE POLLARD, in Australia does not contain any RICE HULLS. In other countries, RICE BRAN is a separate designated product, containing various levels of the above plus often some RICE HULLS. The term RICE POLISHINGS basically refers to that portion of the rice which comes off the exterior of the grain in the final milling process for human consumption. The amount of RICE POLISHINGS produced is small in relation to the other mill products and RICE POLISHINGS are generally included in RICE POLLARD in Australia and RICE BARN in other countries.

RICE BRAN

C.P. about 14% D.E. about 2.90 MCal/kg
T.D.N. about 70% 11.90 MJ/kg.

RICE BRAN, also called RICE MEAL, can be fed as a separate feed or can be used in a number or proprietary pre-mixed horse feeds. RICE BRAN contains reasonably high levels of indigestible silica, (sand) due to the incorporation of RICE HULLS, and whilst it contains high levels of PHOSPHORUS as opposed to CALCIUM, most of the PHOSPHORUS is in the PHYTATE form, necessitating the addition of more than normal amounts of CALCIUM to any ration containing RICE BRAN to overcome any potential CALCIUM deficiency problems.

RICE POLLARD

C.P. about 13.5% D.E. about 3.78 MCal/kg.
T.D.N. about 76% 15.50 MJ/kg.

RICE POLLARD is used, in Australia, as a base for the preparation of a number of ready mixed horse feeds. As an individual horse feed, RICE POLLARD contains a high FAT level of about 19%, has excellent levels of the essential amino acids. The main problem in using RICE POLLARD, as a horse feed, is the severe lack of calcium in the feed, the CALCIUM level being about 25% of the PHOSPHORUS content, making the need to provide a calcium supplement to the animal essential, to ensure a calcium deficiency problem does not to occur.

HIGH PROTEIN HIGH ENERGY FEEDS

DRIED BREWER'S GRAINS

C.P. about 25%. D.E. about 2.75 MCal/kg.
T.D.N. about 63%. 11.30 MJ/kg.

Horses are very rarely, if ever fed WET BREWER'S GRAINS. These contain about 23% DRY MATTER and 77% WATER, but the problem with WET BREWER'S GRAINS is the possibility of deterioration and the development of mould and fungal infections, if kept for any length of time, especially in periods of hot and humid weather. Any such deterioration is likely to produce digestive upsets in the horse. DRIED BREWER'S GRAINS, which is principally the the dried residue, containing 10% moisture, of barley malt left over after brewing, but may contain other grain products, usually from maize and rice, does not suffer from the possibility of deterioration. Little information is available as to the value of DRIED BREWER'S GRAINS for horse feeding. Whilst suitable for feeding to cattle, BREWER'S GRAINS either wet or dry have little use in pig feeding and are of no value in poultry feeding. As both these species are MONOGASTRICES, as is the horse, DRIED BREWER'S GRAINS are probably of little value in horse feeding.

TICK BEANS

C.P. about 26% D.E. about 3.45 MCal/kg.
T.D.N. about 74% 14.20 MJ/kg.

TICK BEANS, also known as HORSE BEANS or FABA BEANS, at 26% protein, is at the lower end of PROTEIN content of the high protein feeds, and there are other feeds available which contain more protein and are generally more economical to buy than tick beans. Tick beans are a palatable and very safe feed for horses, but contain a very low level of the amino acid METHIONINE. TICK BEANS are generally always fed as cracked beans. This can allow oxidation to occur of the feed nutrients in the endosperm after cracking so the beans should be cracked on a daily basis to ensure that any possible oxidation is reduced as much as possible.

SUNFLOWER SEEDS

C.P. about 28% D.E. about 4.00 MCal/kg.
T.D.N. about 70%-80% 16.40 MJ/kg.

The SUNFLOWER SEEDS, before oil extraction, lack both LYSINE and TRYPTOPHAN in the amino acid profile. Sunflower seed is generally only fed in small quantities, generally 0.25 kgs or less, and then usually not as a source of protein but as a conditioner for the horses' coat. Sunflower seed in small quantities will put a shine on any coat, but may darken the coats of palominos or similarly light-coloured horses.

LINSEED MEAL

C.P. about 33% D.E. about 3.40 MCal/kg
T.D.N. about 77% 14.00 MJ/kg.

LINSEED MEAL has long been recognised as a horse feed but, in many instances, purely to put a shine or gloss on the horses' coat, and generally not as a protein supplement. A little linseed added to the feed will always bring a gloss to the horses coat - beware linseed meal may cause darkening in the coat of palominos, so be careful if feeding these horses with this product. As a protein meal, LINSEED MEAL is deficient in both METHIONINE and LYSINE, both essential amino acids, and also suffers from a palatability problem. Whole LINSEED grain SHOULD NEVER be fed to horses, it contains a toxic factor, similar to that in growing sorghum plants, which must be destroyed by boiling.

LUPINS

C.P. about 34% D.E. about 3.36 MCal/kg.
T.D.N about 77% 13.80 MJ/kg.

LUPINS contain more than adequate levels of both PROTEIN and ENERGY but the PROTEIN is deficient in LYSINE and very deficient in METHIONINE and TRYPTOPHAN. There are three common types of LUPINS, recognised by the colour of the flowers, WHITE, YELLOW and BLUE and within each type are varieties which are classed as "BITTER" and "SWEET". Horses will not eat any of the "BITTER" varieties and the "SWEET" LUPINS need to be cracked or soaked before feeding. The analysis of protein and energy contained in the feed can vary dependent on the actual variety of lupins being fed, and also as to whether the lupins are de-hulled or not.

SKIM MILK POWDER

C.P. about 35% D.E. about 4.05 MCal/kg.
T.D.N. about 81% 16.60 MJ/kg.

SKIM MILK powder has been used as the basis of feed preparations for many years. Its use in all animals, except the horse, is well documented and in fact recommended. However in the horse, milk powders of any type are only of value in horses up to two and possibly three years of age. Between two and three years of age, dependent on the horse, LACTASE production ceases in the digestive tract. LACTASE is the enzyme which breaks down the milk sugar, LACTOSE, for absorption and if LACTASE is not present the milk sugar cannot be utilised by the horse. Prior to the disappearance of LACTASE from the digestive tract, the horse can adequately handle milk powder supplements and effectively digest all the food components. Feeding SKIM MILK supplements, in any quantity, to horses over three years of age may even cause scours and diarrhoea. For creep or supplementary feeding of early weaned foals, preparations based on skim milk produce much better growth rates than do supplements, based on soybean meal. Human demand for skim milk powder generally makes it too expensive for horse feeding.

CANOLA MEAL

C.P. about 40%. D.E. about 3.11 Mcal/kg.
T.D.N. about 68%. 12.75 MJ/kg.

CANOLA MEAL, formerly called RAPESEED MEAL, is from the seed of a relatively new oilseed plant developed in Canada from RAPESEED. Rapeseed meal had very restricted value for horse feeding as it contains substances, called GLUCOSINOLATES, which affect the thyroid gland with very adverse results. CANOLA is the new form of rapeseed, containing very low levels of these glucosinolates and is suitable for horse feeding. CANOLA MEAL is able to replace SOYBEAN MEAL in horse rations, as its AMINO ACID profile contains the 10 essential amino acids required by horses.

COTTONSEED MEAL

C.P. about 40-45% D.E. about 3.01 MCal/kg.
T.D.N. about 72% 12.35 MJ/kg.

COTTONSEED MEAL is popular as a horse feed, in areas, close to the cotton growing districts. It is also used as base for a number of prepared feed, e.g. horse mixes etc. Cottonseed meal has two main problems in horse feeding. The first is that the cottonseed meal is deficient in one of the nine essential amino acids, lysine and slightly deficient in methionine. If cottonseed meal is used as part or all of the horse ration, it is essential that lysine and possibly methionine be added to the ration to overcome this deficiency. Cottonseed meal also contains GOSSYPOL, which at certain levels may be toxic to horses. From American studies it seems that cottonseed meal can be fed, at rates of, up to 16% of the ration, by weight, without any toxic affects occurring from gossypol. It would not be advisable to increase the level of cottonseed meal about 16% of the total horse ration as the chronic or mild symptoms of gossypol poisoning are not well defined. There may be a palatability problem, with COTTONSEED MEAL, at feeding levels above 1 kg per horse per day. There is also evidence that the feeding of COTTONSEED MEAL high in GOSSYPOLS, as are produced from by the solvent extraction method, may tie up IRON and make it unavailable to the horse.

SUNFLOWER MEAL

C.P. about 40-48% D.E. about 2.80 MCal/kg.
T.D.N. about 68-80% 11.50 MJ/kg.

SUNFLOWER MEAL is the residue after extraction of SUNFLOWER OIL. This product will have a reasonably high fibre content, up to 38%, due to the presence of some sunflower hulls in the meal. The protein contains twice as much methionine as soybean meal but is very deficient in LYSINE and added lysine needs to be present if the meal is used as part of the ration for growing horses. Sunflower meal has higher fibre levels than most other oilseed meals. SUNFLOWER MEAL may have a laxative effect and there may well be some palatability problems with SUNFLOWER MEAL, fed to some horses. The meal has a very short shelf life.

SOYBEAN MEAL

C.P. about 45%. D.E. about 3.60 MCal/kg.
T.D.N. about 78% 14.76 MJ/kg.

SOYBEAN MEAL is a very valuable feed supplement for horses and is technically ideal for horse nutrition, as it is one of the few high protein supplement which contains all the ten essential amino acids that are required by horses. The feed does however have two technical problems. The first is that the raw soybean contains several heat - labile factors, especially trypsin inhibitors. In the raw soybean direct from the plant, these inhibitors can greatly reduce the nutritional value of the soybean. These inhibitors are removed from the bean by heating as in the extraction process, where the oil content is removed to give soybean oil for margarine manufacture, and the residual is ground to make soybean meal, the inhibitors are destroyed by the manufacturing process. It is important that the heating process used be carefully controlled as overheating will reduce the availability of the amino acids in the meal, and may also cause some palatability problems. Fortunately quality control in the oil seed plants is now of a sufficiently high standard that the overheating problem is virtually a thing of the past. Secondly, 0.5 kg. per horse per day appears to be the upper limit before palatability problems occur. Horses will readily eat up to 1.5 kg of SOYBEAN MEAL for an initial 4 to 6 week period but then suddenly will cease to eat the feed, so in the interests of satisfactory feeding, never feed SOYBEAN MEAL above 500 gram/day for a 450kg horse.

FISH MEAL

C.P. about 50-70% D.E. about 3.10 MCal/kg.
T.D.N. about 72%-98% 12.70 KJ/kg.

FISH MEAL is the most common form of animal protein used in horse feeding. The PROTEIN contains the 10 essential amino acids and the FISH MEAL also contains CALCIUM and PHOSPHORUS in the required ratio which the Ca level double that of P. The price of FISH MEAL prevents its inclusion in most horse rations but it is used in milk replacers and creep rations for foals at rates of up to 10% of the feed. It is essential that any FISH MEAL used for horse feeding is free of bacterial contamination, especially from SALMONELLA, which if present can cause diarrhoea in the horses which can be extremely difficult to eliminate.

COMMON HORSE FEEDS

MAJOR FEED NUTRIENT LEVELS

FEED	C.P. as %	T.D.N as %	D.E/KG. as MCal.	D.E/KG. as MJ.
LOW PROTEIN LOW ENERGY				
OATEN HAY (CHAFF)				
WHEATEN HAY (CHAFF)	8	45	1.90	7.90
LOW PROTEIN HIGH ENERGY				
MOLASSES	2-9	60	3.40	14.00
CORN AND COB MEAL	6	73	3.00	12.30
FATS	0	-	8.50	34.80
MEDIUM PROTEIN MEDIUM ENERGY				
GRASS HAY	6-14	45-50	1.77-2.10	7.25-8.60
MIXED PASTURE HAY	11-17	50-52	2.00-2.20	8.20-9.00
LUCERNE HAY	16-20	50-60	2.30	9.40
ALFALFA HAY	16-20	50-60	2.30	9.40
MEDIUM PROTEIN HIGH ENERGY				
RICE	7-13	74	3.20	13.00
OATS	8-12	70	3.20	13.10
BARLEY	8-14	77	3.50	14.30
SORGHUM	10-12	77	3.60	14.70
MILLET	11	75	3.60	14.80
RYE	12	76	3.84	15.70
WHEAT	8-15	80	3.85	15.80
MAIZE	10-13	84	3.90	16.00
BRAN	14	67	3.30	13.50
POLLARD	16	78	3.42	14.00
WHEY	17	78	3.61	14.80
RICE BRAN	14	70	2.90	11.90
RICE POLLARD	13.5	76	3.78	15.50
HIGH PROTEIN HIGH ENERGY				
BREWER'S GRAINS	25	63	2.75	11.30
TICK BEANS	26	74	3.45	14.20
SUNFLOWER SEEDS	28	80	4.00	16.40
LINSEED MEAL	33	77	3.40	14.00
LUPINS	34	77	3.36	13.80
SKIM MILK POWDER	35	81	4.05	16.60
CANOLA MEAL	40	68	3.11	12.75
COTTONSEED MEAL	40-45	72	3.01	12.35
SUNFLOWER MEAL	40-48	74	2.80	11.50
SOYBEAN MEAL	45	78	3.60	14.76
FISH MEAL	50-70	70-98	3.10	12.70

SUNDRY HORSE FEEDS

BREAD

Some people are able to obtain supplies of reject or old bread from bakeries and shops and often use this for feeding horses. Day old bread has a water content of 20-30% and is fed at the rate of 4 kgs of bread being roughly equal to 3 kgs of grain.

On a dry matter basis, bread has a protein level of about 8% and a D.E. of about 2.5 MCal/kg.

The main problem with feeding bread is the CALCIUM and PHOSPHORUS levels. The Ca/P ratio of bread is 1/1.66 as opposed to the desired ratio of 2/1. Hence, bread when fed to horses, will need supplementation with limestone to correct the lack of calcium. The average horse needs about 23 grams of calcium and 14 grams of phosphorus per day to maintain reasonable body growth and maintenance. To obtain the daily phosphorus needs the average horse will have to eat 21 loaves of bread per day, or in weight some 14.3 kgs. This mean that the horse will be virtually eating nothing but bread to obtain this level of phosphorus. The amount of calcium available in 21 loaves of average bread would only be 8.8 grams so there will be a need for a supplement to be provided of 14 grams of calcium equivalent per day.

Bread may be a reasonable feed for horses provided, it is only fed at no more than one third the total daily ration, say 3 kgs or 4.5 loaves per adult dry horse, provided an amino acid supplement is fed to allow full utilisation of the energy and protein, and provided a calcium supplement is fed to correct the very low level of calcium in the bread. Classical symptoms of calcium deficiency have been produced in horses fed, for some time, on bread without calcium supplementation.

Bread should not be fed to brood mares, foals or horses up to four years of age unless all the corrective measures detailed above are considered, and due allowance made for the greater calcium and phosphorus needs of these horses.

CARROTS

A common horse feed and often given to all types of horses. Carrots have a number of problems. Fresh Carrots, as fed to horses have a water content of 90%, about 1% protein and 10% energy. On a dry matter basis, with all water removed, carrots have a protein level of about 8% and an energy level of about 3.20 MCal/kg. Very few people feed dehydrated carrots to horses.

In order for the average dry adult horse, with a small work load, to be able to get all the protein and energy from carrots, the animal would need to eat 70 kgs of carrots per day. Of this, about 8 kgs would be nutrient and the balance, 62 kgs water.

As we would expect this type of horse to drink about 40 litres of water per day at the most, 62 kgs or litres of water in carrots would be impossible for the horse to digest. Hence as a source of protein and energy in horses, carrots are of little value.

Carotene, the pre-cursor of Vitamin A is also available in carrots, and many people feel that the feeding of these to horses will supply Vitamin A.

Carrots, in general, contain enough carotene in one kg of DRY MATTER, equivalent to 10 kgs carrots as picked from the ground to provide the horse with about 40,000 I.U. of Vitamin A. This is about 40% of the desired level for most performance horses and actively growing animals and hence there is a use for carrots as a means of ensuring the Vitamin A levels of the diet are satisfactory, especially if the horse has no access to green feed.

LAWN CLIPPINGS

Horses are selective grazers and when they have unrestricted access to growing pasture, they are able to pick and choose the feed they eat. However, when confronted with a heap of lawn clippings, the horse is not able to differentiate between various types and qualities of feeds. Secondly, lawn clippings will generally heat up, as in silage making, after about an hour of mowing and ingestion of this heated grass may lead to the animal contracting colic.

There are additional problems in the lawn clippings, they may contain fertilisers, weedicides and insecticides, all of which may affect the horse. There is also the possibility of poisonous plants, pieces of plastic and paper etc. all being contained in the clippings and all of which may produce adverse reactions.

It is most inadvisable to feed such lawn clippings to any horse. If lawns must be used as a source of grazing, let the horse pick and graze over the lawn before mowing.

EGGS

Fresh eggs are occasionally fed to horses and when mixed with the concentrate ration, will be readily eaten.

Eggs contain about 12% protein, energy of 1.90 MCal/kg, all the essential amino acids and most of the necessary vitamins. The presence of the ten essential amino acids is probably the most important reason to consider the feeding of eggs. Based on the cost, as purchased in the local shop, eggs are certainly too expensive as a source of protein and energy. The vitamin content while reasonable is too low in general to look upon eggs as a source of Vitamin B Complex in particular. However, if access is available to eggs at a price less than the normal retail shop price, e.g. home grown on the farm, then the inclusion of 1 or 2 eggs per day in a horses' diet is worthwhile.

SUNFLOWER HULLS

SUNFLOWER HULLS are the outer covering of the sunflower seed which is removed before oil extraction occurs. SUNFLOWER HULLS are often hammermilled to produce a product, known as SUNFLOWER BRAN. In some instances, the sunflower hulls are mixed with the broken seed, and hammer milled to produce SUNFLOWER MEAL. Protein level is about 7%, energy level is about 1.90 MCal/kg, calcium phosphorus ratio is of the order of 4/1. This product is presently being used as the base for a number of proprietary horse feeds due to reduced cost. Sunflower hulls, as is, tend to be unpalatable to horses and requires the addition of molasses to encourage consumption. The hulls also appear to be lacking in some of the essential amino acid and hence the need to add a supplement of these compounds to the feed in order to balance the mix.

SPECIFIC FEEDING PROBLEMS

MOULDY FEED POISONING

Also variously known as LEUCOENCEPHAILITS, ACUTE HAEMHORRAGIC ENCEPHALITIS, CEREBROSPINAL MENINGITIS, FORAGE POISONING, STAGGERS, CORNSTALK DISEASE and MOULDY CORN POISONING, this condition can be due to the feeding of any feedstuff which is affected in any way by any one of many fungi which produce mould in the feed.

Symptoms include lethargy and disinterest, possible paralysis, and internally there may be damage to the parts of the nervous system and the brain.

The condition generally only occurs in areas of hot humid climates, very rarely in areas of dry hot climates and is very difficult to treat as it is necessary to know what type of mouldy feed the horse ate, and in some instances, none of the offending feed is available for examination.

The best solution is NOT TO feed the horse anything which appears to contain any type of fungal or mouldy growth.

EQUINE AFLATOXICOSIS

A condition caused by compounds, called AFLATOXINS, which are produced by specific fungi of the ASPERGILLUS family. The condition has been seen in horses fed contaminated corn and peanut meals. Symptoms of affected horses include damage to the brain, degeneration of fat deposits, bile duct damage, liver damage and heart damage. Death generally results as the condition is currently incurable.

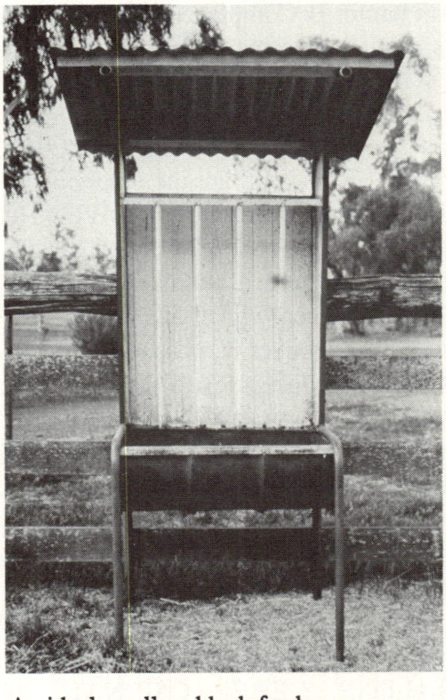

An ideal small paddock feeder –
note half drum to collect leaf before it falls on the ground

21. VITAMIN AND MINERAL CONTENTS OF COMMON HORSE FEEDS

Most horse feeders are not aware that all the common horse feeds contain various levels of vitamins and minerals and, in fact, in the average horse ration, there is probably sufficient VITAMINS and MINERALS to satisfy the needs of the average horse without the use of packaged and prepared vitamin and mineral mixes.

The problem in this regard can be clarified in the following manner:

1. There is no requirement in law that hay, chaff or grains have to carry a label which details the levels of the various food components contained in those feeds. This then leaves the average horse feeder to think that these feeds do not contain anything else other than roughage and possibly protein and energy.
2. Legal requirements generally require that grain by-products and processed horse feeds should be labeled. The label generally contains details as to the protein level, energy measurement and possibly any added minerals and vitamins.
   The many inconsistency in labeling requirements allow the average horse feeder to be excused from thinking that these products do not contain any vitamins and/or minerals. This in fact is not the case, and often these cereal and oilseed by-products are very valuable sources of essential feed components.
3. The attached Table reveals the average vitamin and mineral content PER KILOGRAM of four of the more common horse feeds. The feeds selected are lucerne hay, bran, oaten grain, and soybean meal.

	LUCERNE HAY	WHEATEN BRAN	OATEN GRAIN	SOYBEAN MEAL
Vitamin A (as I.U.)	32000	133	83	N/A
B Complex (mg)	78	1309	1009	2933
C	ANALYSIS NOT AVAILABLE			
D (as I.U.)	2256	0	0	0
E (mgs)	26	3	37	1.5
K	ANALYSIS NOT AVAILABLE			
Calcium (grams)	8.5	1.8	1.0	3.0
phosphorus (grams)	2.0	10.5	3.3	7.2
Ca/P Ratio	4.3/1	1/5.8	1/3.3	1/2.4
Iron (grams)	0.45	0.13	0.08	0.22
Magnesium (grams)	2.3	7.8	1.1	2.7
Potassium (grams)	18.1	11.9	3.8	19.9
Sulphur (grams)	30	N/A	1.1	N/A
Zinc (mgs)	18.3	6.6	23.1	52.7
Copper (mgs)	6.5	13.5	12.1	18.3
Manganese (mgs)	88.0	147.0	60.0	38.7
Molybdenum (mgs)	0.52	0.26	0.17	N/A
Selenium (mgs)	0.32	N/A	0.04	0.55

The levels of vitamin and mineral content of the feeds have been carefully compiled from the references used in the general preparation of this book. Naturally, in the case of all the feeds, the levels detailed here will vary in practice, dependent on growing conditions during the life of the plant and also with the soil fertility and fertilisers used to grow the individual crop.

The Table clearly shows that the feeds analysed contain much more than roughage, energy and protein. In fact, lucerne hay contains all the vitamins and minerals, at levels considered necessary for feeding average horses. The other feeds may lack sufficient quantities of mineral or vitamin in some instances, but in all cases the feeds are not completely deficient in these feed components.

A similar analysis of feed composition would reveal that all the other common horse feeds contain similar vitamin and mineral levels as is presented for these four feeds. There will, of course, be individual variations, between feeds and within feeds, in the various levels of the individual vitamins and minerals, but the horse feeder should keep well in mind the fact that ordinary horse feeds contain many of these compounds.

In terms of the cost of feeding horses, the fact that these vitamins and minerals are already in most of the common feeds means that they are being obtained at virtually nil cost.

MINERALS

CALCIUM AND PHOSPHORUS

Whilst these are two separate and distinct minerals, they are generally discussed together when considering horse nutrition. Both need to be present in certain weights and in a certain ratio so as to allow proper skeletal development and maintenance.

The common horse feeds can be divided into two groups when considering the feeding of calcium and phosphorus to the horse.

GROUP ONE consists of grains, grain by-products and oil seed derived feeds. This includes the following - maize, oats, barley, sorghum, lupins, rice, wheat bran, and pollard, molasses, cottonseed, soybean and linseed meals and sunflower seeds. Also included in this group of feeds are whey and grazing crops of green oats and phalaris. The levels of Ca/P required by a dry adult horse are 23 grams of Ca per day and 14 grams of P per day, present in a ratio of between 6 parts of Ca to 1 part of P, down to 1.3 parts Ca to 1 part P for young growing horses. The range of levels varies from the lowest in whey at a ratio of 1/5.8 to 1/1.65 in sunflower seeds. The most common horse feed, in oaten grain, has a Ca/P ratio of 1/3.3.

All these feeds are then INVERSELY BALANCED for correct horse nutrition and some form of calcium addition is needed to increase the level of that mineral and bring the amounts and ratio of the two minerals back to the desired level.

GROUP TWO consists of most pasture species (with the exception of grazing oats and green phalaris) and hays made from those grasses and clovers. Also in this category is skim milk powder. The ratio of Ca/P in these feeds varies from 1 Ca/1P in the case of paspalum to the highest of 4 Ca/1P in the case of lucerne hay. From a technical angle, all these feeds can be fed directly to the horse with no worry as to the balance of the two minerals. The one exception to this rule is the need to be careful about the excessive level of CALCIUM in lucerne hay when being fed to young growing horses. The high level of CALCIUM, in lucerne or alfalfa hay may lead to the development of bone disorders in young growing horses.

In terms of absolute levels of mineral intake, a horse eating 10 kgs dry matter of paspalum per day would receive 23 grams each of calcium and phosphorus, quite acceptable from a nutritional viewpoint. The same horse on a diet of 10 kgs of lucerne hay per day would receive 95 grams of calcium per day, and 23 grams of phosphorus.

Whilst these CALCIUM and PHOSPHORUS levels, in both the PASPALUM grass hay and the LUCERNE (ALFALFA) HAY are satisfactory for mature horses, the high CALCIUM levels in the lucerne (alfalfa) can lead to bone growth and developmental problems in young growing horses

Ca P Vitamin D

Relationship

Dry adult horse 450 kg (1000 lbs)

DAILY NEEDS

Ca	23 grams
P	15 grams
Vitamin D	2 hours sunlight or sun cured hay

Increase or decrease daily levels IN THE SAME PROPORTION for other types of horses as detailed in text.

Problems may occur in one or more of bone growth, bone maintenance, joint formation, lameness, "big head", soft tissue calcification, excess calcium deposits in ligaments, tendons and blood vessels and possibly death if ratio Ca/P is not correct or absolute basic levels of Ca, P and Vit. D are not maintained.

Based on classifying Ca, P and Vit. D into three categories.

Excess levels, Sufficient or ideal or Inadequate levels

There are 57 different combinations of Ca, P and D which are possible in a horse's ration.

Of these 57 combination

Ca	P	VITAMIN D
0	0	0
+	0	0
+	+	0

where + = excess, 0 = sufficient, - = inadequate

When a simple mixture of lucerne hay and oaten grain is fed to the average horse, any practical mix up to 50%s of lucerne hay per day and 50% of oats per day, by weight, will still provide sufficient calcium and phosphorus from the two feeds to ensure adequate intake. This ration to a 450 kg horse will provide up to 37 grams of calcium per day, 23 grams of phosphorus in a ratio of 1.6/1.

On these types of rations there is no practical need to consider the feeding of any calcium/phosphorus supplement as the basic feed components contain sufficient of the minerals to supply all the animals' daily needs.

IRON

With the exception of maize (corn) and skim milk, all common horse feeds contain more than 40 parts per million of iron. As this is the accepted level of the mineral required by horses, there is no obvious technical reason why iron supplements should be fed. IRON, when fed in larger than normal quantities, in the diet can cause reduced growth rate, diarrhoea, drowsiness, partial shock, affect liver function and affect absorption of other minerals by the horse

MAGNESIUM

All common feeds contain more than adequate levels of magnesium so most horses should therefore be able to get all their magnesium supplies from their natural feeds, with what appears to be one apparent exception.

Horses which are subject to the tying up syndrome, especially when traveling, appear to improve if small levels of magnesium are fed daily in the ration. Epsom salts (magnesium sulphate) is used as a source of magnesium in this situation.

POTASSIUM, SULPHUR, ZINC, COBALT, COPPER, MANGANESE, MOLYBDENUM.

These individual minerals are all required by the horse in very small to minute amounts. All feeds contain reasonable levels of these minerals, and supplementation, of the greater percentage of horses, should not be required.

SELENIUM

Most feeds contain more than adequate levels of selenium, for the horse. Mixed pastures, especially of grasses and clovers, may in certain areas and on certain soils, be low in the levels of selenium, but lucerne grown on the same soils have been shown to test high in this particular mineral. Lucerne appears to be an accumulator of selenium in the plant tissues and no problems of selenium deficiency has been observed in horses fed lucerne or lucerne hay. Specific SELENIUM supplements are required, particularly for foals, in certain areas designated as SELENIUM deficient but these regions are now well known. The use of SELENIUM supplements to horses, in areas where SELENIUM DEFICIENCY DOES NOT EXIST, will produce SELENIUM accumulation within the horse. Too much SELENIUM in the horse is just as bad as too little so be very careful of the problems of over administration of SELENIUM supplements.

IODINE

Feeds, in some very specific areas, may be low in iodine content. Those areas are now reasonably well defined and treatments are available from veterinary surgeons in those specific areas. Fortunately the areas concerned are very small in size and the problem is localised to these districts. Excessive administration of IODINE, to horses, can produce exactly the same symptoms as lack of IODINE in the diet.

FLUORINE

For all practical purposes, there is sufficient fluorine in the average horses' diet to provide all the animals needs and FLUORINE should never be given as a supplement to horses.

VITAMINS

VITAMIN A

Commonly derived from CAROTENE present in green pasture and hays as well as carrots and yellow maize. 2.00 kgs of green feed or hay will provide the average thoroughbred with adequate levels of Vitamin A, in a stabled situation. As the horse has to get at least 2.25 kgs of hay or green feed per day to maintain gut fill and ingesta flow, there should never be any Vitamin A deficiency in horses on this type of diet. Horses, receiving adequate green feed supplies, are also known to be able to store Vitamin A in the liver for up to 9 months and hence any horse, especially performance horses, returning from a spell on pasture, will have more than adequate levels of Vitamin A in the liver reserves. The only practical situation where Vitamin A may be required in horse feeding would be where the rations consists of cereal grains and cereal chaff without any access to green feed, carrots or yellow maize.

VITAMIN B COMPLEX

The horse is known to have a positive Vitamin B balance, that is, the animal makes Vitamin B in its digestive tract and excretes more in the faeces than is consumed in the feed. A detailed study in America in 1967 showed that 20 times as much Thiamine (B1) was excreted in the faeces of the horse as compared to that eaten in the feed. The ratios for some other B vitamins are: Riboflavin (B2) 6 times, Niacin 7 times, and Pantothenic Acid 10 times. Horses, fed diets consisting largely of grains and grain by-products, will have a low intake of the B group vitamins, whilst horses on lucerne or alfalfa hay, pasture hay or green pasture generally have much higher intakes of these compounds. If there is any indication that B group vitamin supplementation is of value to horses, it will only apply to performance horses in peak training, where the horses' demand for VITAMINS of the B GROUP appear to exceed the rate of production and supply from fermentation of celulose or fibre, in the large intestine. There appears no evidence to suggest that Vitamin B supplementation is required to any horse other than those in peak levels of training and performance.

There are practical indications that Vitamin B supplementation to performance horses, which have been stabled for some period of time and not had any reasonable access to green feed do develop bad appetites or feeding problems, which may be stimulated by the addition of some B vitamins to the ration. Often this is a complicated problem involving amino acid balance, protein level and available B vitamins in the ration.

VITAMIN C

Whilst Vitamin C is an essential vitamin for humans, the vitamin can be made in the horses' digestive tract from the energy component of the feed. There is no need for any horse to be fed Vitamin C for normal nutritional purposes. As a specific purpose drug, Vitamin C has been used with some success in the treatment of bleeders. Ascorbic Acid (synthetic Vitamin C) added to the drinking water of race horses prone to bleeding, has sometimes proved effective in treatment of the disease. The Vitamin C is thought to strengthen the walls of the blood vessels and so reduce the likelihood of blood becoming visible at the nostrils after severe physical exertion.

VITAMIN D

Essential in conjunction with CALCIUM and PHOSPHORUS for correct bone growth. Vitamin D, in a horse, is obtained from pasture in the form of Ergosterol which is converted to Ergocalciferol either when the plants are eaten by the horse or in the hay making process. Sunlight also acts on the skin of the horse to form Vitamin D3 which is then transported to the liver and then the kidney where the active form of Vitamin D is produced. Apart from the value of D in bone growth, the vitamin is also essential in the general absorption of the minerals from the digestive tract.

Horses, stabled during the day, may become deficient in Vitamin D. However, if they are being fed reasonable levels of sun cured hay, supplementation with D may not be necessary as the horse may receive sufficient D from the hay.

VITAMIN E

This vitamin is essential for proper cell function and is generally connected with muscle activity. The average thoroughbred horse requires about 300 units per day and that can be readily obtained from 2.2 kgs of lucerne hay. All green feed contains adequate levels of Vitamin E hence any normal horse will not require supplementation of this vitamin. Vitamin E is used, in the performance area, in large doses as a muscle tonic, and may have use in that field, but for the greater majority of horses there is no need, at all, to feed Vitamin E.

VITAMIN K

The horse has a positive balance of Vitamin K, i.e. it produces K in the digestive tract, and excretes more than it takes in as part of the feed.

SUMMARY

Most problems, relating to the level of MINERALS in horse's diets occur when there is a deficiency of roughage or grazing in the ration, when cereal hay and or chaff (oaten or wheaten) form a part of the diet and or when there is an excessive level of grain in the ration.

CALCIUM and PHOSPHORUS is very rarely, if ever, needed as a supplement provided a mixed ration, consisting of up to 50% (by weight) green pasture OR lucerne hay OR pasture hay and 50% (by weight) grain is being fed. If the ration however consists of more than 50% (by weight) of cereal grains and cereal hay or chaff, then some form of calcium supplement will be required to balance the low levels of calcium and the high level of phosphorus in that type of diet.

IRON is available in sufficient quantities in all horse feeds except maize and skim milk. Unless the horses' diet consists solely of these two feeds, and that is most unlikely, then there is sufficient iron in the common feeds to provide the horse with all its needs of iron, some specific anaemias excepted.

MAGNESIUM, horses, subject to the tying up syndrome, especially when traveling, may benefit from small daily doses of magnesium sulphate, in the form of Epsom Salts. All other horses will receive sufficient magnesium from their normal diets.

All other minerals are available in the general feeds at adequate levels to avoid the need for feeding any of them.

VITAMIN AND MINERAL CONTENT OF COMMON HORSE FEEDS

The overall summary reveals that the common feeds used in horse nutrition are able to provide the animals with adequate levels of vitamins and minerals in all but the following cases:

VITAMIN A – only required if the horse has no access to green feed, carrots and or yellow maize.

VITAMIN B – for performance horses or stabled horses which become track sour and go off feed.

VITAMIN D – for horses with no access to sunlight

VITAMIN E – for performance horses only

22. FEED SUPPLEMENTS

To paraphrase Shakespeare

TO SUPPLEMENT OR NOT TO SUPPLEMENT? -THAT IS THE QUESTION.

The horse owner and feeder is continually confronted with numerous commercial products, all designed to make the horse look better, perform better, or simply feel better or so we are told.

Marketing of these products is carried out in a very astute way so as to convince the average horse owner that his or her horse really needs the particular product.

Feed supplements consist of various mixtures of vitamins, minerals, and identified and unidentified substances which may or may not be of value to the horse. These substances are generally fed, as an addition to the normal ration, in small quantities per day to the animal. Daily dose rates, as per the majority of label recommendations, vary from 20 grams per horse per day up to 0.5 kgs per 100 kgs live weight per day, or 2.25 kgs per thoroughbred horse.

WHAT IS A FEED SUPPLEMENT ?

A natural or synthetic compound or group of compounds which, when added to a feed ration, will correct a deficiency or lack of that compound or group of compounds in that ration.

An effective FEED SUPPLEMENT should:-

1. provide any technically necessary feed component required by the horse which is not present in the normal ration.
2. NOT CONTAIN any compound which MAY LEAD TO the development of sub clinical or clinical problems in the horse, either by itself, in combination with the same compound present in the ration already being fed, or acting in conjunction with any other compound, either in the supplement or in the basic ration.
3. correct any specific nutritional deficiencies which can occur, due to the stress of hard training, competition and performance, where the nutritional needs of individual horses MAY not be satisfied by the basic horse feeds.

Just what constitutes a feed supplement CAN VARY with the work load and or performance of the horse

FEED SUPPLEMENTS can be divided into a number of categories, as described in the following.

MINERALS ALONE

the most common are CALCIUM SUPPLEMENTS, IRON and SELENIUM.

CALCIUM AND PHOSPHORUS SUPPLEMENTS

Due to the recognised high PHOSPHORUS levels of grains CALCIUM supplements are commonly available in many forms and under many labels. They are promoted on the need for calcium and phosphorus to act to-gether and in specific amounts to allow proper bone development and maintenance, but if the literature relative to the various products is carefully perused, there is generally no mention of the basic calcium and phosphorus levels that exist in the rations already being fed to the horse. These supplements are generally offered to supply most, if not all, of the horse's daily CALCIUM needs. This approach can be dangerous because, as we have shown earlier in this book, it is possible for most, if not all, horses to be able to obtain all the daily calcium and phosphorus needs from a general mixed ration. Feeding of a calcium and phosphorus supplement to horses on general mixed rations could, in fact, raise the levels of one or both minerals to a level where adverse results may occur. No absolute statement can be made in this regard unless the complete ration being fed to the horse is fully analysed, but the warning is given and horse feeders should be aware of the problem.

CALCIUM AND/OR PHOSPHORUS SUPPLEMENTS WITH MINERAL ADDITIVES

Generally the base of these products are either LIME or DICALCIUM PHOSPHATE, as in the above, with additions of MINERALS such as magnesium, manganese, zinc, iron etc. The comments above again apply with the added fact that most if not all the common horse rations generally contain more than adequate levels of these trace minerals in the base feeds. Supplementary feeding of such trace minerals will, therefore, not provide the animal with anything the horse is not already receiving in the base feed mix.

CALCIUM AND/OR PHOSPHORUS SUPPLEMENTS WITH VITAMIN ADDITIVES

Some supplements are available which are based on either LIMESTONE to supply CALCIUM or DICALCIUM PHOSPHATE to supply both CALCIUM and PHOSPHORUS, plus additions of VITAMIN A and VITAMIN D are common and other VITAMINS and or minerals may also be present at manufacture.

These products suffer from an instability problem in that the VITAMINS, added at manufacture, will be rapidly decomposed by the CALCIUM content of the product and will not be available for use by the horse. While ever STABILITY tests and or USE BY DATES are not required when registering stock feeds,by the appropriate authorities, such products will continue to be marketed.

IRON SUPPLEMENTS

Probably the most common nutritional supplement on the market. There is an incorrect belief, held by many people, that an iron supplement is of value, to all horses, to increase the red blood cell content and, presumably with more red blood cells, the horse will perform better. The full discussion on IRON as a mineral in horse feeding, in earlier sections of this book, emphasises that IRON will not produce any more red blood cells than the horses' body can use in the blood stream and store in the spleen. IRON, in excessive levels in the horse, may well lead to diarrhoea, reduced growth rate, drowsiness, affect liver function and interfere with the availability of both PHOSPHORUS and COPPER, leading to bone disorders and fractures. By far the greater proportion of common horse feeds contain enough iron to satisfy the horse's daily needs.

There appears to be two types of iron supplements on the market. There are those types which, in our opinion, are correctly labeled and indicate use of the iron supplement after severe parasite infestation, after a loss of large quantities of blood as a result of injury or in cases of general anaemia. These products generally carry a recommendation to feed the supplement for restricted periods. The use of such iron supplements on this basis has a logical technical reason.

The second type of labeling on iron supplements is that which promotes the product as being necessary for the continual well being of the horse and recommends daily feeding over long periods of time. The use of an iron supplement in this manner is dangerous, for reasons mentioned earlier, and should not be contemplated.

SELENIUM SUPPLEMENTS

SELENIUM is administered to horses, especially young foals, as either a drench or an injection. The SELENIUM should always be given alone and NEVER in combination with any other mineral or vitamin.

The exact requirements of SELENIUM, as a supplement, needs to be carefully evaluated by competent professionals as there is very little tolerance or margin for error in the dose rates, between fixing any possible SELENIUM problem and creating an equally worse condition of SELENIUM EXCESS.

Whilst SELENIUM acts in conjunction with VITAMIN E inside the horse, the two compounds should not be mixed to-gether at any stage but given to the horse in separate individual doses.

A complete description of the problems of SELENIUM in horse nutrition is detailed in the chapter on MINERALS.

ELECTROLYTES

ELECTROLYTES can be considered a mineral supplement, as four out of the six recognised ELECTROLYTES, namely SODIUM, CALCIUM, MAGNESIUM and POTASSIUM are all minerals.

The needs of each horse for ELECTROLYTES are very specific and the reader should refer to the chapter on ELECTROLYTES for a full appreciation of the topic.

SALT BLOCKS

These are a form of MINERAL SUPPLEMENTATION and are available in many varieties - from pure salt to blocks containing one or more of the minerals, supposedly required by the horse.

The feeding of salt blocks to horses has the following technical problems:

1. There may be sufficient salt and other minerals in the feeds which the animal is already receiving. From previous remarks in this book, it is obvious that the average horse on most common feeds has no need to be supplemented with minerals to ensure adequate health.
2. The additional AD LIB (unrestricted) feeding of minerals at high concentrations insalt blocks may cause excessive consumption of some minerals by the horse with the possibility of some form of toxicity occurring.

3. Rain on salt blocks causes them to become unusable very quickly. Salt blocks should be placed under a cover or roof which keeps the rain off the block and is high enough to prevent horses from injuring their heads on the structure. Feeding of salt blocks, without protection from the weather, means that they have to be picked up from the paddock and put under shelter every time it rains. If this is not done, the salt is quickly dissolved by the rainfall. This is just one more job that has to be carried out on the farm.
4. Despite what some people may believe, not all horses will eat salt blocks. Some horses will not eat free access salt in the paddock, they just do not like that type of feed supplement. If the block is being fed to one horse, it will be possible to work out whether consumption is taking place. If however, the block is available to a mob of horses, only continual observation over long periods of time may give an indication of those that will and will not eat salt blocks.
5. Horses, run in mobs always have the domineering or "bossy" animal, which, in some instances, may prevent other horses in the mob from gaining access to the block. Again observation of the mob, for many hours, will be the only way in which this problem, if it exists, can be sorted out.
6 The concentrations of added minerals to some SALT BLOCKS is so low, that the average horse is really only getting salt, despite the long technical names on the label.
7 Any VITAMINS added to a salt block at manufacture, will be quickly destroyed after packaging and will be of NO VALUE to the horse.

TRACE MINERALISED SALT

Unrestricted feeding of TRACE MINERALISED SALT, to horses, is a common practice in parts of the U.S. The mixture is based on 98% common salt or SODIUM CHLORIDE with trace amounts of the minerals, ZINC, MANGANESE, IRON, COPPER COBALT and IODINE. In SELENIUM deficient areas, this mineral may be added at the rate of 20-40 P.P.M. in relation to the weight of the salt block.

The TRACE MINERALISED SALT BLOCK DOES NOT CONTAIN any CALCIUM or PHOSPHORUS.

Whilst this is a common feeding practice in some areas, particularly low rainfall, low humidity climates, the unrestricted access (AD LIB or free choice) feeding provides NO CONTROL over individual animal intake, suffers from all the problems detailed above of feeding salt block and is a little like the SHOTGUN approach of some mineral/vitamin formulations.

ARSENIC

This has long been used as an appetite stimulant. "Fowler's Solution" is the formula used and in some stables this preparation is commonly used on all horses. The amount of arsenic administered daily is small, and the effects can be variable.

Some horses appear to respond but the reason is not at all clear. Other horses fed normal levels of ARSENIC have suffered quite dramatic adverse effects. Loss of hair, often partial, but sometimes more severe, appears to be a symptom of the reaction of some horses to the supplementation by arsenic. The only cure for these animals appears to be to remove the arsenic completely from the diet and recovery may take up to 12 months before the horse appears normal.

In some instances full recovery may never take place. Even though the affected horse may appear normal after recovery, it is generally not able to stand the stresses and work load of a training programme.

It may well be that the Vitamin B Complex could, in terms of present technical knowledge, be as an effective an appetite stimulant as arsenic, without any of the adverse and possibly dangerous side effects.

VITAMINS ALONE

The packaging of VITAMINS alone, with no other minerals or other additives present, is restricted to VITAMINS of the B COMPLEX and VITAMIN E. Very rarely are VITAMIN A and or VITAMIN D packaged separately and sold to the horse industry. There is no reason, other than a marketing reason, why this can not happen. VITAMINS A and D are packed and available separately and to-gether for other animal species.

VITAMIN B COMPLEX as it is commonly called, is a freely available supplement for horses in any one of a number of formulations, oral liquid, oral powder, and injectable. The term VITAMIN B COMPLEX must convey a magical meaning as the product is extensively used, especially on performance horses.

The main problem is that the B COMPLEX family of VITAMINS contains some nine individual and separate vitamins, some of which are of value to a performance horse and some of which are of NO VALUE at all. The cheaper B COMPLEX formulations generally contain the B vitamins which are NOT required by the horse, despite the long and impressive names. In addition, there is no stated legal requirement as to the minimum number of B VITAMINS which must be in a product which carries the name B COMPLEX. As long as two only B VITAMINS are present, the product can, apparently, be labeled as B COMPLEX.

BIOTIN, one of the members of the B COMPLEX group,is generally sold as a separate vitamin. BIOTIN generally has a very specific use, for strenghening hoof wall and sole tissue, although it does have other valuable uses, especially in performance horses. Secondly, BIOTIN is a very expensive VITAMIN and is much easier marketed as a separate vitamin than in any mixture.

VITAMIN E should always be packed by itself. VITAMIN E, in the presence of most other VITAMINS and MINERALS in a mixture, will degrade and rapidly breakdown. VITAMIN E also has very specific uses within the horse, it is important in the use of fats as an energy source for horses, and is therefore not required to be fed to every horse. As VITAMIN E is also one of the most expensive vitamins to use, its use should be restricted to performance horses and particularly those horses on a diet containing reasonable to high levels of fat.

BREWER'S YEAST

YEAST is being used in horse feeding in two forms, LIVE or MOIST YEAST and DRIED or POWDERED YEAST. LIVE or MOIST YEAST has been tested experimentally in relation to IRON and PROTEIN utilisation.

LIVE YEAST has been shown to have NO VALUE in either increasing the amount of iron absorbed by the horse or in increasing the blood levels of HAEMOGLOBIN and

PACKED CELL VOLUME. LIVE YEAST, added to the ration of performance horses at very small amounts, has been shown to be able to increase NITROGEN RETENTION, within the horse, by up to 10% without increasing NITROGEN and or PROTEIN intake. The increased extraction of nitrogen from the same amount of protein appears to be due to the yeast increasing the microbial population of the large intestine and this then leads to better extraction of the remaining protein within the cell walls, released with additional fibre breakdown.

Yeast has long been recognised as a source of Vitamins of the B Complex. Yeast is especially rich in Thiamine or B1, Riboflavin or B2, Niacin and Pantothenic acid. One tablespoon of DRIED YEAST/day is sufficient to overcome any THIAMINE deficiency which may exist in any stabled, hard fed, performance horse. When compared to other commercial preparations of Vitamin B Complex, yeast may be a very expensive source of these vitamins. Practically it is a reasonable horse supplement but it would be desirable to compare the cost with alternate sources of the B Complex.

VITAMIN/MINERAL MIX

These products are generally a mixture of just about any vitamin and/or mineral that can be put into a product.

Such VITAMIN/ MINERAL mixes are easy to pick, they are the ones with the long list of apparently impressive but confusing names commonly called ACTIVE INGREDIENTS, on the pack.

Most of these VITAMIN/MINERAL mixes are formulated on the "SHOTGUN" approach. If in doubt about the value of a feed component, SHOOT it into the mix. The levels of the various feed components vary tremendously, and often for no apparent reason. Analysis of the daily recommended dose rates shows no pattern of logic, in the formulation, of most of these mixes.

Daily consumption levels, as recommended on the labels, are bewildering when comparisons are made between products and then compared with the known needs of the horse. There appears no technical reason why many of the recommended feeding rates are as stated.

Most VITAMIN/MINERAL formulations have recommended daily feeding rates which, calculated out on the basis of what each individual horse is expected to receive from the supplement, make no allowance for:-

1. individual vitamin and mineral content already in the horses' feed.
2. possible toxicities which may occur in the horse when components in the supplement are added to the same components already in the ration, e.g. the effect of COPPER, ZINC, MANGANESE and MOLYBDENUM levels on the use of each mineral of these minerals and also PHOSPHORUS in the horse.
3. PRODUCT STABILITY, most of the vitamins which have been added to these products, at manufacture, WILL NOT BE AVAILABLE at feeding as these vitamins will have been destroyed by the minerals present in the package, after mixture but before use.

Vitamin A and Vitamin D are two excellent examples of feed components which are readily available to most horses, on a daily basis, yet are in virtually every VITAMIN/MINERAL mix and are also TOXIC to the horse when excessive quantities are present within the horse. VITAMIN A is freely available from green feed or green hay, carrots and yellow maize and VITAMIN D is supplied FREE from sunlight.

VITAMINS A and D are really only needed for horses locked away from sunlight all day and which do not receive green feed or hay. This situation can apply to horses, in winter, in the northern hemisphere but would certainly not apply in the summer. There is the possible need for two separate VITAMIN or VITAMIN/MINERAL mixes, one for winter and one for summer in this part of the world. Problems with VITAMIN D availability can also arise in those horse breeds where colour is of the utmost importance, such as PALOMINOS, DUNS etc. where the horses are sometimes stabled all day to avoid sunlight and retain a desirable coat colour.

VITAMIN/MINERAL MIXES WITH ADDED PROTEIN

Basically, the same comments as are detailed above for VITAMIN/MINERAL mixes, with the exception that some form of protein source, generally an oilseed meal or skim milk, has to be added to the mix as the protein source. These products generally have a protein level in the range of 15-20%. At average feeding levels of about 60 to 300 grams of product per day, the average horse will be receiving only between 1% and 6% of its total protein needs from the supplement. In fact, the daily protein supplied at the recommended feeding rate by these types of supplements, can be readily obtained by feeding one additional kilogram of average lucerne hay per day, or by using a much lesser quantity of higher protein feeds. As discussed earlier, in detail, there is little advantage in feeding excess levels of protein to the horse, most horse feeds contain more than sufficient protein for all needs and purchased protein is always the most expensive part of the horse ration.

CHELATED MINERAL SUPPLEMENTS

A CHELATED MINERAL is one where an inorganic substance, a mineral, is chemically bound to an organic substance, in the form of PROTEIN, CARBOHYDRATE or FAT. The process is also called ORGANIC COMPLEXING.

If the organic compound to which the particular mineral is bound is absorbed faster than the mineral itself, then there will be an advantage in feeding CHELATED MINERALS to a horse. If however the mineral is organically bound to a substance which is less readily absorbed by the digestive tract than the mineral, then the feeding of CHELATED MINERALS will offer no technical advantages.

PHOSPHORUS PHYTATE is a CHELATED MINERAL. PHOSPHORUS PHYTATE is formed when excessive levels of BRAN and CEREAL GRAINS are fed to a horse, the PHYTATE in the bran and the grain binds the balance of the PHOSPHORUS in the ration in such a way that the PHOSPHORUS becomes unavailable to the horse. This is a CHELATED MINERAL which many people have had in their horse rations for years, probably unaware of the fact. However PHOSPHORUS PHYTATE dramatically reduces the availability of PHOSPHORUS to the horse.

To be able to assess whether there is a technical advantage in feeding chelated minerals to a horse, it would be necessary to know the full details of the chelation of each mineral in the supplement.

CHELATED MINERALS are often considerably more expensive than minerals in the inorganic form, so their use should be approached with caution.

SEAWEED MEAL BASED PRODUCTS

Products based on SEAWEED MEAL or KELP are included in this section as they are often promoted as containing a number of minerals in addition to some vitamins. Sales promotion is designed to emphasise the need to feed these vitamins and minerals to the horse. Whilst this type of promotion is technically correct, the approach is incorrect in that no mention is made of the vitamin and mineral content of the feeds which the horse may already be receiving and no mention is made of the possible toxicities which may occur as a result of feeding SEAWEED MEAL.

At recommended feeding rates of 50-100 grams per day, the horse has to consume a lot of other feeds to satisfy appetite. These other feeds will contain vitamins and minerals, in many instances, in amounts sufficient to satisfy the animals average daily needs. The protein levels of these SEAWEED MEAL products, at around 15-20%, will provide insignificant amounts of protein. due to the small weights, of supplement being fed, to the animal and may as well be deleted from the supplement for all the value that the small quantity of protein will do.

In regard to possible toxicities in the horse from feeding SEAWEED MEAL, there have also been reports of GOITRE occurring in horses from the feeding of these types of supplements. Seaweed is generally accepted as having a HIGH IODINE content and goitre in horses can be caused by either high or low levels of iodine in the feed. It is interesting to observe that, whilst these products, containing seaweed meal, are generally promoted and accepted as being high in iodine, the product labels, in some cases, do not indicate any iodine level in the feed.

AMINO ACID SUPPLEMENTS

All feeds with the exception of green pasture, hay made from that pasture, soybean meal and canola meal are deficient in one or more of the ten essential amino acids that the horse requires on a daily basis.

Amino acid supplements are currently available, either as a mixture of amino acids alone, or amino acids combined with vitamins and minerals, and may be used to balance the deficiency of one or more of the essential amino acids in the base feeds. It is important, if using amino acid supplements, to ensure that the amino acid which may be deficient in the normal ration is, in fact, in the supplement being fed. Some amino acid supplements do not contain the amino acids that are generally deficient in grains and grain based feeds. The feeding of these types of supplements, with a grain based ration, will only reduce the availability of the protein in the ration rather than increase such availability to the horse.

Careful evaluation of the contents of the supplement are necessary to ensure that the amino acids present will in fact balance the deficiency in the feed.

DO NOT USE AN AMINO ACID SUPPLEMENT UNLESS YOU ARE CERTAIN IT WILL BALANCE THE OTHER AMINO ACIDS IN THE RATION.

AMINO ACID supplements are generally available in two forms, injectable and oral. The injectible forms are recommended to be given twice weekly, in the jugular vein, with the possible problems at some stage of "needle shy" horses. The oral form, mixed with the feed, is the preferred form of administration.

Amino acid supplements should only be used after the ration has possibly been re-assessed to contain the optimum levels of pasture, lucerne hay and soybean meal. All these feeds contain all ten essential amino acids and generally at a much cheaper cost than the feeding on of a amino acid supplement.

DIGESTIVE ENZYME PREPARATIONS

These consist of a number of products, all of which contain one or more ENZYMES which are able to decompose CELLULOSE or FIBRE, within the horse's digestive tract.

The principle behind the use of ENZYME preparations, as a feed supplement, is to assist the natural enzyme production of the horse with FIBRE and CELLULOSE rupture and decomposition in the digestive tract of the horse. In the absence of such ENZYME preparations, which has been the common situation for all horses until about 1987, FIBRE and CELLULOSE is partially broken down in the stomach and small intestine and completely broken down in the large intestine by natural enzymes produced in the SALIVA and DIGESTIVE TRACT.

The idea of FIBRE and CELLULOSE breakdown, earlier in the digestive tract, is to allow better release of the CARBOHYDRATE type energy and other food nutrients, at the start of the digestive tract and, in theory, providing more chance for absorption of a greater percentage of these feed components within the stomach and small intestine and so get better feed utilisation and, presumably, less waste than is the situation without using the enzyme in the feed.

There is some scientific doubt as to whether these DIGESTIVE ENZYME preparations actually do what they are supposed to do and very little research work has been published on the subject. Some people, who are using these DIGESTIVE ENZYMES in a practical situation, are claiming good results in increased horse performance.

As is often the case in horse feeding, one has to ask the question - WHAT OTHER FEEDING AND OR MANAGEMENT CHANGES WERE MADE AT OR ABOUT THE SAME TIME AS THE DIGESTIVE ENZYMES WERE BEING FED. Past experiences lead to a very cautious approach when told by some how wonderful something is for the horse. Often the reason for the change is NOT WHAT the horse person thought, but some other nutritional or management change made at or about the same time.

CONTROLLED ENERGY RELEASE PREPARATIONS

Based on a chemical know as SODIUM HYDROGEN MONTMORILLONITE or BENTONITE, sometimes MINERALISED EARTH and "DRILLER'S MUD", and used in the U.S. beef cattle feedlot industry.

BENTONITE is a naturally occurring clay, mined out of the ground, which has the ability, when moistened, to be able to expand to about six or seven times its size. It has very practical applications when incorporated into the walls of dams, preventing loss of the wall and is also used by water drillers, who pump the BENTONITE down the shaft, where it swells with the soil and makes continual cleaning of the drill hole a lot easier.

In feedlotting beef cattle, BENTONITE has been shown to prevent digestive upsets and other problems which are common in cattle fed high grain rations to appetite capacity and with very restricted exercise.

In horse nutrition, BENTONITE added to the ration, swells inside the horse's stomach and "soaks up" the energy component of the digesta, immediately after feeding, and then slowly releases that energy to the bloodstream over the next few hours rather than the horse receiving a large amount of energy, into the bloodstream, within minutes of eating a hard feed. This changed pattern of energy absorption, by the stomach and small intestine, has the practical implications of quietening or calming or slowing down the behaviour of a horse which was previously a little hard to control.

Some of the commercial products contain not only the BENTONITE clay, but also has additives in the form of various digestive enzymes, micro-fine limestone for calcium supplementation, amino acids, methionine and lysine, both of which are lacking in all cereal hays, chaffs and cereal grains, and folic acid a member of the Vitamin B Complex. Stability problems, in the mixture, after packing probably mean that the AMINO ACIDS and the vitamins are destroyed before use and the same fate possibly occurs to the digestive enzymes.

BENTONITE or BENTONITE based products are of some value in feeding to those horses on a high grain diet or horses with "spooky or flighty" temperaments. Before feeding this clay, it would be advantageous to carefully evaluate the energy level of the ration in relation to the horses work load. It could well be that reduction in the energy level may produce the same end result as feeding this product with previous high energy levels.

If you get a response to feeding BENTONITE, then you are most likely OVERFEEDING ENERGY in relation to the horses' needs. Reduction of ENERGY INTAKE and elimination of BENTONITE from the diet will probably improve the performance of the horse and reduce feeding costs quite considerably.

BENTONITE also has a place in the ration of the horse with persistent DIARRHOEA which cannot be controlled, even after veterinary attention. The swelling ability of the clay will slow down the digesta movement and some reasonable success stories have been achieved in these type of situations.

HIGH PROTEIN SUPPLEMENTS

HIGH PROTEIN SUPPLEMENTS are generally in the protein range of about 10 to 40% CRUDE PROTEIN, with energy levels of 1.90 to 3.20 MCal/kg and usually, some or most of the vitamins and minerals required by the horse, are added to the product which is generally promoted as being able to provide the horses with most, if not all, his daily needs.

The products appears to be based on two major components, either seaweed meal or soybean meal, with the addition in some instance of molasses and cod liver oil.

Any type of good green pasture and or hay made from that pasture will have a protein level in the range of 14%-22% sufficient for any horse.

The problem of lack of PROTEIN in a ration will only come when the ration is based on very dry, mature pasture which has seeded. Even then, on some pasture types, the protein level of the mature pasture will be above 12% which means that those horses which may require higher protein levels than 12%, FOALS, WEANLINGS and YEARLINGS can get all the additional protein they need from good pasture or lucerne hay fed as a supplement.

A PROTEIN DEFICIENCY problem will exist on an ALL CEREAL RATION but that is only one problem of many problems which can occur on this type of ration.

With very few exceptions, most horses are able to obtain sufficient protein from normal horse feeds, there really is no reason, from a technical angle, to consider feeding a protein supplement when your horse has access to common horse feeds. Should your horse, for any one of a number of reasons, require a higher level of protein to the ration, increasing the amount of good quality lucerne hay will be the cheapest and best method.

HIGH FAT SUPPLEMENTS

These products are predominately based on SOYBEAN and RICE BY-PRODUCT but there is no reason why similar products could not be developed from other oilseed meals or the components of present pre-mixed horse feeds with added fat.

Soybean Based Products can be subdivided into two categories:

A. Those based on soybean grain as harvested in the field

B. Those based on soybean meal as obtained from the oil crushing plants after the oil content has been removed.

PROCESSED WHOLE SOYBEAN

Sometimes known as FULL FAT, as no fat has been removed before processing the beans, direct from the paddock, are subject to a heat extrusion process which destroys the trypsin inhibitor in the bean and produces a product palatable to horses.

This process retains the fat (oil) content of the beans. Protein analysis generally is in the range of 35-40% and fat levels are around 18%, giving an energy value of about 6.20 MCal/kg.

SOYBEAN MEAL PRODUCTS

Commonly called SOYBEAN MEAL refer chapter on COMMON HORSE FEEDS.

Suggested feeding rates for both soybean products are about 200 to 500 grams per day. It is inadvisable to exceed 500 grams/day. In the initial stages of feeding products, based on SOYBEAN MEAL, it is possible to get the horses' intake up to 1 or 1.5 kgs/day. After about 4 or 6 weeks, at this level of feeding, a palatability problem will occur and the horse may well completely reject the soybean product. If the initial daily feeding level does not exceed 500 grams, then the palatability problem does not appear to occur.

As the average large horse needs about 1.6 kgs of protein per day, this maximum level of feeding will only provide 180 grams of protein or 11% of the animals daily protein needs. The same thoroughbred horse will need, in reasonable work, 5.50 kgs of energy per day and at 500 grams of this type of feed supplement, the amount being eaten will provide about 34% of the horse's daily expected energy needs. Whilst the feeds are very concentrated, consideration needs to be taken of the other horse feeds available and the protein and energy levels of such feeds, as well as the need to maintain gut fill and ingesta flow.

The horse is certainly not going to satisfy his appetite on 0.5 kgs of SOYBEAN supplement when, in fact, he needs about 10 kgs of feed per day. The greater proportion of the ration, some 9.5 kgs, will contain protein and energy and it is up to the individual horse feeder to work out if he can get the same feed components from the other feeds, at a cheaper price.

A number of SUPPLEMENTS are promoted as HIGH FAT, to provide extra ENERGY to the horse.

One must ask the question IS MORE ENERGY REALLY NEEDED BY THAT HORSE?

One of the major problems of feeding horses is the provision of too much ENERGY, from normal feeds, in the ration in relation to the horses' workload, so why add extra ENERGY to the ration if it is not required ?

There is the additional problem that FATS require a large amount of OXYGEN to be broken down into components which can be used by the horse. If the horse happens to be an animal which is expected to produce muscle energy in an ANAEROBIC situation, in the absence of oxygen, as in a racehorse, standardbred, showjumper, cutting horse etc., then the addition of high fat supplements to the ration will adversely affect the performance of the horse.

Unless there are very specific technical reasons for feeding FATS, i.e. a horse which produces all its muscle energy in an AEROBIC situation, it is generally much better to stay with CARBOHYDRATE ENERGY from GRAINS.

HIGH FAT RATIONS AND POSSIBLE VITAMIN OVERDOSE.

The FAT SOLUBLE VITAMINS A, D, E, and K are stored in the horse's body within the fat reserves, especially those fat reserves connected with the liver.

It is well known that levels of these VITAMINS, fed in excess of the horse's daily needs are stored within these fat reserves and that a build up of the levels of VITAMIN A, D and K can produce undesirable problems in the horse. Sometimes, these excessive levels of the FAT SOLUBLE VITAMINS, can lead to adverse changes of a permanent nature, rendering a horse of no further economic use and also occasionally causing death. As far as can be determined from the technical literature, any such cases of VITAMIN A and D toxicity which have been documented have been with horses fed low fat rations but with what would be considered overdoses of the fat soluble vitamins in feed supplements.

The big question mark over the feeding of any type of supplement containing VITAMIN A and or D, in particular, to any horse also receiving a high fat ration at the same time, is whether the high fat ration will encourage the retention of vitamins A and D, within the fat depots in the body. There is the technical possibility that this may occur and could lead to earlier and more intensive manifestations of the problems of VITAMIN A and D EXCESS and the subsequent adverse effects on the horse.

There is no current information available to prove the case one way or the other but those considering feeding HIGH FAT rations would need to carefully consider the possible effect on VITAMIN A and D toxicities.

POSSIBLE PROBLEMS FROM USE OF FEEDS SUPPLEMENTS

FEED SUPPLEMENTS should be fed because they add something to the ration and thereby complement the general ration to be a complete feed, at the same time, not producing any adverse reactions and or toxicities in the horse.

FEEDS SUPPLEMENTS should NOT BE FED:-

1. if the name sounds attractive.
2. if the label and or the package catch's the eye.

3. if they are cheaper than any other.
4. if you cannot understand exactly what is in them.
5. if you cannot work out how much of each micro-ingredient, your horse is getting each day, you may be feeding the horse a very expensive dose of starch or limestone.
6. if you do not know EXACTLY what supplements your horse needs and WHY?
7. if you are unable to determine whether any possible toxicities may occur.
8. because someone else said so.

This probably means that many horses should NOT BE RECEIVING supplements or are receiving the wrong supplement.

So if the feeders persist in adding all these "goodies" to the feed, without having all the answers to the eight points listed above, the following is a list, of some of the things that can happen if the wrong feed supplement is being fed.

BONE GROWTH AND STRUCTURAL PROBLEMS
from
IMBALANCE OF CALCIUM/PHOSPHORUS RATIO
INSUFFICIENT CALCIUM AND OR PHOSPHORUS
EXCESS VITAMIN D
EXCESS SELENIUM
EXCESS IRON
EXCESS MOLYBDNEMUM

EXCESS ENERGY PROBLEMS
from
TOO MUCH FAT IN THE RATION
OVERFEEDING ENERGY

POOR GROWTH PROBLEMS
from
UNDERFEEDING PROTEIN
DEFICIENCY OR EXCESS OF IODINE
OVERFEEDING OF VITAMIN A
OVERFEEDING OF VITAMIN D
EXCESS SELENIUM

POOR GENERAL PERFORMANCE
from
LACK OF VITAMIN B1
INSUFFICIENT OR INCORRECT ELECTROLYTES
OVERFEEDING OF VITAMIN A
EXCESS IRON
EXCESS MOLYBDENUM

FEED SUPPLEMENTS

THE INTERRELATIONSHIP OF THE FEED COMPONENTS WHICH ACT IN COMBINATION WITH OTHER FEED COMPONENTS includes:-

LACK OF ONE OR MORE OF THE 10 ESSENTIAL AMINO-ACIDS
FAT AND CARBOHYDRATE ENERGY USE
COBALT AND VITAMIN B12
CALCIUM/PHOSPHORUS and VITAMIN D
SELENIUM AND VITAMIN D
IRON AND PHOSPHORUS
COPPER AND MOLYBDENUM
SALT AND ELECTROLYTES
NIACIN AND PANTOTHENIC ACID (vitamin and amino-acid).

THE PROBLEM IS TO EVALUATE EACH HORSE'S NUTRITIONAL REQUIREMENTS so that the horse gets what it needs for its level of activity, without any possible problem occurring from either too little or two much of any food component or from an adverse interaction of two or more food components.

There are many commercial feed SUPPLEMENTS available to the horse owner. It is not the intention to critically analyse each preparation as this would be too large a subject for this publication.

Rather it is the intention to look at and detail the horse's needs in terms of vitamin and mineral supplementation and to analyse and describe the types of feed supplements that are technically desirable from the horses' viewpoint, for particular feeding situations.

The use of feed supplements by horse owners appear to be based on the following criteria:

1. No consideration is made of the vitamin and mineral content of the pasture, or other feeds, being given to the horse.
2. The premise that, if a small quantity of something is good for the horse, a larger quantity will be better.
3. That there will be no problem with any form of sickness in the horse, due to larger excessive doses of any product.
4. Promotional material and product labeling is such as to make the horse's owner believe that the animal must have a particular product.
5. The common horse feeds such as lucerne hay and chaff, cereal hays and chaff, all the grains oilseed meals etc., DO NOT HAVE LABELS which clearly indicate the actual vitamin and mineral content of those feeds, which include all the additives which are present in feeds supplements.

Some of the present feed supplements available for horse feeding do, in fact, have a label which can contain details of up to 24 separate feed components.

Our "normal" horse feeds listed earlier, pastures hays and grains, in fact, could also have attached to each of them a similar label, in most instance providing values for up to 24 separate feed components.

The average horse feeder, however, on reading the label on one of these supplements can but not be impressed by the composition of the product. What is written on the label may not mean a thing to the purchaser, but the long list of impressive and hard to pronounce names quickly gives the impression that the product must do some good for the horse.

In reality, the following matters need to be considered:

1. How many of the components in the purchased supplement are already available to the horse in his basic feeds ? As shown earlier, the basic feed stuffs can contain considerable quantities of the compounds detailed on the labels of proprietary feed supplements.
2. What is the actual amount of each compound that the horse receives in the daily recommended dose? While the content on the label may appear to be impressive, insome instances, when the actual daily dose of individual feed components are worked out, the quantity being fed is so small as to be useless to the horse.
3. Can you understand the various ways of measuring the many components in these feed supplements.International units, milligrams and micrograms are commonly used as well as percentages and grams. It is quite simple if you want to make a label look impressive to quote content in milligrams on the label instead of grams. The label value is much bigger but the horse will not get any more of the component in his ration. It is also good marketing to use as many different units of measurement on the label as possible, this really impresses the potential buyer. There is no legal requirement to standardise the methods of expressing the measurement of micro-nutrients in feeds supplements
4. Is it possible to change the ration you are feeding to obtain the desired vitamins and minerals from other common feeds at a cheaper price than buying a tin or bag of prepared supplement ? Remember, all these minerals and vitamins are already in the basic horse feeds and are probably costing you nothing, you have already paid for the protein and energy level, which are the items which determine the price of bulk feeds. Feed supplements vary considerably in cost when looked at on a per horse per day basis, and this will be covered in more detail in later sections of this book.
5. Is the advertising literature presented with the product correct. The best practical example of this is a product which, as a complete horse feed, puts great emphasis on the fact that the calcium and phosphorus ration is in the feed at 1.5/1. Whilst this is technically desirable, the actual daily feeding rate recommended for the product shows that the horse is receiving less than half the required physical level of the two minerals. Horses on this feed must eventually suffer bone problems from an insufficient intake of the two minerals.
6. Has consideration been taken of the vitamin and mineral content of the basic feeds and will the feeding of an additional supplement raise the levels of one or more of the feed components to the degree where some form of sub-chronic illness or adverse affect may occur to the horse.
7. Have you placed confidence in something in a tin or a bag as a means of correcting problems in the horse which in fact are not related to the contents of the pack or bag?

The horse may suffer a straight protein or energy deficiency, he may need a good drench to clean out the internal parasites, or he may too "toey" and simply need the energy level of his feed being reduced or his work rate increased. Supplements will not correct these problems so it is imperative that the horse owner gets the priorities right in the first place.

"IF A SMALL QUANTITY OF SOMETHING IS GOOD, A LARGER QUANTITY MUST BE BETTER"

There is no scientific basis for this type of approach in horse nutrition. Unfortunately horses cannot talk. If they could, they would probably tell most horse feeders to throw away most of the supplements presently being fed. Humans are able to communicate to someone if they feel the adverse affects of a particular feed or drug. The poor horse is not able to tell his feeder if he is feeling unwell, or has a stomach ache. We all use the techniques of an "experienced" horseman to attempt to tell when the animal is "off colour". Unfortunately, in many situations the symptoms we try and observe and occasionally notice, in the horse, have often been at a sub-clinical stage for some time before the feeder notices any changes in the animal.

No research work has ever been carried out to show that some of the massive mixed doses of vitamins and minerals that are often given to horses are of value to the animals. In fact, there is a considerable amount of practical evidence which shows that the feeding of high levels of vitamins and or minerals to horses is dangerous. The use of daily supplements of multi-vitamin and mineral mixes does not serve any technical purposes in the great majority of horse feeding situations.

"NO GENERAL PROBLEMS WILL OCCUR WITH THE OVERFEEDING OF VITAMINS AND MINERALS"

This attitude to the feeding of vitamins and mineral supplements is incorrect. Many vitamins and minerals when fed in quantities higher than the desired levels to the animals, may, or will produce undesirable effects in the horse.

VITAMIN A.

Levels of Vitamin A in a diet greater than 160,000 International Units per day can cause adverse affects in the horse. Scientific studies have documented such cases. The effects of combined daily intakes of Vitamin A, supplement plus base ration, above this level, may have a depressing effect on growth rate, with resultant development of many types of abnormalities in muscle, bone, tendons and ligaments.

VITAMIN B COMPLEX

There is no available technical knowledge which shows adverse effects occurring in the horse from feeding higher than normal levels of this group of vitamins.

VITAMIN C.

As for B there does not appear any problems known at the present time that can be caused by excessive levels of Vitamin C in the horse's diet.

VITAMIN D.

When fed in large doses, or in small doses combined with the effects of sunlight, this vitamin has been proven to have a number of undesirable effects on horses. The average thoroughbred, at 450 kgs, has an accepted Vitamin D daily need of 3000 International Units. Mares fed 10 times this daily level of Vitamin D during pregnancy, produces foals which die shortly after birth. These deaths were caused by the Vitamin D causing calcium to be deposited in the main blood vessels in the region of the heart. The build up of the calcium deposits caused a restriction in the blood vessels internal diameter and rupture of the blood vessels occurred, due to pressure build up.

Unfortunately the experiment did not show whether this same effect would occur at levels of Vitamin D supplementation less than 10 times the accepted rate. It may well be that Vitamin D levels at only 5 times the accepted rate, or even less, may also produce similar symptoms.

Growing horses, fed higher than normal levels of Vitamin D, have developed ossification of the joints and depositions of CALCIUM within the blood vessels, reducing overall blood supply. This simply means that excess calcium is laid down at and around the area of the joints and within the blood vessels. The joints become stiff and may eventually cease to function effectively. There are also various reported cases where excess feeding of Vitamin D has caused calcium deposition in and around the kidneys and lungs.

VITAMIN E.

There is no known evidence to suggest adverse affects from feeding high doses of Vitamin E to horses. On the contrary Vitamin E at levels up to 15 times the accepted feeding rates have been used to attempt to increase muscle performance and work output in performance horses.

VITAMIN K.

Vitamin K, should not, in any circumstances, be fed to a horse, unless under strict veterinary supervision.

VITAMINS

DEFICIENCY OF LACK OF, MAY CAUSE PROBLEMS

A	B1	Folic Acid
Biotin ?	C ?	D

NO KNOWN GENERAL DEFICIENCY IN HORSES

B2 Riboflavine	B6 Pyridoxine	B12
Choline	Niacin	Pantothenic Acid
K	B15	B17
	P	

EXCESS LEVELS IN RATIONS MAY CAUSE PROBLEMS

A	D

? Indicates possible problems in specific cases. Refer to text for detailed explanation.

CALCIUM AND PHOSPHORUS

Feeding of high levels of CALCIUM and PHOSPHORUS need to be carefully monitored. It is essential that the amounts of both minerals consumed daily by the horse, (the total of ration content plus fed supplement content) have the amount of CALCIUM EQUAL TO OR EXCEEDING THE WEIGHT OF PHOSPHORUS. If this fact is appreciated and monitored, then the CALCIUM/PHOSPHORUS RATIO will always be correct. It is desirable that each horse receive the correct amount of both CALCIUM and PHOSPHORUS as excessive levels of PHOSPHORUS in the ration can markedLy depress and reduce CALCIUM absorption by the digestive tract. High levels of CALCIUM will increase water consumption and electrolyte demand as the body attempts to excrete the excess CALCIUM via the urine. Excess CALCIUM can also produce the condition commonly called NUTRITIONAL SECONDARY HYPERPARATHYROIDISM.

IRON

Overfeeding of iron has been shown to be unable to increase the levels of HAEMOGLOBIN and PACKED CELL VOLUME, in healthy horses and to cause decreases in growth rate and produce skeletal problems in young horses. Excess iron may also tie up or render useless the PHOSPHORUS and COPPER in the animals' body, causing poor mineralisation of bone to occur. The end result of this type of problem can be bone disorders, leading to breakdowns and possibly even fractures.

MAGNESIUM, POTASSIUM, SULPHUR, COPPER, MANGANESE.

These are all required by the horse in minute amounts and satisfactory levels are available in most mixed feeds. The small amount of scientific work, available at this time, to show the effects of feeding any of these minerals in daily doses larger than normally required, indicate no known problems.

ZINC

At excessively high daily dose rates of 90 grams of zinc fed to foals, bone and joint problems develop. The symptoms include stiffness lameness, enlarged ends on the long bones and general increased levels of zinc in other body tissues. It is most unlikely in practice that anyone would feed such high levels of zinc to a horse, but the problem exists that the trial did not determine the maximum level of zinc supplementation that could be fed without causing these symptoms to occur. High ZINC levels in the diet can also cause a COPPER DEFICIENCY, which is permanent in effect as it WILL NOT respond to treatment.

MOLYBDENUM

Excessive levels of MOLYBDENUM in the diet can cause low levels of PHOSPHATES and COPPER to occur in the horse, leading to all types of bone deformities, skeletal problems and possibly RICKETS.

SELENIUM

Commonly used in combination with Vitamin E for muscle "toning" and conditioning. EXCESSIVE levels of SELENIUM in the diet will cause SELENOSIS, also know as BOB TAIL DISEASE or ALKALI DISEASE. Symptoms include, loss of appetite, hair falling out, especially in mane and tail, hoof wall destruction, blindness and possibly paralysis. SELENIUM EXCESS problems are IRREVERSIBLE.

IODINE

Goitre can be produced from not only iodine deficiency but also from the OVERFEEDING OF IODINE. There are known cases where goitre has been found in horses, being fed supplements, based on seaweed meal and other cases of goitre have been related to the use of some drugs in horses. Iodine is a very "touchy" mineral and as most feeds contain small levels, the mineral is best deleted from any supplement being fed to the horse. This comment does not apply to those very small restricted localities where known iodine deficiency exists. These areas are well defined and your local veterinary surgeon will be able to advise you on this matter.

FLUORINE

Fluorine in levels greater than the accepted NATURAL LEVELS in all feeds, about 0.04%, will cause lesions to develop on the bones, may cause weakening of the bones with the likelihood of fractures occurring and can also produce general unthriftness in the horse.

The feeding of fluorine in any form of supplement to the horse is to be discouraged. There appears adequate levels of fluorine in normal horse feeds for all reasonable needs.

MINERALS

DEFICIENCY OR LACK OF, MAY CAUSE PROBLEMS

Calcium	Ca	Selenium	Se ?
Phosphorus	P	Iodine	I ?
Iron	Fe ?		

NO KNOWN GENERAL DEFICIENCY IN HORSES

Magnesium	Mg	Cobalt	Co
Potassium	K	Manganese	Mn
Sulphur	S	Molybdenum	Mo
Zinc	Zn	Fluorine	F
Copper	Cu		

EXCESS LEVELS IN RATIONS MAY CAUSE PROBLEMS

Iron	Fe	Phosphorus	P
Zinc	Zn		

? Indicates possible problems in specific cases. Refer to text for detailed explanation.

VISUAL EFFECTS FROM FEEDS SUPPLEMENTS

We really know so little about the actions and interactions of the various feed components and how they affect the differing growth rates and performance criteria that we ask of horses,that it virtually impossible to be able to measure the effect of many supplements on the performance of horses.

What we can say is that, in theory, this or that or something else is required for the average horse.

What we cannot say, with any degree of authority, is whether this or that is required for the particular horse, on a particular feeding programme, at a particular stage of its career.

The effects of changes in feeding regimes very rarely happen overnight and some may take months to come to fruition. One therefore has to be very wary and cautious of any claim that a particular product is so much better than any other because someone saw a response.

Firstly most responses from changed feeding practice take some time to become visible.

Secondly some responses from changed feeding are not visible to the naked eye.

Thirdly what other change, if any, occurred at the same time as the new supplement was fed ?

Fourthly if a marked visual response is obvious, I would be very worried as to what was wrong before hand as all sorts of other problems could now occur. If this is the situation, it would be desirable to get professional assistance to sort out what was wrong before.

If the supposed visual response was based on the fact that the horse ate the supplement, the owner has fallen for the oldest "three card " trick in the horse feeding business. There are a number of flavours available which can be readily added to horse feeds to make them palatable, you could even get a horse to eat a full ration of flavoured sawdust, but it will not do him much good.

IT WOULD BE IN THE READER'S INTERESTS TO REFER TO CHAPTER 16 LABELING REQUIREMENTS OF HORSE FEEDS.

23. PREPARED FEEDS

Prepared, or pre-mixed commercial, feeds are convenience foods for horse owners, and maybe horses. They generally consist of a variety of mixes, mostly grain and or oilseed bases to which is added vitamins, minerals and other feed components, whilst some also include chaff or chopped hay. Prepared feeds are basically the all-purpose, one bag feeding mix.

They are a distinct and different feed to the vitamin and mineral supplements, described in the previous chapter, in that these prepared feeds are generally fed at levels of about 50% to 100% of the horses' daily total needs, supplemented with hay and/or grazing where applicable.

Some prepared feeds are marketed as a complete horse ration, whilst others may require some form of supplementation as recommended on the label by the manufacturer.

ADVANTAGES OF PRE-MIXED PREPARED HORSE FEEDS

1. the horse owner only needs to have one bag of feed, very suitable for the one horse owner or where restricted storage space is available.
2. the horse owner does not have to make up feeds each day from a number of different components.
3. if produced by a reputable manufacturer, will be of continual and consistent physical quality and technical standard.
4. formulations are based on standard data for average horses and with feeds from reputable manufacturers, there will be little chance of any adverse consequences happening to the horse.

DISADVANTAGES OF PRE-MIXED PREPARED HORSE FEEDS.

1. generally more expensive on a kilogram basis than if purchasing individual feeds and mixing your own.
2. rarely is there any indication of energy level of the feed on the product. As energy levels of feed are one of the most important aspects of horse feeding, there is no easy or reliable way in which the feeder is going to known whether the energy level in the prepared feed is correct for the particular horse at the particular time in the training and or competition programme.
3. being a standard fixed formula, feeding adjustments are unable to be made for individual horse differences and or requirements.
4. can contain feeds which will not readily be eaten by horses, if provided as a separate feed. Cottonseed hulls and sunflower hulls are two feeds with little technical value for horse feeding and which horses find most unattractive if fed as individual feeds. However mixed to-gether, add a little molasses and that is the basis of a number of prepared horse feeds currently being sold.
5. physical content of the feed can vary from mix to mix, possibly affecting the performance of the horse. This does occur with product from those companies

who are using least cost mixes and are more concerned about producing a feed at the cheapest price to meet the requirements of any registration obligations, rather than a feed of consistent physical composition and quality, which is most important in horse feeding.

6. due to the physical texture of the feed preparations, there is a possibility that some horses, especially fast eaters, may suffer digestive problems when consuming prepared feeds and any such horse, eating these products, will chew the feed a lot less and as a result will require attention to the teeth more frequently.

TYPES OF PREPARED FEEDS.

Prepared feeds are generally available in three forms:

a) Meal type produced on chaff and cereal products with additives.
b) Grain type, based on some type of cereal grain, grain by-product, oilseed meal, with additives.
c) Pelleted feeds generally on the same or similar base but in pellet form as a convenient way of feeding and reducing feed waste.

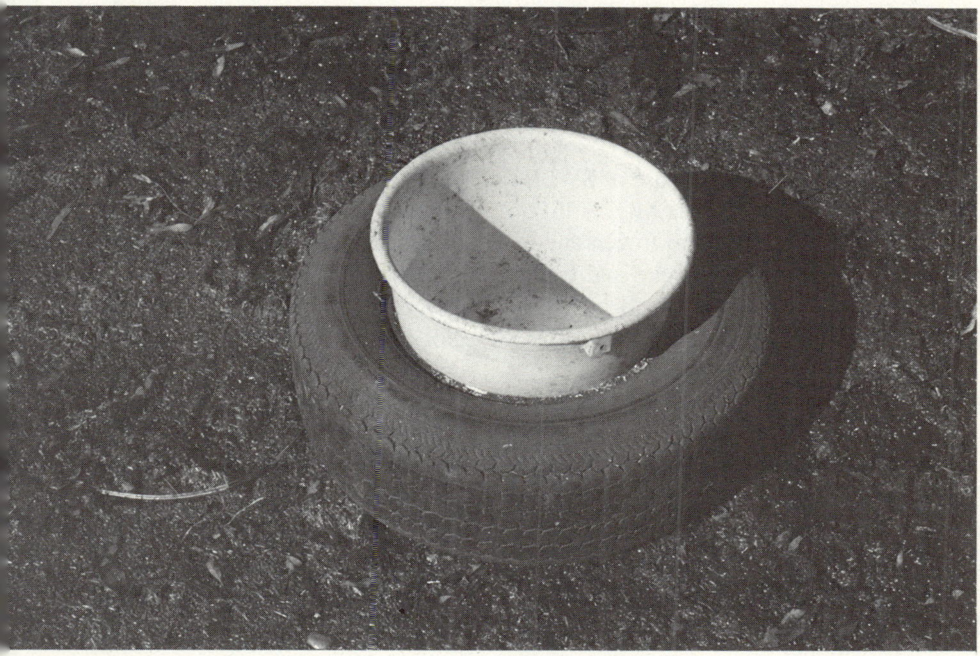

Cheap, effective and safe home made feeder.

It is highly likely that any prepared feed will contain one or more of the following MOLASSES, FAT and BENTONITE.

MOLASSES, at levels of around 1%-2%, by weight, is added to these types of feeds to act as a "binder" to assist in even distribution, throughout the feed, of any vitamin and or mineral additives. These additives are generally incorporated in the feeds at very small quantities, and the MOLASSES helps to "stick" these very small quantities to the larger grain, bran or similar particles, preventing separation, either in the bag or in the bottom of the feed bin. This level of MOLASSES also reduces the possible dust problem and assists in palatability and is not high enough to cause reduced consumption problems which can occur with some horses, given feeds with high molasses content.

FATS, in this instance OILS, are often added to prepared feeds at the rate of up to 3%, by weight of the ration. The FATS (OILS) act as a "binder", as described above, but also impart a shine or gloss to the feed which certainly makes it look more attractive to the purchaser. The gloss or shine, produced by the addition of FATS to prepared feeds, certainly cannot be of any significance as far as the horse is concerned as the horse has a "BLIND SPOT" in a circle of about 1.2 metres from its nose, so is unable to see exactly what it is eating at any time.

BENTONITE, in very small quantities, is also added to prepared feeds for the same "binding" purpose. BENTONITE lacks both the palatability aspects of MOLASSES and FATS and does not produce a shine on the feed as does FATS, but in the hot humid areas, as in the tropics and sub tropics, BENTONITE is the only additive which can be used as both MOLASSES and FATS, added to horse feeds, can produce all sorts of stability and palatability problems.

Various premixed feeds, commonly called SWEET FEEDS, are now becoming available for the horse market. SWEET FEEDS contain reasonably high levels of MOLASSES, usually in the range of 5-10%, incorporated for palatability, to act as a binder in the feed, reduces any dust problem and allows even distribution of any mineral/vitamin mix which has been incorporated in the feed.

The effective and satisfactory use of SWEET FEEDS depends very much on the climate and the season of the year. If the MOLASSES level is too high in cold winter climates, it is possible for the fed to become frozen and in hot humid climates, the high temperatures can cause the MOLASSES to cake and become unpalatable, due to the development of mould in the feed. There may well be a palatability problem with the high levels of MOLASSES for some horses with SWEET FEED. Not all horses like molasses.

A – MEAL TYPE FEEDS,

BASED ON CHAFF AND CEREAL GRAINS.

These pre-mixed feeds are often designed to provide the horse with the complete ration in the one bag. They will normally consist of at least 50% roughage, in the form of chaff with grain making up the greater proportion of the balance of the mix and other additives being incorporated. These feeds are generally designed to provide the horse with all its needs, the feeding of hay and or pasture being optional.

B – GRAIN TYPES

GENERAL PURPOSE

Generally formulated to be fed in conjunction with pasture and or hay. These products can be based on any grain or mixture of grains, dependent on local availability and consumer preferences. OATS, BARLEY, MAIZE, and small amounts of SUNFLOWER are the main grains used. It is important to remember that no matter what grain is being used, the chemical composition of ENERGY available from those grains is the same to the horse. Human personal preferences, for a particular grain for horse feeding has no sound technical basis.

Grains in these mixes are generally crushed, rolled and or possibly steamed, so it is wise to ensure that the product is reasonably fresh to avoid any nutrient loss by oxidation.

RICE BY PRODUCT BASED

These consist of a series of formulated products based on rice pollard and sometimes broken rice. The feeds concerned have additives of salt, lime, dicalcium phosphate, soybean meal, lupins and other normal horse feeds. Basically the feeds are prepared products designed to supply the horse with the complete ration in a specified quantity of feed per day as per the manufacturers' recommendations.

The rice by-product is supposed to have an energy fraction which is "less heating" than the energy fractions of other horse feeds. No actual evidence is presented to back up this claim but the product is recommended for feeding to those horses which may become agitated of "fizzy" on oats or maize. Our practical experience would tend to indicate that this may be true due to the fact that the principle source of energy in the product comes from the oil (fat) content of the rice pollard. This contains 18-19% oil which is only effectively converted to muscle energy when the horse's energy utilisation system is working in an AEROBIC environment. As it is usually only endurance horses and horses with similar levels of physical activity which use energy AEROBICALLY, the FAT or OIL content of these rice based feeds is really not available for effective use by most other types of horses.

Eventing horses fed rations containing high levels of fat in the range detailed above, have been sluggish, lazy and not performing to expectation as when carbohydrate energy constituted most of the energy supplies in the ration.

C – PELLETS

For a full description of the advantages and disadvantages of pellets, refer to the chapter of COMMON HORSE FEEDS and the section on LUCERNE PELLETS.

Apart from the good and bad points detailed there, compounded pellets, consisting of a number of ingredients have two main disadvantages. Firstly, once the pellet is made, it is not possible to be able to differentiate exactly what is in the pellet. Secondly, the green colour, in some compounded pellets, is obtained from the same dye which is used to put the green colour in some samples of lucerne chaff.

Reputable feed manufactures do not do other than incorporate fist grade ingredients in any pellet, but, as in any industry, there will always be someone who will use second or third grade feeds and green dyes. It is up to the purchaser to be aware of the problem, and act accordingly.

PROBLEMS WITH PREPARED FEEDS

VARIABLE QUALITY

If the prepared feeds are an equivalent cost, on a per kilogram basis, as the cost would be of making a similar ration from base ingredients, then the feed manufacturer is doing one of two things.

Firstly, they may be using in the prepared feeds, base feedstuffs which would not normally be fed to horses due to low nutritional values and/or palatability problems. These base ingredients are therefore cheaper to purchase and the palatability problems are overcome by the addition of MOLASSES and possibly artificial flavourings. There has been, and probably always will be, the feed manufacturer who prepares feed from second grade material such as poor quality grain, cereal mill offal that is not suitable to be sold as bran or pollard, grain and other sweepings collected from the mill floor etc. cottonseed hulls and sunflower hulls.

Whilst, hopefully, these types of feed manufacturers are in the minority, there is no way in which the person buying the bag of prepared feed can be sure of the exact ingredients and base components. Whilst each and every bag of prepared feed normally has to have a label indicating the feed nutrients present in the product, there is often no requirement for the label to indicate exactly what the base ingredients are in each and every bag.

Quality control is also sometimes lacking in prepared feed manufacture. Whilst some of the larger manufacturers may have, in plant, analytical laboratories, and, in fact, analyse each batch of feed to ensure conformity with the label requirement, many of the small feed manufacturers are not so equipped and do not have access to such analytical facilities. There is, therefore, no guarantee that the feed you may purchase does, in fact, contain what is stated on the label in terms of either base ingredients or technical levels of various nutrients.

Secondly, due to the large quantities of base ingredients that the manufacturer may purchase, they may be able to buy the base feedstuffs at a reduced price compared to the horse owner who buys only in one bag lots, exactly the same as BULK BUYING at the butcher's shop or supermarket.

INCORRECT LABELLING

There have also been reported situations where in fact, prepared feeds have been labeled incorrectly.

Prepared feeds are generally produced in various forms, e.g. foal mix, mare mix, growing horse mix etc. with differing technical specifications.

There have been instance where labels have, in fact, been changed so that the feeds with lower levels of feed nutrients are misrepresented as feeds which should contain much higher levels of the feed nutrients. Hopefully this practice is not widely spread, as it not only misleading advertising, but in fact unscrupulous business, and certainly does not help the honest operators in their general business dealings.

PRICE/BAG or PRICE/KG.

Prepared feeds are generally very competitively priced when compared to the common base feeds. It is however necessary to know the weight of the bag of prepared horse feed compared to the other substitute feeds. Shrewd marketers will pack less weight per bag in some instances, so that the product will sell at a price comparable on a per bag per basis to other feeds. Beware of the pitfalls of buying feed on a per bag basis.

INADEQUATE TECHNICAL FEEDING LEVELS

Generally, on a technical basis, any prepared feed, which is registered and therefore carries a label or a product description on the bag, should contain all the necessary components which appear on the label. Analysis of the recommended daily feed levels for some such feeds however, show that the availability to the horse of some feed components, are less than the desired daily needs, at the recommended feeding rates. In one product, much emphasis is placed on the fact that the calcium/phosphorus ratio is correct. Analysis of the actual quantities, the horse would be expected to receive of both CALCIUM and PHOSPHORUS, in grams per day reveals that the horse will receive, from the feed, a daily intake of only 50% of actual needs of both minerals.

This calculation is not the sort of thing that the average horse feeder can carry out in the produce store, even if he carried a hand calculator. The point is proven that there is a multitude of assessments that need to be carried out by horse feeds to ensure that the best technical mixture is being fed at the least cost.

To those people who are using prepared feeds for their horses, it is desirable to buy feed on a weekly basis and to ensure that, if at all possible, the feed is freshly made. Oxidation of the protein and energy components of the grains etc. and breakdown either by oxidation or by interaction of the added vitamins and or minerals may mean that prepared feeds which are more than say 14 days old after mixing, may not contain most of essential feed components, as stated on the label.

SECTION THREE

Economic Aspects

24. PRINCIPLES OF LEAST COST HORSE FEEDING.

Many rations have been suggested, in the past, to be fed to the many types of horses and most are based on experiences handed down from generation to generation with at times little regard for the cost of the rations or the technical basis of the feeds.

The aim of this section of the book is to show a simple technique which can be used to formulate various rations which will not only provide the horse with the correct feed components for the particular purpose but, will also do so at the least cost to the horse feeder. These calculations, which can be done by any person with a small calculator, do have a variation in results, due to some assumptions made in the method of calculation. This variation will not matter, in practice, as the range of feed nutrient levels, in the various feeds, are averages only and there is the possibility of considerable variation existing in actual sample details. For those who are interested in more accurate feed formulation methods, there are a number of well designed computer programmes now available for this purpose.

RATION FORMULATION has to start on some technical basis and whilst there are two different technical feeding standards available for horses, the American N.R.C. and the English A.R.C., the horse feeding industry appears to prefer to use the N.R.C. figures as base data rather than the A.R.C. details.

HORSE FEEDING RATIONS can be worked out on the following basis:-

1. DAILY DRY MATTER INTAKE.

Using this method, assumes that the horse is eating the same amount of DRY MATTER/DAY as used for the ration calculations.

e.g. our 450 kg (1000 lb) horse, at rest, would need about 2.0% of its body weight as DRY MATTER RATION/DAY, with a range of from about 1.5%, if the horse is a poor eater to about 5% if the horse is a very active animal in full training.

In absolute figures, our reference horse has an expected average feed consumption, in terms of DRY MATTER of 9.00 kgs (20 lbs), with extreme ranges of 6.75 kgs (15 lbs) to 22.50 kgs (50 lbs).

This is a possible VARIATION in daily feed intake, based on average figures of 150%.

If you are using this method of assessing a horses' requirements for ration formulation, you need some idea of the DRY MATTER INTAKE OF YOUR HORSE. Hence the need to:-

A – weigh all feeds.

B – FEED to APPETITE satisfaction, clean feed bins will not mean a thing, if the appetite is not satisfied and the horse's digestive tract will not operate effectively unless full of ingesta all the time.

C – if supplementary feeding on pasture, the best practical method of determining DRY MATTER intake is to stable the horse for about two or three days for complete hand feeding, feed the normal weight of grain/concentrate/chaff mix and allow unrestricted access to the best lucerne (alfalfa) hay you can buy. Weigh daily hay intake and this will then be very similar to the amount of DRY MATTER which the horse is getting from grazing. You may well get some very surprising results.

D – Having established the DAILY DRY MATTER INTAKE, the ration is then formulated in PERCENTAGE TERMS. e.g. 12% Crude Protein, 50% energy, 0.3% calcium etc. or in absolute amounts e.g. 1.00 kg (2.20 lb) protein, 450 MCal energy, 26 grams CALCIUM etc.

2. DAILY NUTRIENT REQUIREMENTS/HORSE

This method of ration formulation works on the principal of determining the amounts of each individual nutrient which the horse needs/day in absolute terms as kgs and grams or lbs and oz., and compiling a ration around these details.

The problem with this method of ration formulation is that you also have to know the horses' DRY MATTER INTAKE of your feed each day. A ration can be readily compiled but it will be of little use if our reference horse above is fed a ration of 9kgs (20lbs) when in fact its appetite and work requirements require 26 kgs (50 lbs) of feed /day. APPETITE and work activity are positively correlated with increasing DRY MATTER intake, as activity increase so does feed consumption.

To those that think this daily feed consumption of 26 kgs of DRY MATTER is not possible, this is an actual example on an advanced level performance horse and, remember, horse feeding is about individual animals, not averages.

If we were to compile a ration, based on EXPECTED DAILY FEED REQUIREMENTS, in say 9 kgs (20lbs) of dry matter and our horse really is eating 15Kgs (33 lbs) dry matter, the following can happen:-

1. the horse is underfed by about 6 kgs (13 lbs) or 66% of bulk.
2. the extra bulk can be provided by increasing the amount of hay or other roughage in the ration but this hay or other roughage will contain some feed nutrients which will upset the balance of all the figures we have just calculated so the whole ration has to be re-calculated.
3. we can add bulk to the ration, by some inert substance such as sawdust, but even if horses would eat sawdust, it will upset the digestive functions of cellulose and fibre in the large intestine

and we still will need to go back and re-calculate as a definite fibre problem has arisen.

Even after we have formulated the ration, we need to consider some things which need attention.

MAXIMUM AND MINIMUM LEVELS.

Some feed components require special consideration in some feeds.

LYSINE is desirable in the feeds of growing horses, ZINC and PHOSPHORUS can be dangerous when fed above certain levels of the ration and need to be considered in relation to COPPER levels, COTTONSEED MEAL cannot be fed at more than 15% of the ration, on a DRY MATTER basis, due to the presence of a toxic component, etc.

PALATABILITY

PALATABILITY is all important, it is no use having a technically correct and balanced ration, if the horse will not eat it Two of many examples are SOYBEAN MEAL, which appears to have palatability problems, at long term ration levels higher than 500 grams/ 450 kg horse/day and MOLASSES, which is magic to some horses but others are really put off eating any feed containing molasses.

Which ever method you select for ration formulation, you will need to know two things.

1. WEIGHT OF HORSE

2. DRY MATTER INTAKE/DAY

It would also be advisable to have some idea of the weight of the horse in relation to one or other of the two CONDITION SCORING SYSTEMS detailed earlier in this book and some idea of the extra DRY MATTER the horse eats at various stages of exercise.

On the other hand, there is really no need for you to do any of this. You can do what horse people have been doing for years, a bit of this, a bit of that, because you like the look of some particular feed or someone told you it was a good thing etc.

You will not have all the hassles of trying to sort out the feeding technology in relation to the horse. You may strike it lucky and, just by chance, get a balanced ration from all the bits. You are, however, not going to know when the ration is correctly balanced and you can probably upset the ration simply by the addition of one new feed or supplement.

The other possible problem is you will be probably be spending more on the costs of feeding than you should, but if you have money to throw away pushing the "wrong" feed down a horses' throat that is your decision. The horse will only excrete, via urine or faeces, the excess feeds (your money) or will suffer some type of problem, many described earlier in this book, in either a sub clinical or clinical condition which will cost more money, either in inadequate growth and or performance, in veterinary fees, to fix the problem and the cost of the loss of the use of the horse during the period it is affected by the nutritional disorder caused by incorrect feeding.

In the competitive horse world, however, if you are in there to win prizes, trophies, races and ribbons or to sell the best yearlings in the thoroughbred and standard bred world, you will probably find that those who are most successful are no longer feeding a bit of this and a bit of that.

Technical details of all the common horse feeds have already been discussed in previous chapters. Feed prices and the subsequent economic factors will now be considered.

Horse feed prices can vary considerably from place to place. The criteria to be considered are -

(a) cost per kilogram of the feed.
(b) cost per kilogram of energy in the feed.
(b) the relative cost of the protein content in the feed.

The reason we are interested in the cost per kilogram of the feed is that horses feed intake is related to the animals' body weight. Each horse, at rest, requires about 1.55kgs, (3.5lbs) of DRY MATTER for each 100kgs (224lbs) of body weight to maintain adequate gut fill so that digestive disturbances do not occur. As all common feeds, with the exception of grass and pasture, contain about 10% moisture, this translates in practical terms to about 1.75kgs of feed per 100kgs. of body weight.

A normal thoroughbred of 16 hands weighing about 450kgs would have a daily feed intake of about 7.9 kilos of feed on the basis of the feed containing 10% moisture.

The minimum roughage level that most horses can utilise, without the problem of digestive upsets occurring, is generally recognised at 0.5% of the animals body weight.

This absolute minimum base level of roughage intake is essential to allow continuous movement of ingesta in the digestive tract and correct digestion of the food nutrients. A horse at 250kgs needs a minimum of 1.25kgs of roughage per day

300	1.50
350	1.75
400	2.00
450	2.25
500	2.50

These are the MINIMUM WEIGHTS of roughage that should be fed to horses of the stated weights. The balance of the horse's feeding requirements is usually made up to the required daily DRY MATTER weight, by the addition of grain, grain by-product, oilseed meals and or prepared horse feeds. There is no reason why the horse cannot be fed rations containing 100% roughage, that would be an exact duplication of what grazing horses are doing all the time. In fact, with some horses, such rations of 100% roughage, obtained from either pasture and or hay intake, is sufficient to provide the horse with all its feed nutrient requirements.

Rations which contain greater than 50% roughage, either as pasture and or hay ARE recommended for the greater majority of hand fed horses. With correct ration formulation, such rations of 50% roughage/50% grain, by weight, will provide feed nutrient levels which will satisfy the technical requirements of all but the performance horse performing medium to hard strenuous work. In fact, with some horses, the 50/50 roughage/grain (by weight) ration may well provide too much energy for the type of activity and work being performed by the horse. In order to get the best results from such horses with low to medium work loads, it could well be necessary, from a technical angle to reduce the level of grain and increase the level of roughage in the daily feed.

Table 1 details a range of horse feeds available. The table consists of the commonly used feeds and is not meant to include each and every feed that can or is being used in horse nutrition. The table is designed to show how to evaluate the important points in assessing the costs of the stated feeds.

COST PER KILOGRAM.

As the table reveals, there are vastly differing bag/bale weights and differing prices. The first true measure of the cost of any feed or or feed supplement is the cost per kilogram. This is simply obtained by dividing the cost of the bag/bale by the weight of the bag/bale. This calculation reveals a range in per kg. cost of from 18 cents for lucerne hay to $2.22 for skim milk powder.

The second important indicator in costing horse feeds is the cost of the ENERGY component of the ration. On a percentage basis there is more energy in any ration than there is any other horse feed nutrient. Energy costs will always be determined in an individual market by the price of the cheapest grain on an ENERGY DENSITY basis. Two examples will illustrate the point.

In Australia, the price of feed grains is determined by the price of feed wheat. Since the type of energy available, in all grains, is chemically identical and since the feed wheat market in Australia, largely for pigs and poultry, is the largest grain stock feed market, this determines the price of other feed grains. In the U.S.A., the price or cost of energy in stock feeds is a little more complicated but is partially determined by both the stockfeed wheat market and the market for oaten grain, for human consumption. Generally OATS, from a stock feed angle has always been cheaper to purchase than wheat, oats contains less energy and more fibre, but the increasing demand for oaten grain for human consumption, as oaten bran has, in some parts, forced the price of oaten grain up to levels where oats is no longer an economic horse feed. That is not to stop any person who wants to feed oats from doing so, it just means in these circumstances, of the demand of oaten bran products for human consumption, less expensive rations could be formulated, if other grains, notably barley were substituted for oats.

The third important measure is the protein content in the ration and relative cost per kg of protein content is important when the feeding of horses are considered. The cost of PROTEIN is always the most expensive part of any ration so correct ration formulation can lead to the provision of the correct or desired amount of protein in the ration at the least cost. These principles apply, especially to the formulation of rations for young growing horses and brood mares. In both these categories the higher protein needs of the animals can lead to very expensive rations if the calculations are not correctly performed.

The basis of the calculation of the relative cost of energy and protein is as follows:

DETERMINATION OF RELATIVE COST OF ENERGY.

There are two methods which can be used.

Firstly, select a common horse feed, which contains reasonable levels of energy and low levels of protein. Two such common feeds are available, MOLASSES and FATS.

MOLASSES contains an energy level of about 3.40 MCal/kg and a very variable protein level, ranging from 2% to 9%. However as most of the PROTEIN in MOLASSES is in the form of NON PROTEIN NITROGEN, it is of little value to the horse so can be ignored, from a horse feeding angle.

As table ? shows molasses at 20 cents per litre (1 kg.) containing 3.40 MCals of energy will provide energy at a cost per MCal of 5.80 cents.

FATS or OILS contain about 8.50 MCals/kg of energy and NO PROTEIN. With a cost of FATS at 150 cents per litre, energy is being provided at a cost of 17.64 cents/MCal.

On this particular produce market, MOLASSES is a more economical source of energy than FATS, about 33% of the cost of energy derived from fats.

To calculate the cost of ENERGY, using the ENERGY COST of MOLASSES, 1 kg of average OATS contains 3.20 MCals of energy per KG of grain. At an energy cost, derived from MOLASSES of 5.80 cents/MCal, the 3.20 MCal of energy in the one kilogram of oats has a RELATIVE VALUE of 5.80 x 3.20 or 18.56 cents.

A practical problem immediately arises, in that the purchase price of one kilogram of oats is only 18.00 cents and no consideration at this stage has been taken of the protein value in the oats, about 100 grams of protein/kilogram of oats.

We can then say that either the protein level in the oats comes for nothing or else energy, purchased as molasses, is more expensive than energy purchased in grain.

SECONDLY, there is no common horse feed which contains protein but NIL energy. So to determine the cost of energy it is necessary to take the most common source of energy in horses, namely grains, and to derive a relative energy cost from the quoted prices.

In practical terms, most grains contain 10% protein. There are variations, in the protein level of grains as discussed earlier, but such variations are generally small and are therefore of little consequence in the practical formulation of horse rations, tending to cancel each other out.

The method of relative costing assumes that the protein in the grain (assumed 100 grams/kg of grain) is available at no cost to the horse. This is a satisfactory assumption as all horse feeds with the exception of four contain protein levels in excess of 10%.

The four concerned are molasses and fats (vegetable oils) both pure energy sources and cereal hay and cereal chaff. The two cereal feeds, oaten and wheaten, are generally accepted as containing 8% protein. This low level is just sufficient to maintain an adult horse in reasonable condition, for any length of time, and the technical factors of horse feed formulation require that these cereal hays and chaffs need to be supplemented with a a number of feed additives to raise ration levels to desired amounts.

As protein is always the most expensive of the two components, protein and energy, any protein which is available at least cost will always ensure the feeding of the cheapest ration.

Taking OATS, as an example, 1kg costing 18 cents and with 3.20 MCals of energy will have a cost MCal of energy of 5.62 cents, (18 cents divided by 3.20). Remember, in this calculation, the 10% protein level, or 100 grams of protein/kg of average oats, is assumed to be available to the animal for nothing.

It is possible, using this technique, to find out the cheapest grain to feed to the horse as an energy supplement. Using the same principles of calculation and the prices detailed maize has an energy cost/MCal of 6.11 cents, barley of 6.00 cents and sorghum of 5.85 cents. Based on the assumptions used in these calculations, ENERGY supplied from OATS is the cheapest source. The difference between the most expensive and the least expensive energy sources from grains amounts to some 0.49 cents or 9% difference. It is most likely that in the practical situations, there will be more than a 9% difference in the energy levels of various grain samples.

The ENERGY COST/MCal selected for the balance of the calculations will, therefore, be 6.00 cents/MCal, with the exception of MOLASSES and FATS which do not contain any protein where the separate calculations reveal that MOLASSES, at 20 cents/litre provides energy at the same cost as BARLEY at 21 cents/KG. BARLEY will still be the cheaper feed as in the 6.00 cents/MCal cost is the "hidden" value of 100 grams of protein/kg of feed.

CALCULATION OF COMPARATIVE ENERGY AND PROTEIN COSTS OF COMMON HORSE FEEDS

	$ BAG	KGS WEIGHT	COST PER KG.	PROTEIN %	ENERGY MCal/kg	CENTS/KG MCal	TOTAL ENERGY VALUE	TOTAL PROTEIN VALUE	C.P. -	CENTS/KG C.P. -10
GRAINS										
Maize	15.50	65	23.85	10	3.90	6.11	-	-	-	-
Oats	9.00	50	18.00	10	3.20	5.62	-	-	-	-
Barley	12.60	60	21.00	10	3.50	6.00	-	-	-	-
Sorghum	11.60	55	21.09	10	3.60	5.85	-	-	-	-
OILSEEDS										
Cottonseed Meal	15.40	50	30.80	42	3.01	6.00	18.06	12.74	32	39.8
Linseed meal	17.68	40	44.20	33	3.40	6.00	20.40	23.80	23	1.03.0
Sunflower seeds	20.20	35	57.71	28	4.00	6.00	24.00	33.71	18	1.87.0
Soybean meal	28.40	50	56.80	45	3.60	6.00	21.60	35.20	35	1.00.0
Full Fat Soybean	33.20	25	1.32.80	32	6.20	6.00	37.20	95.60	22	4.34.0
GRAIN BY-PRODUCT										
Bran	7.65	45	17.00	12	3.30	6.00	19.80	-2.80	2	?
Pollard	9.10	55	16.50	13	3.42	6.00	20.52	-4.02	3	?
HAYS & CHAFF										
Lucerne Hay (Alfalfa)	4.50	25	18.00	18	2.30	6.00	13.80	4.20	8	52.0
Lucerne Chaff (Alfalfa)	11.00	39	28.20	18	2.30	6.00	13.80	14.40	8	1.80.0
Cereal Hay	3.50	22	15.90	8	1.90	6.00	11.40	4.50	-2	?
Cereal Chaff	11.75	45	26.11	8	1.90	6.00	11.40	14.71	-2	?
OTHERS										
Tick Beans	46.80	75	62.40	26	3.45	6.00	20.70	41.70	16	2.60.0
Lupins	23.00	60	38.40	34	3.36	6.00	20.16	18.24	24	76.0
Skin Milk	44.40	20	2.22.50	35	4.05	6.00	24.30	1.98.20	25	7.92.0
Molasses	50.00	250L	20.00	0	3.40	5.86	-	-	-	-
Fats (Oils)	1.50	1L	1.50.00	0	34.80	17.64	-	-	-	-

NOTE Molasses and Oils are in LITRES, (1 litre weighs 1 kg.)

As soon as the price of MOLASSES/litre rises in relation to the price of barley/kg, and MOLASSES can sell for up to 60 cents/litre, MOLASSES becomes an expensive source of energy. The most expensive source of energy is that derived from FATS, 17.64 cents/MCal OR nearly 200% more expensive than CARBOHYDRATE energy from grains, even allowing for the "hidden" value of 100 grams of protein/kg.

DETERMINATION OF THE RELATIVE COST OF PROTEIN

The RELATIVE COST of PROTEIN is then obtained, using COTTONSEED MEAL as an example, as follows:-

1. Determine the total RELATIVE COST of the energy component of each feed. ENERGY CONTENT x ENERGY COST IN MCals. 3.01 x 6.00 = 18.06
2. Subtract 18.06 cents, the value of the energy in each kilogram of cottonseed meal, from the cost of that kilogram of cottonseed meal, namely 30.80 cents 30.80 minus 18.06 = 12.74
3. This value 12.74 represents the RELATIVE COST of the PROTEIN CONTENT in the cottonseed meal. This 12.74 does not represent the ABSOLUTE COST as the value of some 100 grams of protein, or 10%, is included in the RELATIVE ENERGY COST of ENERGY in grains.
4. The PROTEIN level of cottonseed meal is assessed at 42% so deduct 10 from this, to allow for the protein value of grains, include in the RELATIVE COST of energy, to obtain a figure of 32.
5. Divide the PROTEIN VALUE 12.74 by 32 to obtain 39.8, and this figure is the RELATIVE COST of PROTEIN.

REMEMBER-ENERGY is ENERGY no matter what feed it comes from, it all acts exactly the same inside the horse.

PROTEIN, provided it contains the ten essential amino acids required by the horse is the same no matter what the base feed. Unfortunately these essential amino acids are only available in pasture, lucerne hay and chaff, canola meal and soybean products. The proteins in all the other feeds lack one or more of the ten essential amino acids and hence need to be supplemented either by feeding in combination with pasture, lucerne hay, canola meal and soybean meal products or else by addition of an amino acid supplement.

COST COMPARISONS

The following tables, derived from data in the table on Page 321 ranks the feeds from the least expensive to the most expensive, in terms of COST/KG of weight and

RELATIVE COST of PROTEIN.

ABSOLUTE COST/KG.		RELATIVE COST OF PROTEIN	
FEED	COST	FEED	COST
CEREAL HAY	15.90	BRAN	?
POLLARD	16.50	POLLARD	?
BRAN	17.00	MAIZE	0
LUCERNE HAY	18.00	OATS	0
OATS	18.00	BARLEY	0
MOLASSES	20.00	SORGHUM	0
BARLEY	21.00	COTTON SEED MEAL	39.8
SORGHUM	21.09	LUCERNE HAY	52.0
MAIZE	23.07	LUPINS	76.0
CEREAL CHAFF	26.11	SOYBEAN MEAL	1.00.0
LUCERNE CHAFF	28.20	LINSEED MEAL	1.03.0
COTTONSEED MEAL	30.80	LUCERNE CHAFF	1.80.0
LUPINS	38.40	SUNFLOWER SEEDS	1.87.0
LINSEED MEAL	44.20	TICK BEANS	2.60.0
SOYBEAN MEAL	56.80	FULL FAT SOY	4.34.0
SUNFLOWER SEEDS	57.71	SKIM MILK	7.92.0
TICK BEANS	62.40	CEREAL HAY	??
FULL FAT SOY	1.32.80	CEREAL CHAFF	??
FATS (OILS)	1.50.00	MOLASSES	00
SKIM MILK	2.22.50	FATS	00

To some explanations, on the above table.

1. These details are applicable to this set of price data. Both sets of figures, will change as the price of the various feeds change, both between suppliers and between seasons.
2. In terms of straight COST/KG of physical product, it is interesting to note that CHAFFING or CHOPPING CEREAL HAY or LUCERNE (ALFALFA) HAY adds about 60% to the roughage costs of the feed bill, for no additional technical advantage.
3. All energy costs are assumed at 6.00 cents/MCal which is the average price of energy in grain, including a 10% "hidden" protein component. Energy is readily available in horse feeds and is always a lot cheaper to feed than protein.
4. Based on these cost figures, FATS are about three times the price for ENERGY, compared to carbohydrate energy contained in grains.
5. BRAN and POLLARD have a negative RELATIVE PROTEIN COST. This means that the energy in these two feeds is costing much less than 6.00 cents/kg.

This does not mean to rush out and use BRAN and POLLARD as energy sources, refer Chapter 20 COMMON HORSE FEEDS for the problems with these two mill by-products.

6. The RELATIVE COST of PROTEIN in the grains is NIL. The value has already been taken up in the RELATIVE COST of ENERGY.
7. The RELATIVE COST/KG of PROTEIN can vary from about 40 cents/kg up to nearly 800 cents/kg or eight dollars, dependent on the protein supplements selected.
8. Both CEREAL HAY and CEREAL CHAFF will be expensive as a source of PROTEIN, simply because PROTEIN supplements will have to be added to raise the level to one suitable for most types of horses.
9. The PROTEIN levels of MOLASSES and FATS are both nil from a horse feeding angle so no RELATIVE COST can be determined in these instances.

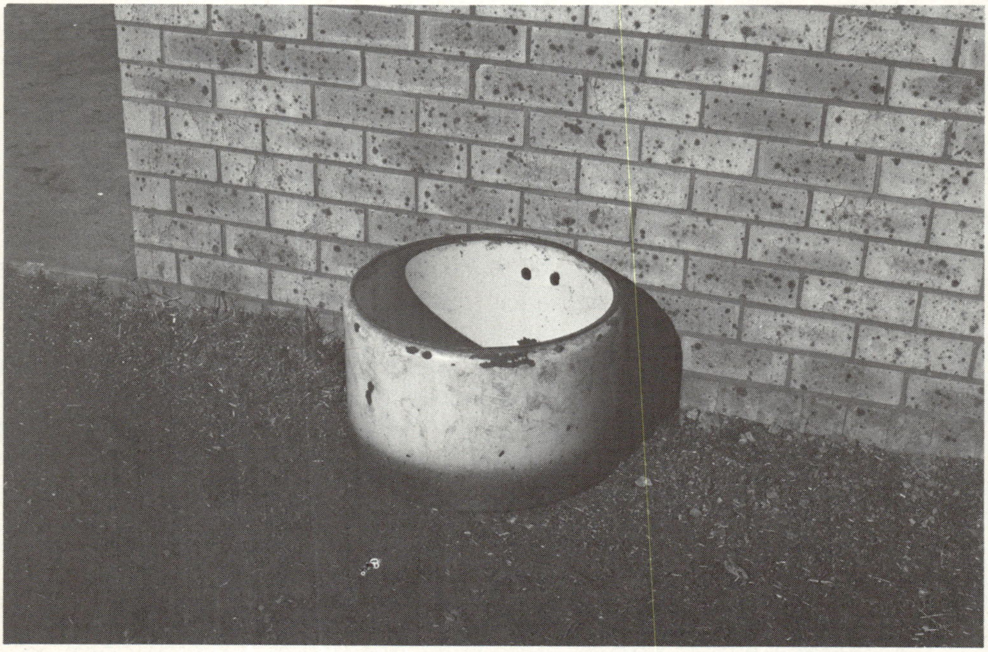

An undesirable paddock feeder – leg injuries may occur.

25. FEEDING ADULT HORSES

For the purposes of this book, an adult horse is defined as any horse over 3 years of age.

These horses only require sufficient nutrients to:-

1. maintain body function.
2. repair any damaged body tissues.
3. provide energy for the appropriate level of physical activity.

As such these types of horses, with low work loads, have the simplest nutritional requirements. Once the level of physical activity increases to any degree the ENERGY component of the ration becomes very important.

ADULT HORSES WITH LOW ENERGY NEEDS

Adult horses, with low energy needs, will include any horse over 3 years of age which is either, AT REST, i.e. basically doing nothing, or horses with LIGHT WORK LOADS, where the level of physical activity may or may not be on a daily basis and is sufficient to cause some mild sweating on the neck and a possible increase in breathing rate at the completion of work, but which quickly returns to normal on cessation of physical activity.

Feeding guidelines can be summarised as follows:

PROTEIN - sufficient needed to maintain body tissues only - crude protein ration level can be in the range of 8-10%. Protein IS NOT required for growth, pregnancy or lactation and as these types of horses have low energy demands, the feeding of excess protein, for conversion to energy in the animal, is not pertinent as energy obtained from protein is an expensive form of energy for horse nutrition. As most average quality, mixed pasture will contain at least 10-14% crude protein, any adult horse, at rest, will get all its protein needs from grazing.

ENERGY - this type of horse will require ENERGY to allow continual body function, known as MAINTENANCE ENERGY REQUIREMENTS, plus a supply of ENERGY to allow the required level of physical activity to take place.

MAINTENANCE ENERGY requirements can be calculated from mathematical equations developed from scientific research.

One such equation - EQUATION 1 - to determine the amount of ENERGY required for maintenance, on a daily basis, is

MAINTENANCE ENERGY (KCal of D.E.) = 1.375 + 30 X BODYWEIGHT.

A second equation - EQUATION 2 - again for determination on a daily basis, which is used is.

MAINTENANCE ENERGY (MCal of D.E.) = 1.4 + 0.03 BODYWEIGHT.

For horses which weigh above 600kg, generally draught or heavy horses, this equation tends to overestimate energy needs so the equation suggested for use, in this instance is:-

MAINTENANCE ENERGY (MCal of D.E.) = $1.82 + 0.0383W - 0.000015W^2$

For those people who are not mathematically inclined, the following table provides MAINTENANCE ENERGY LEVELS, for horses, in the body weight range of 150 to 650 kilograms.

NOTE. BODYWEIGHT refers to the weight of the horse and is not to be confused with LIVEWEIGHT which is generally taken to mean BODYWEIGHT PLUS GUT FILL, the gut fill sometimes weighing up to 100 kgs in a big thoroughbred horse.

With the exception of the column providing weights in pounds (lbs.), all figures in this table are expressed in METRIC units, ENERGY levels being in KCals or MCals per KILOGRAM NOT per POUND.

The table clearly shows a close relationship between the two formula even though one expresses energy in terms of KILOCALORIES and one in MEGACALORIES.

The table assumes that the average horse will eat 2% of its body weight/day as DRY MATTER and that, as pasture, that dry matter will contain average energy levels of 2.10 MCals/kg.

NOTE some horse nutritionists contend that the DRY MATTER intake of a resting horse will vary between 1.5% and 3%, of body weight, the figure of 2% has been selected as an average and MAY have to be adjusted for specific horses.

BODY WEIGHT		MAINTENANCE ENERGY REQUIREMENTS		D.M.	PASTURE ENERGY	EXCESS ENERGY
		EQUATION 1	EQUATION 2			
KGS	LBS	KCal	MCal	2%	MCAL	MCAL
150	336	5875	5.9	3	6.3	0.4
200	448	7375	7.4	4	8.4	0.5
250	560	8875	8.9	5	10.5	1.6
300	672	10375	10.4	6	12.6	2.2
350	784	11875	11.9	7	14.7	2.8
400	896	13375	13.4	8	16.8	3.4
450	1008	14875	14.9	9	18.9	4.0
500	1120	16375	16.4	10	21.0	4.6
550	1232	17875	17.9	11	23.1	5.2
600	1344	19375	19.8	12	25.2	5.4
650	1456	20875	20.7	13	27.3	6.6

The result show that any adult horse, at rest or with very small work loads, should be able to obtain all its energy needs from average quality mixed pasture.

ENERGY NEEDS TO MAINTAIN BODY TEMPERATURE.

For a healthy horse, BODY TEMPERATURE range is very critical. For a horse, at rest or performing very light work where little SWEATING is involved, the range is in the order of 37.5 to 38.0 degrees CENTIGRADE (99.5 to 100.4 degrees FAHRENHEIT) a range of less than 1%. THis means, that on all but the very hot days, the body temperature of the horse WILL ALWAYS be greater than that of the air temperature. In fact there will be some horses who are in climatic regions, where their body temperature WILL ALWAYS exceed the air temperature.

ENERGY is a form of HEAT, it is measured in units of heat, so the average horse will require some additional energy in the feed to maintain body temperature at the desirable and, in fact, necessary level. The exact amount of energy required for this purpose, IS NOT KNOWN. It is simply not possible to measure, in practical situations, the amount of energy which the horse requires to maintain body temperature as there are so many variables involved.

These include :-

1 – whether the horse is rugged or not and if so how many rugs.

2 – MINIMUM DAILY TEMPERATURES, not AVERAGES; the horse has to provide for the coldest time of the day not the average.

3 – type of energy in the feed, the more roughage and hence fibre in the feed, the more energy will be needed to digest that roughage in the large intestine and the less energy will be available for maintaining body temperature.

VITAMINS AND MINERALS – required only for maintenance and allowance. These horses do not have the demands for vitamins and minerals as exist with performance horses because they are not producing the physical work as required of a racehorse or an eventer. Pasture will provide all the needs of this type of horse for vitamins and minerals, exactly the same as pasture has been doing for the many years, before horses became domesticated.

OTHER SUPPLEMENTS - Electrolyte needs will be satisfied from those electrolytes present in the pasture. These horses are not doing any physical work or sweating to the extent that electrolyte loss will affect performance, so electrolyte supplementation is not required.

PROVIDE THE STOCKING RATE OF THE PASTURE IS REASONABLE AND THE PASTURE IS NOT USED AS A "PARKING LOT", ANY ADULT HORSE, AT REST, OR WITH LOW WORK LOADS CAN GET ALL ITS NUTRITIONAL REQUIREMENTS FROM PASTURE. In winter, during periods of low temperature, a SMALL SUPPLEMENT OF GRAIN, say 0.25 to 0.75 KGS, could be desirable to provide extra energy to satisfy the increased needs for body temperature maintenance.

SUPPLEMENTARY HAND FEEDING ON PASTURE GRAZING.

MAY be necessary for any one of the following situations.

1. OVERSTOCKING- too many horses on too small an area.
2. LOW WINTER TEMPERATURES – to allow the horse to maintain body temperature in the required very narrow technical range.
3. "FRIENDLY FEEDING" – to quieten the horse, make it easier to catch not really necessary from a technical nutritional angle but certainly helps management.

The main problem is to discourage the horse from substituting purchased feed for paddock feed, and this is often a human problem, not a horse problem.

From our table of COMPARATIVE FEED COSTS, and other information in the book, the best technical feeds, for supplementary feeding, when also grazing on pasture, will either be lucerne hay or a good mixed pasture hay, except possibly in winter time. These hays contain all the feed nutrients the horse needs and will be cheaper on a PER KILOGRAM basis than any of the other feeds, including pre-mixed commercial feeds.

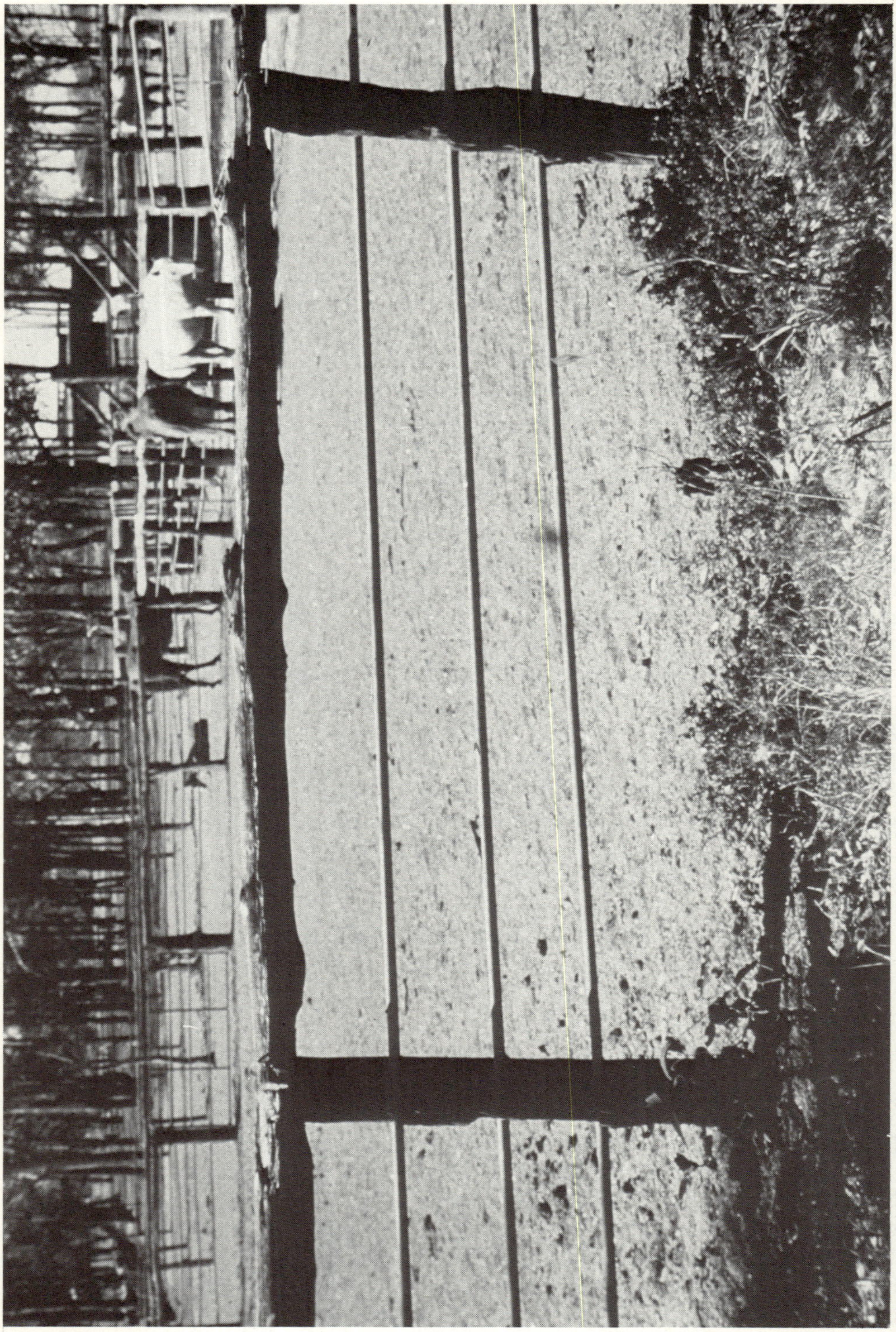

The complete hand feeding situation – not a blade of grass in sight.

FEEDING ADULT HORSES

There is no technical need, other than in the cold periods of winter, to provide a "hard feed supplement", but if there is an emotive need from the human angle, to quieten the horse, a simple home mixed supplement of one third of each, of medium energy feeds by weight of BRAN, OATS and LUCERNE CHAFF, fed at the rate of no more than 0.75kg/day for a 450 kg horse will be sufficient. This supplement will provide 2.20 MCals of energy at a daily cost of just under 18 cents/kg. This level of EXTRA ENERGY will be low enough as to not affect adversely most horses.

There will be no need to worry about CALCIUM SUPPLEMENTATION to counteract the low CALCIUM level of the BRAN. The CALCIUM level of both the pasture and the hays will be sufficient to balance that CALCIUM deficiency.

PRE-MIXED COMMERCIAL FEEDS, at the time of preparing this table of costs, were selling in the order of 28-38 cents/kg retail., some 44% to 111% dearer than the supplementary mix detailed above. For these pre-mixed feeds to be used they would have to be the approximately the same price as the BRAN, LUCERNE CHAFF, OATEN GRAIN MIX unless cost of feeding is no object, or there is restricted storage space for only one bag, instead of three.

The other problem with pre-mixed commercial feeds is the UNKNOWN ENERGY level. Such feeds, including SWEET FEEDS would appear to have energy levels in the range of 2.20 to 3.50 MCals/kg. Those pre-mixed feeds, containing energy levels at the lower end of the range, 2.20 MCals/kg will be high in fibre and will be no better than roughage, either hay or pasture, in providing energy to the horse. Those pre-mixed feeds which contain energy levels at the higher end of the range will be of two types. Those which contain reasonably high levels of grain, will have energy sources readily available to the horse and the only consideration will be cost/kg. Those pre-mixed feeds, commonly called SWEET FEEDS, which contain levels of MOLASSES in the order of 5-10% will be of little value in providing energy in cold climates and low temperatures. This is especially so, for maintenance of body heat, as there is the physical problem of the freezing of MOLASSES in such low temperatures.

Should these horses be grazing any tropical or sub tropical pastures where an OXALATE problem may occur, CALCIUM supplementation, as described earlier in this book, will be desirable.

These feeding recommendations also satisfy the following technical criteria

1. BRAN never more than 10% of the ration, can cause diarrhoea.
2. POLLARD is excluded, no reasonable technical need.
3. SUFFICIENT GRAIN in the suggested small supplement, enough to reward and satisfy the horse but not enough to produce problems from excess energy in the ration and in sufficient work and exercise for the horse.
4. The ration does NOT CONTAIN any CEREAL HAY and or CEREAL CHAFF, for the following reasons:-imbalance of CALCIUM and PHOSPHORUS, lack of VITAMIN A pre-cursors, high FIBRE or LIGNIN content. If there are worries about possible dust problems, from feeds other than cereal chaff or hay, refer to section on HEAVES in the chapter on NUTRITIONAL DISORDERS.
5. No consideration has been taken of feeding any protein and or fat supplements. These adult horses at rest or doing very little work DO NOT REQUIRE the addition of such supplements to their rations.

STABLED HORSES WITH LOW WORK LOADS

Such horses will require full hand feeding which, from a technical and economic viewpoint, can be adequately satisfied by lucerne (alfalfa) hay and or pasture hay, any additional energy required for body temperature maintenance, in cold winters, can be provided as discussed above. There is no reason why pre-mixed feeds, from reputable manufactures cannot be used, they are generally low in energy, most do not even show the energy content on the bag, saves storage space, the horse likes these products and feeding is easy, but it will be about 60% more expensive than feeding on hays.

LED IN OR IN HAND HORSES.

Horses which are shown IN HAND or in LED IN CLASSES have very little physical activity and in fact should be fed the same as any other horse with LOW WORK LOADS or energy requirements.

Three problems immediately occur if such horses obtain all their feed from pasture and or hay, despite the fact that this is the least cost and technically desirable method of feeding.

1. GRASS BELLIES

This is the situation where the size of the ABDOMEN containing most of the digestive tract is larger than is normally desired by show ring judges. It is purely a subjective ideal, the horse does not "look right" with a GRASS BELLY. The "increased" size of the BELLY or abdominal cavity is a result of the content of fibre or cellulose in the feed, and the need for that fibre to remain in the large intestine for some time for efficient digestion.

A conflict immediately arise between the following points:-

1 the need for the horse to have a certain level of roughage in the diet, for efficient digestive tract operation.

2. to overcome this people feed what appear to be low fibre diets so the horse has less fibre to digest and, in theory, will not have as big a GRASS BELLY.

AVERAGE FIBRE LEVELS OF SOME COMMON HORSES FEEDS, DRY MATTER BASIS, ARE:

DRY ROUGHAGES		GRAINS ETC.	
LUCERNE (ALFALFA) HAY	30.0%	BARLEY	7.0%
PASPALUM HAY	34.0%	MAIZE	2.5%
CEREAL HAY	30.0%	OATS	12.0%
BLUEGRASS HAY	31.0%	GROATS	2.5%
FESCUE HAY	26.0%	SOYBEAN MEAL	7.0%
RYEGRASS HAY	23.0%	WHEAT	2.6%
		BRAN	11.0%
		POLLARD	6.0%

GREEN ROUGHAGES

Any green growing plant will have about 3-8% LESS FIBRE than the figures quoted above for HAYS of the same species.

GRASS BELLIES will occur when feeding pre-mixed feeds. These feeds contain fibre levels, in the range of 15-30% and sometimes more, dependent on the composition of each individual mix, especially if there is any amount of chaff, cottonseed hulls, sunflower hulls or similar "BULK" in the ration. Roughage, as detailed above, also contain fibre levels in the order of 20-30% and GRASS BELLIES are a direct result of the horses' need to digest roughage.

Whilst grains etc. have a fibre level, about one third or less, compared to the dry roughages, these grains also contain much higher levels of energy. REMEMBER LOW FIBRE LEVEL = HIGH ENERGY LEVEL.

3. the need to ensure that the horse DOES NOT receive excess levels of energy in the ration which can make the horse uncontrollable and or ill. Horses are funny animals, especially when fed levels of energy, in excess of their daily needs. Such a horse, when worked or trained in familiar surroundings will show very little visual evidence of signs of slight excess energy problems. Major excess energy problems will become very obvious with the horse developing FOUNDER, COLIC or some similar disturbance. Take the horse with slight excess energy problems out to a show, where the surroundings are different and the horse will then generally misbehave in some manner. How many times have you seen a LED IN HORSE misbehave in a show ring class ?.

The solution to GRASS BELLIES ?. The answer is a combination of feeding and management practices.

1. let the horse have as much green feed as possible. Green feed contains less fibre, in general, than the hays made from that green feed.
2. if a "hard feed" supplement MUST be fed, select those with the lowest fibre BUT remember energy level will also increase as fibre level decreases and the last thing required is a horse affected by too much energy in the ration.
3. exercise the horse. If the horse is unable to be ridden for any one of a number of reasons, lunge the animal, let it run in paddock but give it plenty of exercise. Develop your own aerobics for horses. Exercise will do wonders for reducing GRASS BELLIES.

For those, trying to eliminate a GRASS BELLY from a LED IN HORSE, which is being fed a ration with reasonable levels of energy (grain) supplement, confined to a stable for management reasons and or for for coat condition and which does not get exercised, you do have a potential problem for which there is no general answer.

2. COAT CONDITION

The easiest and simplest, and generally the cheapest way to get a shine on any horse's coat is to feed either up to a tablespoon of COOKING OIL or SUNFLOWER SEEDS in the ration each day. Eggs are also useful.

3. HUMAN PROBLEMS

Simply the fact that the horse MUST be fed something. We often do not know why but we still want to persist with supplementary feeding. Up to 0.5 kgs of something/day will not matter, but go over that level and you will not help either yourself or your horse.

ADULT HORSES WITH MEDIUM TO HEAVY ENERGY NEEDS

It is possible to get into all sorts of arguments about whether the work load, or physical activity of the horse can be considered LOW, MEDIUM or HARD.

WORK LOAD directly determines ENERGY REQUIREMENT, the more physical activity the horse performs, the more energy it requires in its ration. The better that working or performance horse is trained, exercised and conditioned, the better that horse will be able to utilise the energy provided in the ration, muscle function ability increasing with repetitive exercise.

In order to remove the human emotive element from our calculations, the following figures provide an indication of the amount of energy expended in various activities.

ENERGY EXPENDED AVERAGE HORSE/HOUR,

	as KCals	as MCals.
AT REST	625	0.63
WALKING	200	0.20
SLOW TROTTING AND CANTERING	2300	2.30
FAST TROTTING, MODERATE CANTERING	5650	5.65
FAST CANTERING, GALLOPING, JUMPING	10500	10.50
MAXIMUM EFFORT (RACING)	17500	17.50

NOTE: these figures are not meant to indicate that a horse can race at maximum speed for one hour. They are to be used to calculate the energy needs, created by exercise and or work, over and above maintenance levels needs in the ration.

From the above figures, it is possible to calculate the MAINTENANCE and EXERCISE ENERGY DEMANDS of a horse on a PARTICULAR day.

MAINTENANCE ENERGY 24 hours x 0.63 MCals — 15.12 MCals

EXERCISE ENERGY

SAY	30 minutes SLOW TROTTING requires	1.25 MCals
	30 minutes MODERATE CANTERING requires	2.82 MCals
TOTAL ENERGY REQUIRED FOR THAT DAYS ACTIVITY		19.19 MCals.

Our figures show that a 450Kg horse should be able to obtain from pasture and or pasture hay of average to good energy levels something like 18.90 MCals of energy, or nearly enough energy to perform all this work. Allowing for variations in feed composition and training programmes, this horse, in theory, really does not need any energy supplements to perform this daily work rate.

However a second set of data, derived from the research work from which the MAINTENANCE ENERGY FORMULA M.E. (in MCal) = 1.4 + 0.3 X body weight, provides much increased energy requirements for the performance horse

Without going into all the calculations involved in a complex mathematical formula, the ADDITIONAL ENERGY REQUIREMENTS FOR WORK are suggested as follows:-

GAIT or PACE	MCals/hour
WALK	0.25
SLOW TROT	6.50
MEDIUM TROT	9.50
FAST TROT/SLOW CANTER	13.7
MEDIUM CANTER	19.5

On a 450 kg horse, doing a reasonable amount of physical activity, in fact the exact same level of activity as the horse described above, the THEORETICAL ENERGY needs would be:-

MAINTENANCE ENERGY		15.00 MCals
EXERCISE ENERGY		
SAY	30 minutes SLOW TROTTING requires	3.25 MCals
	30 minutes MODERATE CANTERING	9.75 MCals
TOTAL ENERGY REQUIRED FOR THAT DAYS ACTIVITY		28.00 MCals.

This system of energy calculation provides for the horse to receive 28.00 MCals of energy as opposed to 19.19 MCals as determined earlier.

This is an assessed ENERGY REQUIREMENT INCREASE of some 8.81 MCals or 46% over that energy calculated as being required for maintenance and work.

The next question is why the additional ENERGY NEEDS and where does that energy go?

ADDITIONAL ENERGY DEMANDS

As far as practical situations are concerned, feeding of energy needs to consider the following additional factors.

VARIATION IN PHYSICAL ACTIVITY.

The horse will not necessarily perform at this level of physical activity each and every day. This may be the hardest days work, in say a fortnight, other days may have much less work loads and there is probably at least one day of light work or nil physical activity. It is therefore necessary to average out the horses' energy needs over a number of typical days or training and or competition.

ENERGY REQUIRED FOR FIBRE DIGESTION

Energy is required for from the fermentation and breakdown of cellulose in the large intestine of the horse to again produce energy in the form of VOLATILE FATTY ACIDS and HEAT. VOLATILE FATTY ACID type of energy is able to supply some, between 40 and 60%, of the energy needs of a horse at rest. However the rate of production of this VOLATILE FATTY ACID energy from the large intestine, is not fast enough to support any reasonable level of physical activity. That energy, required for physical activity or work, has to come from ENERGY reserves or stores in the body, in the form of CARBOHYDRATE and FAT. The higher the FIBRE level in the ration, the more VOLATILE FATTY ACIDS that will be produced and also the more HEAT that will be generated in the decomposition of that fibre.

ENERGY LEVEL IN THE RATION.

ENERGY level in the ration is the total of
ENERGY present as CARBOHYDRATE.
ENERGY present as FAT.
ENERGY present as FIBRE which is broken down to form VOLATILE FATTY ACIDS.

CARBOHYDRATE type energy requires very little energy use to be converted to GLYCOGEN for muscle use.

FAT type energy HAS TO be converted through a multi-stage process, in the presence of oxygen, (AEROBIC), to GLYCOGEN for muscle use and reasonable quantities of energy are required for this purpose.

VOLATILE FATTY ACID type energy has to come from fermentation of fibre in the large intestine and this requires large amounts of energy which are NOT AVAILABLE for muscle use.

Each ration will vary in not only total energy level but also in the percentage of that total energy made up by the three energy sources.

If the amount of ENERGY FED to the horse is INSUFFICIENT to meet the physical demands for maximum performance, the horse will not work as required.

If the amount of ENERGY in the ration is well in excess of the horses' needs, additional heat will be produced, within the horse, as the excess energy is converted from body fat reserves to muscle energy or produced as excess heat in fermentation in the large intestine. The end result of all this will be increased SWEATING by the horse to maintain body temperature, within the narrow accepted range. This increased SWEATING will in turn, lead to increased ELECTROLYTE and WATER LOSS and the need to take corrective action to correct these problems.

ENERGY AVAILABILITY

The amount of ENERGY required, in a very short period of time, for MEDIUM to HARD physical exercise is such that the horse is unable to absorb sufficient from the digestive tract, during exercise to fulfill its needs. ENERGY for physical activity will come from stored energy reserves, within the horses' body, either in the form of CARBOHYDRATE or FAT forms.

AIR TEMPERATURE

The horse, in winter will have higher energy needs, at the same level of physical activity, in order to keep warm than will its summer requirements be, refer to the discussion on energy needs of ADULT HORSES WITH LOW WORK LOADS.

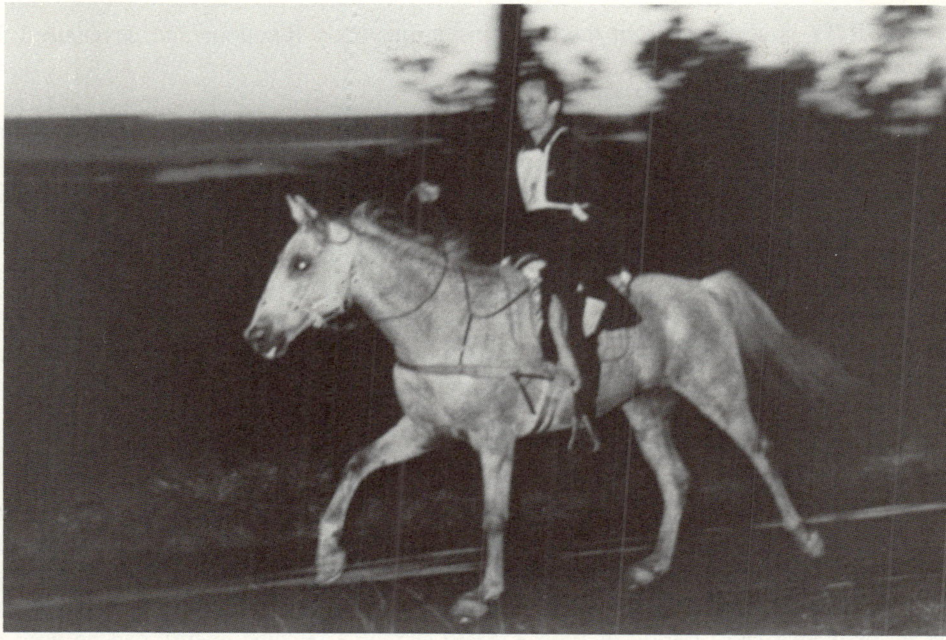

Top class endurance horses perform well on rations of 50-55% energy. The secret is in the training programme of the horse.

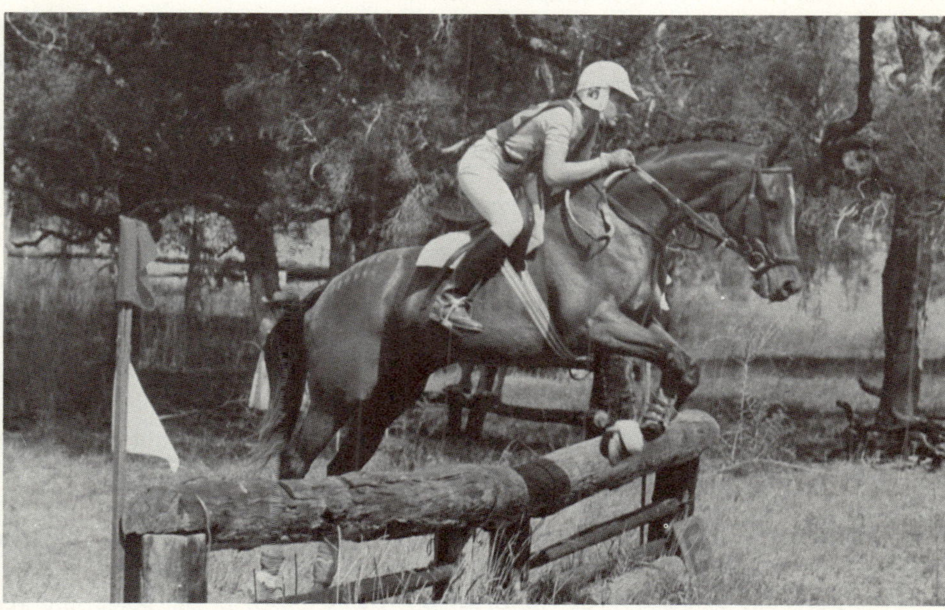

Eventers are difficult horses to feed – beware tying up and similar problems after dressage phase and before or during the cross country phase. Very specific feeding programmes are needed to overcome this problems

ENERGY LOSS

ENERGY is also lost from the horse in various body functions and never used for muscle activity.

A – in excreta, both URINE and FAECES.

B – as HEAT, rising from the skin of the horse, and in association with sweating, responsible for cooling the horse in periods of hard physical work.

C – is energy used within the body as part of body function, to break down cellulose (fibre) in the large intestine, to utilise body glucose stores for muscle energy and to convert body fat reserves to muscle energy.

It has been suggested that, with horses at maximum levels of physical activity, ONLY 50% OF THE ENERGY IN THE RATION IS USED FOR MUSCLE ACTIVITY, with some 50% of the ration energy being used within the horse for purposes other than muscle activity or being lost from the horse as heat, in urine and faeces.

AEROBIC-ANAEROBIC MUSCLE ENERGY USE

The effective use of ENERGY in the performance horse depends on the speed of the exercise and the length of time that exercise takes. AEROBIC MUSCLE energy use, where energy is used in the presence of OXYGEN, takes place at slow paces and over long periods of time. ANAEROBIC MUSCLE energy use occurs in the absence of oxygen and occurs at fast paces over a short period of time. CARBOHYDRATE type energy can be used as muscle fuel, by the horse in both AEROBIC and ANAEROBIC situations. Energy, derived from FATS can only be used in AEROBIC conditions.

Of all the possible horse activities listed above, the only ones where some degree of AEROBIC muscle activity is likely to occur are those where the length of hard physical activity exceeds at least two and possibly three minutes, namely TRAIL RIDING, ENDURANCE, EVENTING, POLO, POLO-CROSSE, STANDARDBRED RACING, and the longer THOROUGHBRED races.

AMOUNT OF TRAINING

The more training and conditioning the horse receives for its particular physical activity, the more efficiently its' muscles will be able to effectively utilise the energy, either in the feed or stored within the body.

WEIGHT OF RIDER

It is important to remember that any ridden horse has to produce not only enough muscle activity, and hence ENERGY use, to move itself about but also additional muscle activity, at the same time, to carry the rider. This requires extra ENERGY in the feed, and when you place a 75 kg (168 lb or 12 stone) rider on top of a 450 kg horse, the extra weight to be moved immediately increase by 16% or one sixth.

These problems of ADDITIONAL ENERGY DEMANDS, in the horse, are very difficult, or IMPOSSIBLE be measure, and rely on the ability of the horse feeder to observe, assess, determine and "measure" from experience.

PRACTICAL ENERGY NEEDS FOR PERFORMANCE HORSES

In order to determine the ENERGY needs of a particular horse and therefore the ENERGY LEVEL of a ration, there is really no THEORETICAL DATA which PROVIDES ALL THE INFORMATION REQUIRED IN THE ONE SET OF DATA TO ALLOW REASONABLE ENERGY RATION CALCULATIONS TO BE MADE.

The mathematical equations suggested to calculate ENERGY use, in horses with medium to heavy work loads, are very technical and require some interest in mathematics to use correctly. Further these equations relate to constant speed only and very few horses ever go at a set constant speed.

METHOD 1 THEORETICAL ASSESSMENT

" PERCENTAGE PLUS "

One suggested method of determining ENERGY used for MEDIUM to HEAVY work load activities is to increases MAINTENANCE ENERGY requirements by 50% and 100% respectively.

MEDIUM WORK

If we take our 450 kg "reference horse", as an example, it will require, from previous tables, about 15 MCals/day for maintenance energy.

ADD 50%/day for medium work	7.50 MCals
TOTAL EXPECTED ENERGY NEEDS/DAY	22.50 MCals

Compare this energy intake to another way of theoretical measurement, previously outlined.

ENERGY REQUIRED FOR MAINTENANCE	15.00 MCals
ENERGY REQUIRED FOR MEDIUM LEVELS OF WORK	
1 HOURS SLOW TROTTING AND CANTERING	2.30 MCals
TOTAL ENERGY REQUIRED	17.30 MCals
ENERGY SURPLUS	5.20 MCals

required for those energy uses which are difficult, if not impossible to measure, particularly HEAT LOSS and additional rider weight.

HARD WORK

If the same horse is doing hard levels of physical activity

ENERGY REQUIRED FOR MAINTENANCE	15.00 MCals
ADD 100%	15.00 MCals
TOTAL ENERGY AVAILABLE	30.00 MCals
ENERGY REQUIRED FOR HARD WORK	
1 HOURS FAST TROTTING and MODERATE CANTERING	5.65 MCals
TOTAL ENERGY REQUIRED	20.65 MCals
ENERGY SURPLUS	9.35 MCals.

METHOD 2. THEORETICAL ASSESSMENT

"SPEED ASSESSMENT"

This system is based on the previous table which assigns various levels of ADDITIONAL ENERGY USE to differing types of gaits or paces, refer table ??

Again referring to our 450 kg "reference horse"

MEDIUM WORK

ENERGY REQUIRED FOR MAINTENANCE/DAY	15.00 MCals
ENERGY REQUIRED FOR MEDIUM WORK	
1 HOURS SLOW TROTTING AND CANTERING	2.30 MCals.
TOTAL ENERGY REQUIRED	17.30 MCals.
This horse should have a DRY MATTER intake, at rest, of 9 kgs/day.	
9 KGS ROUGHAGE at 2.10 Mcals/kg provides	18.90 MCals
PLUS	
say 50% extra DRY MATTER INTAKE	
(increased appetite due to work)	9.45 MCals
TOTAL ENERGY POSSIBLY AVAILABLE	28.35 MCals
EXTRA ENERGY AVAILABLE FOR	
ADDITIONAL ENERGY NEEDS	11.05 MCals

If this horse was on a ration of 50% roughage and 50% grain, the energy level of the ration would increase from 28.35 MCals, provided by roughage and if appetite is increased by exercise, up 50% to 35.77 MCals if the grain was OATS and 39.82 MCals if the grain was maize, providing SURPLUS ENERGY, over and above MAINTENANCE and ENERGY, of 18.47 MCals or 106% on oaten grain and 130% on maize grain.

At this stage of the analysis, it is sufficient to say that providing over 100% extra energy, in the ration, is probably not very desirable. This theoretical calculation can, of course, be changed, (a) by reducing the allowance made for expected increase in DRY MATTER intake due to exercise and (b) by having a greater percentage of roughage and less grain in the ration.

HARD WORK

ENERGY REQUIRED FOR MAINTENANCE/DAY	15.00 MCals
ENERGY REQUIRED FOR HARD WORK	
1 HOURS FAST CANTERING AND GALLOPING	10.50 MCals
TOTAL ENERGY REQUIRED	25.50 MCals

From the previous calculations, this horse could be expected to receive 28.35 MCals/day from a diet of good quality roughage alone.

This the only leaves an ENERGY SURPLUS of 2.85 MCals, or 10% of the total ration, for ADDITIONAL ENERGY NEEDS. This would appear to be far too little, considering the increased work load of this horse, and the energy which will be dissipated and lost from the body as heat in the sweating and cooling process.

If the ration fed to this horse is 50% roughage and 50% grain as above, daily energy needs are expected to be 25.50 MCals and daily energy supplies 35.77 MCals if the grain is oats and 39.82 MCals if the grain is maize.

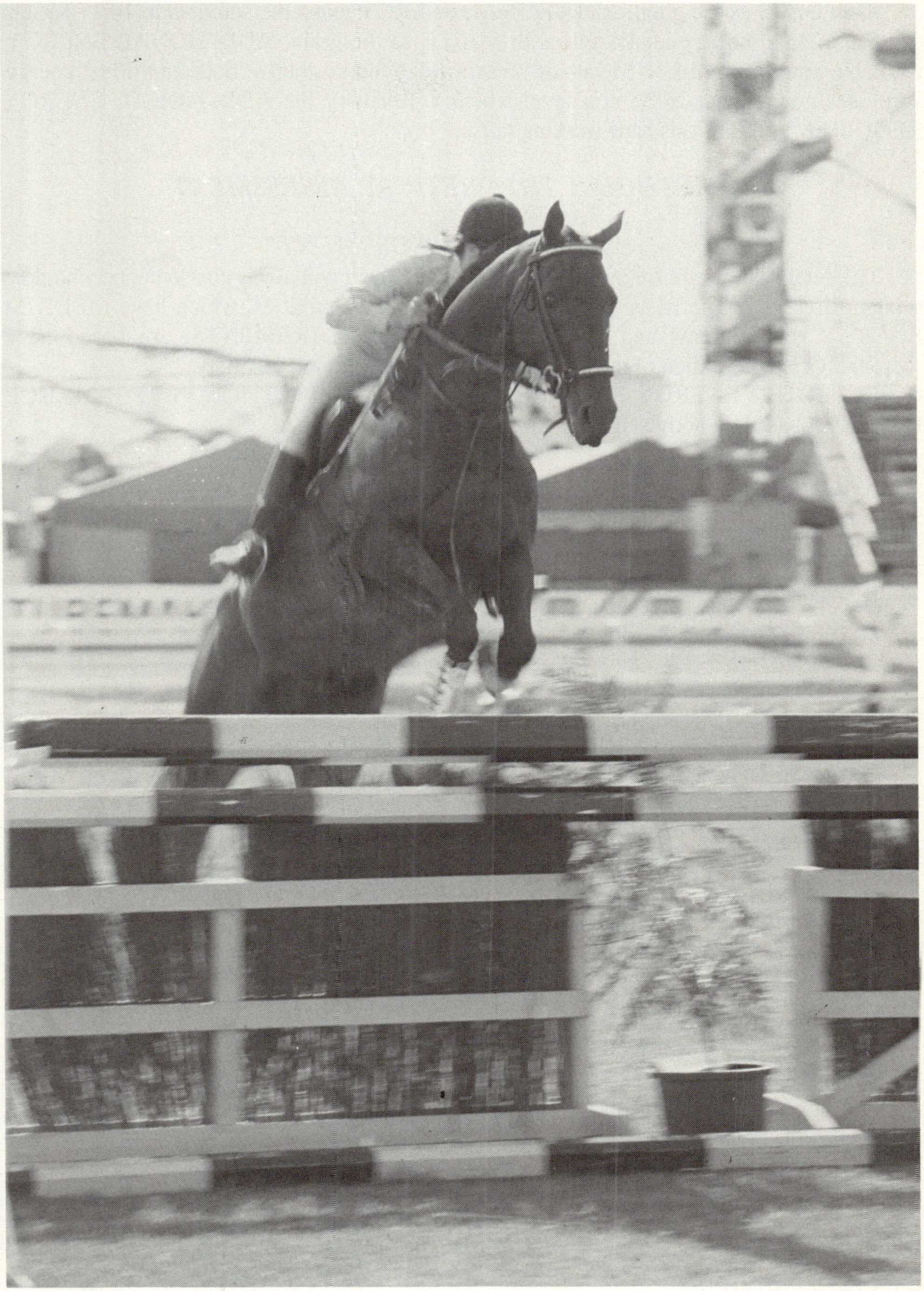

Show jumper with medium to heavy work loads – varying nutritional needs for each horse.

With OATS as the grain, ADDITIONAL ENERGY available amounts to 10.27 MCals or 28% of total energy intake and with MAIZE as the grain, ADDITIONAL ENERGY available amounts to 14.32 MCals or 36% of total energy intake, both additional energy surpluses now appear to be at a level which will satisfy the ADDITIONAL ENERGY REQUIREMENTS of this hard working horse.

METHOD 3 THEORETICAL ASSESSMENT

"ACTIVITY ASSESSMENT"

The details below are for average circumstances, there will always be someone who does things differently. The basis of the separation of horse activities, which have MEDIUM ENERGY requirements and HEAVY ENERGY REQUIREMENTS, are based on a reasonably clear definition of the MCals required per day for each activity.

EXPECTED ENERGY REQUIREMENTS OF COMPETITION PERFORMANCE HORSES – based on bodyweight of 450kgs

ACTIVITY	MINUTES / DAY	MCals REQUIRED/DAY	MAINTENANCE ENERGY/DAY	TOTAL ENERGY /DAY
MEDIUM LEVELS OF WORK AND ACTIVITY				
HACK	60	2.00	15.00	17.00
PONY CLUB	60	2.00	15.00	17.00
PLEASURE	60	3.00	15.00	18.00
DRESSAGE	60	3.00	15.00	18.00
ROPING	30	3.00	15.00	18.00
DOGGING	30	3.00	15.00	18.00
CAMPDRAFTING	30	3.00	15.00	18.00
CUTTING	40	3.20	15.00	18.20
REINING	40	3.20	15.00	18.20
HARD LEVELS OF WORK AND ACTIVITY				
SHORT SPRINT	15	4.50	15.00	19.50
BARREL	15	4.50	15.00	19.50
TRAIL	120	6.00	15.00	21.00
ENDURANCE	60	6.00	15.00	21.00
EVENTING	60	6.00	15.00	21.00
JUMPING	60	6.00	15.00	21.00
POLO CROSSE	40	6.00	15.00	21.00
RACING				
INTERVAL TRAINING	30	6.00	15.00	21.00
THOROUGHBRED	20	5.00	15.00	21.00
POLO	40	7.20	15.00	22.20
RACING				
STANDARDBRED	30	7.50	15.00	22.50

Let us assume that we have a "super horse" which can perform all these activities and that it weighs 450Kgs, a reasonable sized thoroughbred or similar.

If we go back to our previous figures, this horse eating 13.5 kgs/day (9 kgs for maintenance and 4.5 kgs additional appetite due to work) would receive:-

AS GOOD QUALITY ROUGHAGE 28.35 MCals

AS 50% GOOD QUALITY ROUGHAGE AND 50% OATS 35.77 MCals

AS 50% GOOD QUALITY ROUGHAGE AND 50% MAIZE 39.82 MCals

HACKS AND PONY CLUB HORSES

DAILY ENERGY NEEDS 17.00 MCals

POSSIBLE DAILY ENERGY SUPPLIES

as roughage, 28.35 MCALS, as 50/50 roughage and oats, 35.77 MCals and as 50/50 roughage and maize, 39.82 MCals.

WESTERN PLEASURE, DRESSAGE, ROPING, DOGGING, CAMPDRAFTING, CUTTING AND REINING HORSES.

DAILY ENERGY NEEDS 18.00 MCals

POSSIBLE DAILY ENERGY SUPPLIES

as roughage, 28.35 MCals, as 50/50 roughage and oats, 35.77 MCALS and as 50/50 roughage and maize, 39.82 MCals.

SHORT SPRINT and BARREL RACING HORSES

DAILY ENERGY NEEDS 19.50 MCals

POSSIBLE DAILY ENERGY SUPPLIES

as roughage, 28.35 MCals, as 50/50 roughage and oats 35.77 MCals and as 50/50 roughage and maize 39.82 MCals.

TRAIL RIDING, ENDURANCE, EVENTING, JUMPING, POLOCROSSE, INTERVAL TRAINING, THOROUGHBRED RACING.

DAILY ENERGY NEEDS 21.0 MCals

POSSIBLE DAILY ENERGY SUPPLIES

as roughage, 28.35 MCals, as 50/50 roughage and oats, 35.77 MCals,
as 50/50 roughage and maize, 39.82 MCals.

POLO HORSES AND RACING STANDARDBREDS.

DAILY ENERGY NEEDS 22.50 MCals

POSSIBLE DAILY ENERGY SUPPLIES

as roughage, 28.35 MCals, as 50/59 roughage and oats, 35.77 MCals,
as 50/50 roughage and maize, 39.82 MCals.

What can we currently learn from these three different systems for calculating ENERGY NEEDS FOR EXERCISE.

At this stage very little, no clear pattern is emerging which will allow any reasonable practical benchmarks to be provided.

PRACTICAL EXAMPLES OF ENERGY USE

Instead of working from theory to practice, let the situation be reversed and work from practice to theory. After all it has been said, with regard to horse nutrition, that all theory does is prove correct what some people have already been doing anyway, either by accident, good luck or good management.

METHOD 4. PRACTICAL ASSESSMENT

In a number of successful racing and eventing stables it is common practice to feed rations which contain between 40 and 50 MCal of energy/day.

If we use the figures for energy consumption detailed earlier.

ENERGY REQUIRED FOR MAINTENANCE	15.00 MCals
ENERGY REQUIRED FOR EXERCISE based on 30 minutes/day trotting and 30 minutes/day cantering	4.07 MCals
TOTAL ENERGY NEEDED FOR MAINTENANCE AND EXERCISE ONLY	19.07 MCals.
ADDITIONAL ENERGY available for HEAT PRODUCTION AND OTHER USES 20.03 TO 30.03 MCals	

METHOD 5. PRACTICAL ASSESSMENT

This is a specific example on one horse with a large appetite. This eventer weighs very close to 500Kgs and in full training consumes 14kgs of oats and 12 kgs of hay per day.

On a DRY MATTER BASIS

TOTAL ENERGY AVAILABLE in the ration	
12.32 kgs OATS at 3.20 MCals/kg	39.42 Mcals
10.56 kgs HAY at 2.10 MCals/kg	22.17 MCals
TOTAL DAILY ENERGY SUPPLIES	61.59 MCals
ENERGY REQUIREMENTS	
MAINTENANCE for 500 kgs	16.40 MCals
EXERCISE AND WORK	19.07 MCals
TOTAL ENERGY NEEDS FOR WORK AND MAINTENANCE	35.47 MCals
ADDITIONAL ENERGY available for HEAT PRODUCTION AND OTHER USES	26.12 MCals.

METHOD 6. PRACTICAL ASSESSMENT

There is a common rule of thumb principle which is used by some people as an indicator of the amount of grain to feed horses.

MEDIUM LEVELS OF WORK 1.00-1.50 kgs grain/hour of work.

HEAVY LEVELS OF WORK 2.00-2.50 kgs grain/hour of work.

It is assumed under this system that the horse gets all or most of its MAINTENANCE ENERGY from roughage.

For a 450 kg horse.

MEDIUM LEVELS OF WORK

ENERGY AVAILABLE IN THE RATION		
9.00 KG ROUGHAGE (MAINTENANCE) X 2.10 MCals	=	18.90 MCals
4.50 kg ROUGHAGE (EXTRA APPETITE) X 2.10	=	9.45 MCals
1.25 KG GRAIN X average energy of 3.40	=	4.25 MCals
TOTAL ENERGY IN FEED		32.60 MCals
ENERGY REQUIRED		
MAINTENANCE ENERGY	=	15.00 Mcals
ENERGY required for 0.5 hours slow trotting and 0.5 hours medium cantering	=	4.00 MCals
TOTAL ENERGY REQUIREMENTS	=	19.00 MCals
ADDITIONAL ENERGY available for HEAT PRODUCTION AND OTHER USES		13.60 MCals

HARD LEVELS OF WORK

ENERGY AVAILABLE IN THE RATION	
ROUGHAGE as above	28.35 MCals
2.25 KGS GRAIN at average level of 3.40	7.65 MCals
TOTAL ENERGY AVAILABLE IN FEED	36.00 MCals
ENERGY REQUIRED	
MAINTENANCE ENERGY as before	15.00 MCals.
1 hour/day fast cantering	10.50 MCals
TOTAL ENERGY REQUIRED	25.50 MCals
ADDITIONAL ENERGY available for HEAT PRODUCTION AND OTHER USES.	10.50 MCals

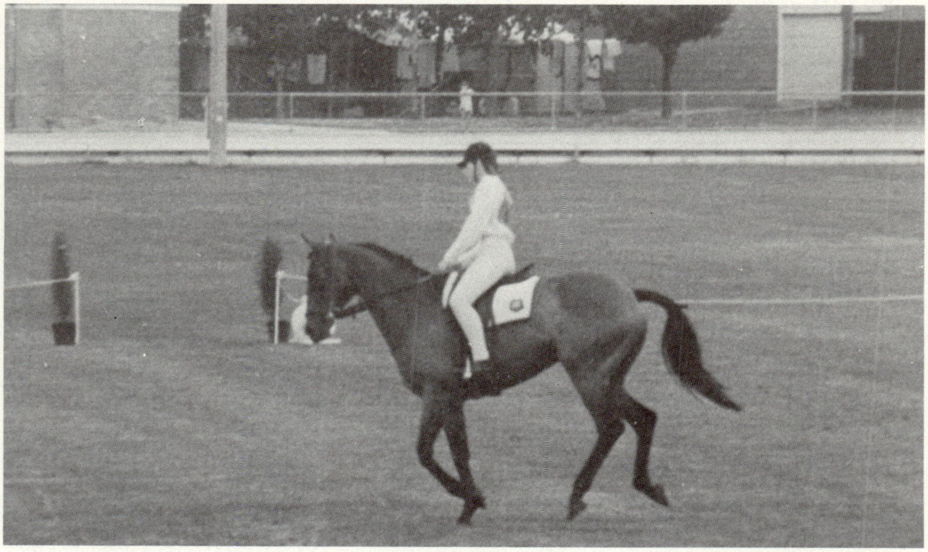

Dressage horse – dependant on age, standard of training and ability of the rider, energy levels in the ration will vary considerably.

The previous results will now be tabulated, in an attempt to derive some practical commonsense indicators to determine ENERGY NEEDS OF performance horses.

ENERGY ASSESSMENT METHOD	ADDITIONAL ENERGY REQUIRED AS % OF MAINTENANCE AND EXERCISE NEEDS	AS % OF TOTAL RATION
PERCENTAGE PLUS		
medium work	30%	23%
hard work	45%	31%
SPEED ASSESSMENT		
medium work	64%-130%	38%-46%
hard work	11%-56%	10%-36%
ACTIVITY ASSESSMENT		
hacks, pony club	66-135%	40%-57%
western pleasure, dressage, roping, dogging, cutting, reining, campdrafting.	57-121%	37%-55%
short sprint, barrel racing	54%-110%	31%-51%
trail riding, endurance, eventing, jumping,interval training, polo-crosse, racing.	35-90%	26%-47%
polo, standardbreds	26-77%	21%-43%
PRACTICAL 1	100-150%	50%-60%
PRACTICAL 2	74%	42%
PRACTICAL 3		
medium levels	71%	42%
hard work	42%	30%

ENERGY NEEDS OF ADULT PERFORMANCE HORSES

1. There is no simple method of calculating ENERGY NEEDS of performance horses.
2. Each of the above methods requires
   A – some idea of the ENERGY CONTENTS OF THE FEEDS in mathematical terms
   B – an indication of the MAINTENANCE AND EXERCISE NEEDS of the individual horses.
3. All methods, except the ACTIVITY METHOD, require the weight of the horse, to be known.
4. There is currently no technical method of separating the energy value of the feed, within the horse, into the energy types, CARBOHYDRATE, FATS and VOLATILE FATTY ACIDS.
5. Horses which perform at fast paces over short period of time, should only be fed CARBOHYDRATE type energy. Fat type energy is only of value to horses

whose work is at a slow pace and over long periods of time.

6. There is no clear cut changeover points where one or another type of energy becomes important in supplying the horse's needs.
7. ADDITIONAL ENERGY is required, over and above maintenance and exercise needs, for a number of functions in the horse, associated with exercise.
8. DRY MATTER intake increases with exercise, the percentage increase varying with horse to horse and activity to activity.
9. For horses with medium to high energy needs, the amount of fibre in the ration needs to be reduced as high fibre level affects energy utilisation. Poor quality hay will take a lot more energy to digest and produce more heat during the digestive process than will good quality hay.
10. Too much energy in the ration can lead to increased heating in the body, hence to INCREASED SWEATING and hence to INCREASED ELECTROLYTE EXCRETION, leading to reduced performance unless changes are made to increase appropriate electrolyte supplementation.
11. The AVERAGE PERFORMANCE HORSE should receive ENERGY LEVELS in the ration, about 40-50% greater than the ENERGY NEEDED for MAINTENANCE AND EXERCISE.
12. The problem is there is no AVERAGE PERFORMANCE HORSE.
13. Appropriate ENERGY LEVELS IN THE RATION will depend on many factors, all detailed above. Due to the variation in horse activities, individual horse differences, human preferences and the technical inability to be able to measure, at this present time, a number of factors which affect ENERGY USE and therefore RATION ENERGY LEVEL, the correct ENERGY LEVELS IN THE RATION will continue to be determined by TRIAL AND ERROR. There is a considerable amount of information available however, which will reduce the TRIAL TIME and the ERROR RATE if the horse owner is interested.

INCREASING RATION ENERGY LEVELS

It is necessary to be careful with ration ENERGY level when taking a horse from the paddock or grazing situation into a training programme. Whilst, it MAY be possible with some horses to remove the horse completely from a ration of grass and or hay and transfer immediately to a ration of 2 to 3 kgs of grain plus hay and chaff, this is generally not desirable. Whilst grazing, the microbial population in the digestive tract, the large intestine in particular, is organised to handle a high fibre diet. Reduce the fibre level and increase the energy level of that diet as will occur, in this situation and the microbial population has to have time to change. This takes a minimum of three weeks and possibly longer.

If the ENERGY LEVEL of the ration is increased TOO RAPIDLY, the use of such energy by the horse MAY NOT be ideal, leading to the occurrence of any of the many problems which can occur due to excess levels of energy in the ration. ALWAYS INCREASE RATION ENERGY LEVELS IN CONJUNCTION WITH INCREASED PHYSICAL ACTIVITY.

As a general rule, increase GRAIN LEVELS in the ration at 0.5 to 0.75 kgs/day, on a weekly basis, until maximum desired grain intake is achieved. To be even safer, start with OATS the low energy grain, when at full grain intake start to replace some of the OATS with grains of a higher energy level, e.g. BARLEY and or MAIZE etc.

LEVEL OF ROUGHAGE IN THE RATION

The MINIMUM LEVEL OF ROUGHAGE in any horse ration has to be 25% of total DRY MATTER weight. This is essential to allow correct intestinal tract movement, and roughage level should not be allowed to drop below this level.

A common ROUGHAGE LEVEL, in the ration, is 50% of the total ration weight.

If we again look at our 450kg "reference horse", doing medium to hard work, it should have a DRY MATTER intake in the region of 13.5 kgs and on a 50/50 roughage/grain basis this could provide

50% by weight, 6.75 kgs ROUGHAGE at 2.10 MCals	14.17 MCals
50% by weight 6.75 kgs MAIZE at 3.80 MCals	25.65 MCals.
TOTAL ENERGY AVAILABLE	39.82 MCals

Allowing for all sorts of variations, in feed analysis etc. this ration can provide a total of 40.00 MCals, which if you refer back to our previous calculations, will theoretically provide sufficient energy for most horse activities.

Unless there are specific and defined reasons, ROUGHAGE level should be kept at 50% OF ration weight. To reduce roughage level and increase grain level, could well lead to production of excess HEAT, which you cannot see or measure and this in turn will lead to increased SWEATING to keep the horse cool,immediately increasing ELECTROLYTE DEMANDS and possibly changing desired ELECTROLYTE supplement content.

TYPE OF ROUGHAGE IN THE RATION

LUCERNE -ALFALFA- hay and/or or pasture hay and/or chaff would form the technical basis of any ration for a horse with medium or heavy work loads. When compared to cereal hay/chaff, these roughages have the following advantages:-

a) Complete amino acid profile - cereal hay lacks three important amino acids.

b) Protein level generally of 12-14% - cereal hay has a low protein level of about 8%

c) CALCIUM and PHOSPHORUS levels and ratios are much more suited to the requirements of an adult horse.

d) Will contain CAROTENE, the precursor of VITAMIN A, there is very little such CAROTENE in CEREAL HAYS/CHAFFS, as they are generally cut when the seed head is well past the "boot stage".

e) much more digestible fibre and hence lower heat production, lower additional energy requirements, less sweating and less electrolyte loss, as a result of and from fibre digestion in the large intestine.

ELECTROLYTES

There will be a need for these horses, with medium to heavy work loads, to have some type of electrolyte supplementation. The nature of their work is such that HEAT will be generated, and SWEATING will take place. ELECTROLYTE LOSS will be inevitable and may be above the necessary levels, if the horse is feed excess levels of energy in the ration.

The amount and composition of any electrolyte supplement will be determined, on an individual horse basis, and will depend on:-

1. AEROBIC or ANAEROBIC MUSCLE ACTIVITY
2. AIR TEMPERATURE

3. MINERAL CONTENT OF THE RATION, (4 of the electrolytes are also minerals.)
4. previous electrolyte supplement history
5. individual horse differences.

PROTEIN

PROTEIN is only required, in these horses to maintain and repair existing tissue. No protein is required to produce new tissue as the horse is skeletally mature. Ration protein levels need to be in the range of 8% to 12%. If the total ration protein contains the 10 essential amino acids, the protein level can be at the lower end of this range. If however, the ration protein does not contain the 10 essential amino acids, then the ration protein level will need to be at the higher end of the range. Any ration containing more than 25% by weight of grains MAY have AMINO ACID balance problems. There are practical observations that tend to indicate that performance horses, fed protein levels in excess of 12-14%, do not appear to use energy efficiently and tend to go 'sour', i.e. do not perform to their expected ability in relation to the energy intake in the ration.

Apart from the maintenance of the existing tissues, these adult horses require PROTEIN for REPAIR of tissue, especially muscle tissue. These types of horses, often suffer some type of soft tissue damage during training and or competition, which is not able to be detected by the human eye. These problems, however, can be detected by the levels of some of the enzymes, the results of which are obtained from BIOCHEMICAL analysis of blood, refer to the chapter on BLOOD TESTS.

MINERALS

On properly formulated rations, of feeds of average or better quality, and based on the roughage being lucerne(alfalfa) and or mixed hay or grazing, there will be a very restricted need for these types of horse's to have any MINERAL supplements, in other than the unusual circumstance. The main MINERAL problem will occur when the grain level of the ration exceeds 40% of the total ration weight. Up to this level the calcium SURPLUS in the roughage will normally balance the calcium DEFICIENCY in the grain. Over this level, CALCIUM supplements will probably have to be fed to balance the excess levels of PHOSPHORUS in the ration.

If however the roughage contains any amount of cereal hay and or chaff to-gether with grain, a CALCIUM DEFICIENCY problem will be present and will need correction.

VITAMINS

VITAMIN A – not required if the roughage component is reasonably fresh lucerne hay, which is naturally green, or the horse is getting a decent green pick. Definitely required as a supplement to the ration if cereal hay/chaff forms any part of the roughage.

VITAMIN B COMPLEX - has been shown to be of value to a performance horse and would be worthwhile feeding a B supplement to this type of animal. The need for VITAMINS of this group, for these types of performance horses appears to faster than the rate of production from the large intestine, hence the need to consider a B supplement.

VITAMIN C – not required, except, possibly, in the case of "BLEEDERS".

VITAMIN D – only needed if the animal has no access to direct sunlight or hay

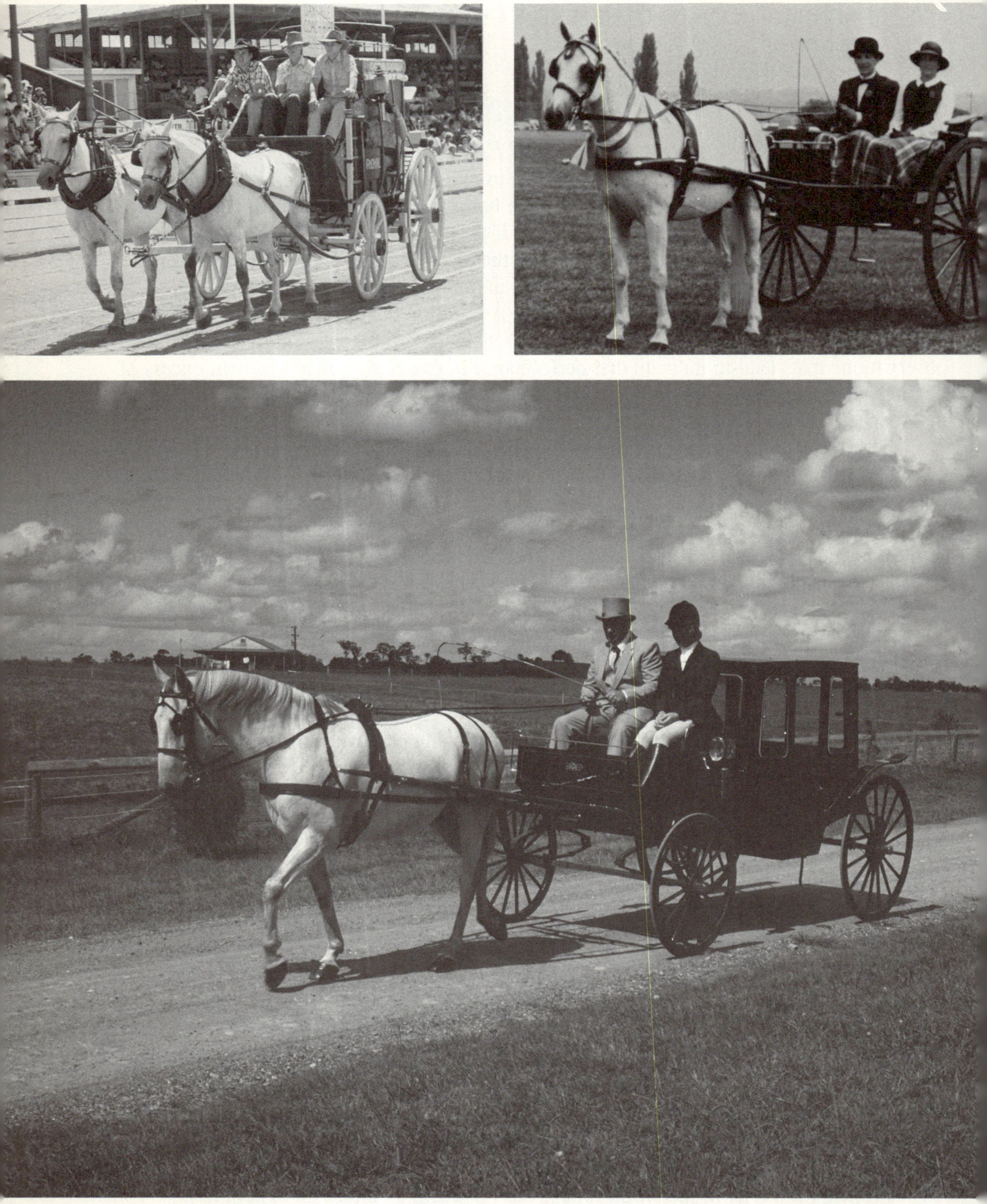

The feeding of harness horses will vary tremendously depending on the work load.

VITAMIN E – of value for muscle function and can be fed at rates up to 15 times the normal accepted level, no know problems at this time at this high dose rate.

VITAMIN K – of no value

OTHER CONSIDERATIONS

To some, this ration may seem too simple, especially those who feed a little of this and a little of that. The ration contains basically two feed components, grain and lucerne (alfalfa) hay/chaff, but is able to provide the horse with all the necessary feed components required, is technically correct and is produced at the least cost whilst meeting all the nutritional needs of the animal. Probably the only addition to the ration would be the tablespoon of an oilseed based product to improve the condition of the coat.

NOTE: Horses on rations with the levels of energy detailed above, should not be fed very high energy rations on days of nil or restricted work. This will most likely produce the classical symptoms of azoturia and/or ty-ing up. On days of nil or restricted work, such horses should have the lucerne hay content of the ration increased slightly, up to 50%, and the balance of the ration should be made up as a BRAN MASH. There are various recipes for a bran mash, one is detailed as follows. Mix 0.5 kgs bran with sufficient boiling water to produce a wet but not liquid mixture. Place a bag over the mixture and feed to the horse when cool. Sometimes small quantities of MOLASSES are added to the Bran mash.

Horses on high energy diets can be fed in this manner on days of reduced work load or exercise and returned to the high energy diet the following day with no adverse results provided of course the normal training programme is maintained when the energy level of the ration is again increased.

"SOUR" HORSES

A reasonably common problem with performance horses, after being in training for some period of time. Symptoms of "SOUR" horses include going off feed, reduced performance, changed temperament, generally always occurring on high grain diets and after some months in training. Possible reasons include:-

1 – Protein levels above 12-14%, and or amino acid imbalance. 2-Work load not hard enough for the energy content of the ration, solution is to either reduce the energy level or increase the work load.

2 – Possible vitamin B problem in that the horse appears to have a greater daily demand for vitamin B complex than can be produced in the horses' digestive tract. Supplementation by Vitamin B complex will overcome this problem.

3 – Body salts may be lost in sweat and not being replaced quickly enough from the ration. The use of electrolytes as an addition to the feed will overcome this problem.

4 – Muscles may not be functioning at their correct peak, due, not to the lack of energy but, to the possible lack of vitamin E and/or selenium. Results have been obtained in performance horses by feeding vitamin E, combined with very low levels of selenium at rates of up to 4500 International Units E per day - normal dose around 300 I,U, per day without any adverse results. Vitamin E is important for cell respiration and a deficiency of vitamin E will mean body cells especially the muscle cells will not function normally.

5 – Be careful of the excessive levels of VITAMIN A and or D, from feed supplements.

6 – dehydration due to sweating and self imposed reduced water intake may be important. There are a number of veterinary authorities who feel that MILD

DEHYDRATION of performance horses, unable to be detected by the PINCH TEST, but possibly predicted by closely observing the horses' water intake BEFORE the event, is a very important factor affecting the performance of some horses. Every effort should be made to ensure that the horse will consume adequate quantities of water - for a normal thoroughbred in training – at least 30 and possibly 40 litres per day.

Water intake can be increased by one or more of the following factor methods:

(A) ensure that body salts are at the correct level by use of electrolytes.

(B) use a proprietary MILD diuretic formulation which will have a slight flushing effect on the kidneys and encourage the horse to drink more – needs to be followed by increased electrolyte supplementation.

NOTE. this is different to the use of severe diuretic treatments, such as kidney balls, kidney flushes etc. which in theory "clean out" the kidneys and remove all the "bad" products. "Cleaning out" the kidneys really means that the feeder has been giving the animal feedstuffs and/or supplements which have been of no value in the horses' training programme, have accumulated in the kidneys and need severe action to get these or related compounds out of the horses' body. In this situation the problem is a basic one in that the horse has not been worked hard enough to allow it to utilise these accumulated compounds or the compounds are of no value to the horse and should not have been fed in the first place. In either instance the trainer who has to continually resort to the use of heavy kidney flushes to "clean out" the horses should re-evaluate either the training schedule or the feeding programme or both.

(C) add a flavouring to the water, refer CHAPTER ON WATER.

PRE-MIXED COMMERCIAL RATIONS AND PERFORMANCE HORSES

The problems of feeding PRE-MIXED COMMERCIAL RATIONS to PERFORMANCE HORSES are as follows:-

1. PROBLEM OF FIBRE DIGESTIBILITY

The types of FIBRE in pre-mixed commercial rations can vary from the best quality lucerne (alfalfa), to virtually indigestible hulls of some of the grains, cottonseed, sunflower rice, etc. The roughage or FIBRE component of rations of performance horses MUST BE the most digestible fibre available, otherwise excess HEAT is generated in breaking down the fibre, reducing the expected performance of the horse.

2. NO KNOWLEDGE OF ENERGY LEVEL

Very few of these rations ever provide any indication of the total energy level of the ration. There is generally a legal obligation, under most stock feed registration acts, to indicate the level of fat in a ration but NOT carbohydrate energy. As energy is the most important feed component, in rations, for mature performance horses, lack of any indication of the energy level, in the ration, is the same as driving blind, you really have no idea where you are going.

FEATURES OF SUB-CHRONIC OR LESS THAN DESIRABLE PERFORMANCES IN A HORSE.

PROBLEM	*POSSIBLE CAUSE*	*POSSIBLE CURE*
Horse misbehaves or hard to handle	Too much energy	Reduce energy content of feed or increase workload
Horse just cannot reach desired level of performance	Internal parasites (worms)	Drench
	External Parasites (Lice)	Treat
	Low Protein ration level	Increase ration protein level
	Amino-acid imbalance	Correct amino-acid imbalance and/or change rations
	Ca/P/Vit D ration and/or daily amounts incorrect	Correct levels and or ratios
	Vitamin A excess	Delete feed supplement containing Vitamin A
	Not drinking enough water	Add salt or electrolytes to ration
	Feeding excess iron	Cut iron supplements
	Feeding excess zinc	Cut out supplements containing zinc
	Feeding excess iodine	Do not feed supplements based on seaweed
Horse suffering fatigue after exercise	Tying up – excess lactic acid in muscle	Decrease grain level in ration or increase work load, feed electrolytes
	Muscle tremors & horse reluctant to move	Add calcium to ration
	Fatigued for days Possible potassium deficiency	Add minute amounts of potassium or appropriate electrolytes
	Flutter or thumps hindquarters move with heart beat Excess Ca, K & losses	Add appropriate electrolytes
	Total exhaustion	Condition better, make sure amino acid balance is correct and horse has appropriate electrolytes
Horse sweats with energy or is bad traveller	Electrolyte problems	Small daily quantity of nervours epsom salts or electrolyte mix of correct type
Horse mildly lame	Sub chronic founder	Reduce energy level or increase work load
Horse "off colour" – not passing faeces	Large intestine	Get vet surgeon and then feed better quality roughage

NOTE:

1. The above are *NOT* definite diagnosis, only an indication of what the problem may be.
2. The horse may suffer more than one problem at the sametime.
3. Seek expert help rather than do something that may make the horse worse.

3. NO KNOWLEDGE OF TYPE OF ENERGY

Whilst the level of FAT in the ration should be on the bag or label, FAT as an energy source is of little value to horse whose muscle energy production is in an ANAEROBIC environment. Similarly for those horses whose muscle energy production is in an AEROBIC environment, FAT is of value in the ration.

4. COST

Pre-mixed commercial feeds are generally always more expensive than buying your own individual feeds and mixing your own rations. often 60-60% more expensive. That can work out to a lot of money over a year.

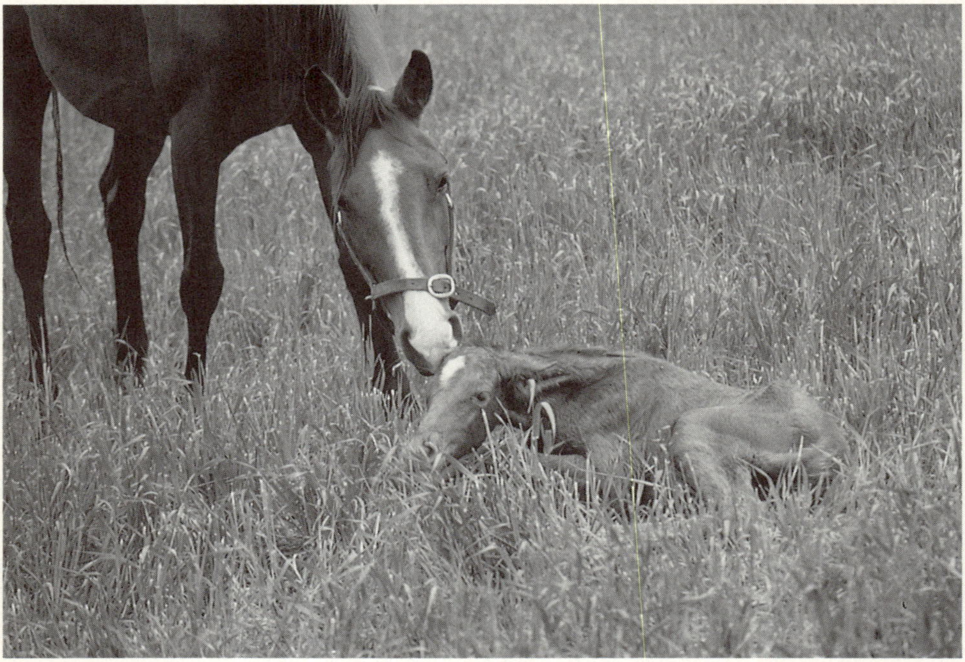

The end result of breeding.

27. FEEDING BREEDING HORSES

BROOD MARE, FOAL AND STALLION

The feeding of the brood mare has to be considered in terms of what are three completely different nutritional situations. Even though it may be the exact same mare, the varying nutritional demands of pregnancy and lactation produce a technical situation where the nutrient demands can change, often quite markedly, dependent on the state of the pregnancy of the mare.

1 THE MAIDEN MARE
2 90 DAYS or 3 MONTHS PRE-FOALING
3 FOALING TO 120 - 150 DAYS WEANING
4 MID PREGNANCY WEANING TO 90 DAYS PRE-FOALING.

NOTE: ALL FIGURES USED REFER TO A MARE WITH A BODYWEIGHT OF 450 KG (1000 LB) and adjustments will need to be made for mares of differing body weights.

PHASE 1 THE MAIDEN MARE

A brood mare has always to be bred for the first time. Prior to the actual service by the stallion, the mare could have had a prior feeding and or training history which may or may not be known. Whilst there are many factors which can affect the ability of the maiden mare to conceive satisfactorily, it is the intention, in this chapter, to investigate only the NUTRITIONAL FACTORS, involved in successful conception.

Nutritional management of maiden brood mares, for maximum conception rates, requires the dry mare to be in average to slightly above average body condition at mating but having been gaining weight for at least 6 weeks prior to mating. Numerous studies have shown that this approach to increasing mare weight, commonly called FLUSHING, will assist to stimulate the reproductive hormone production of the mare, so essential for OVULATION and FOETAL DEVELOPMENT. When the overall conception rate of horses is in the range of 55-65%, anything which will help to increase the likelihood of the mare getting in foal is of value.

For mares which are FAT or in good condition all the time, there appears little need to be worried about increasing their body weight in the six weeks before mating, such a practice would probably make them over fat and less likely to conceive. With these types of mares they either have to be taken down in condition, or made lose some weight, some months before mating is even contemplated and then allowed to gain weight or alternately left as they are, BUT they should never be in a situation of losing weight just prior to or at mating. The problem FAT MARES, which are difficult to get in foal as those mares which are able to alternate between fat and thin, either due to hormonal and or feeding problems. If the FAT and THIN problem is due to feeding, then get the mare onto a reasonable plane of nutrition, if the FAT and THIN problem is hormonal seek the advice of a veterinary surgeon.

One of the big problems in mating maiden Thoroughbred and Standardbred mares is the habit of racing females on the Saturday, sending them to the stud on the Sunday and expecting them to get in foal within the next three weeks. Whilst this may occur with some such mares, there are also some mares which have taken up to 3 or 4 months to "LET DOWN", or adjust from the racing environment and normal oestrus behaviour which will allow effective conception. The female is being asked to leave a stabled environment, being fed a performance ration, physiologically conditioned by training to produce muscle energy, possibly still under the effects of anyone of a number of drugs used in racing stables to go to an environment where physiological muscle use does not matter, no protection is afford from the weather, the feed is from pasture and possible hay with little or no grain and the primary objective is for her to now have a normal oestrus cycle, produce an egg and conceive.

Some mares find this immediate change of environment and use too much and simply take some time to adjust.

Maiden mares, off the racetrack, to the stud should:-

1 be sent to stud at least 6 weeks before the intended mating.

2 be "TAKEN DOWN" or "LET DOWN" from the stabled ration of grain etc. to the stud ration over a period of at least 3 weeks by replacing the stable ration with the stud ration.

3 if possible be provided with at least the shelter of a roof, in some part of the paddock, for the initial three week period until the mare gets used to not having the comfort and warmth of a stable.

4 be continually observed to see whether in fact she commences to show the external signs of the OESTRUS CYCLE. If such signs are NOT seen within the first 28 days after being at the stud, immediate veterinary examination is desirable.

The feed requirements for the first 8 months of pregnancy, in a maiden mare, are very small over and above the feed needed for the mares' own bodily needs as the amount of FOETAL development in the first eight months of pregnancy is very small, in terms of nutrient demands.

The maiden brood mare can be treated an as adult horse with low workload for the first 8 months of pregnancy, refer chapter on FEEDING ADULT HORSES.

PHASE 2 90 DAYS PRE-FOALING

In the last 80-90 days of pregnancy, the foetus increases considerably in size, some 60% of the total weight being developed in that last 90 days before foaling. This rapid weight gain is shown in the following table.

AVERAGE THOROUGHBRED FOAL

WEIGHT at 240 days	16.00-18.75 kg	36-42 lb.
WEIGHT at birth	37.00-47.70 kg	85-107 lb
WEIGHT INCREASE LAST 90 DAYS	21.00-28.95 kg	49-65 lb
WEIGHT INCREASE % IN LAST 90 DAYS as % of BIRTH WEIGHT	57% to	61%

Increasing quantities of protein and energy are required to allow the foetus and associated tissues to fully develop.

PROTEIN requirements for the last 90 days of pregnancy are generally assessed at an additional 10 kg of total protein fed over 90 days. This translates to an increase in the protein content of the ration of 0.11 kgs protein per day or from 8-10% to 9.5 to 11.5%.

ENERGY requirements for the last 90 days of pregnancy are generally assessed at 55 MCals (220 MJs), which works out at an average daily increase, in the mares' energy needs of 0.61 MCals/ day. In practical terms this amounts to an increase in the mares' daily ration of 0.33 kg of reasonable hay, 0.22 kg/day of oats or 0.20 kg/day of maize

With the rapid growth of the size of the foetus during this last 90 days of pregnancy, there can be some reduction in the capacity of the digestive tract, due to the enlarging foetus taking up more space in the abdominal cavity. This could have an effect on digestion and absorption of food nutrients so it is worthwhile ensuring that mares, in the last 90 days of pregnancy, receive top quality roughage, which will be readily digestible in the large intestine and not old, stemmy, mature hay which can take considerably longer to pass through the digestive tract.

The main nutritional problem in the last 90 days of PREGNANCY is the amount of both CALCIUM and PHOSPHORUS in the ration.

The mare should be grazing a mixed pasture, with a plant population consisting of 50% legumes and 50% grasses. In most instances this pasture., if fertilised correctly will contain adequate levels of both CALCIUM and PHOSPHORUS. The exact same situation will exist if the mare is being fully hand fed on hay made from similar mixed pasture.

If the grazing is grass only or the hand feeding is grass hay only then there will be no problems in the CALCIUM and PHOSPHORUS levels, provided:-

1. the soil contains adequate levels of soil PHOSPHORUS. There are vast areas of the world where PHOSPHORUS deficiency, for pasture growth, exists and this lack of soil PHOSPHORUS will be reflected in the PHOSPHORUS content of the grasses and or legumes grown on those soils and eventually eaten by horses. The simplest way to counteract this problem is by the sowing of improved pasture species and the application of the fertiliser superphosphate. If this choice of action is not possible then the feeding of a PHOSPHORUS supplement is required.
2. grazing green cereal crops.some grazing cereal crops, oats, barley and wheat can have extremely low CALCIUM levels and very high PHOSPHORUS levels. This imbalance may be of such magnitude that if adequate correction cannot be made, it may be wise not to allow grazing of pregnant mares on such green cereal crops, unless the actual CALCIUM and PHOSPHORUS content is determined by laboratory analysis.

If the mares' ration consist mainly of grazing and or hay based on LUCERNE (ALFALFA), then a PHOSPHORUS DEFICIENCY PROBLEM will exist. All legumes, including LUCERNE (ALFALFA) have very high levels of CALCIUM and very low levels of PHOSPHORUS, often ending up with a CALCIUM/PHOSPHORUS ratio of about 6/1. As this Ca/P ratio has to be reduced to 1.5/1, the feeding of such lucerne (alfalfa) hay and or pasture to brood mares, especially in the last 90 days of pregnancy, MUST be accompanied by an appropriate PHOSPHORUS supplement or else the feeding changed to mixed pasture hay and or grazing.

POSSIBLE PHOSPHORUS SUPPLEMENT

If the additional protein and energy required, in the last 90 days of pregnancy, by this mare, is in the form of a mix of equal thirds by weight of grain, bran and GRASS hay, then the normally excessive levels of PHOSPHORUS in the grain and bran can be usefully used to balance a PHOSPHORUS deficiency when mares are grazing PHOSPHORUS deficient pasture or being fed a ration based predominately on lucerne (alfalfa) hay. DO NOT use lucerne or alfalfa hay in this mix, its natural high level of CALCIUM will negate any additional PHOSPHORUS value in the grain and bran.

FAILURE TO RECOGNISE AND CORRECT THE PRE-FOALING CALCIUM AND PHOSPHORUS PROBLEM

Visually, as far as the mare is concerned, during the last 90 days or pregnancy, absolutely nothing externally and visible will change.

However internally the mare will be drawing upon her own CALCIUM and PHOSPHORUS supplies, predominately from bone, to make up the deficit in the ration so that the foal can develop as correctly as possible. The short term result of this will be REDUCED MILK PRODUCTION in the mare and LOWERED FERTILITY at subsequent matings.

As far as the new born foal is concerned, the extent of any CALCIUM and or PHOSPHORUS problem in the mares' ration pre-foaling may occur in one of two ways.

1. the foal may be born with leg and or joint problems.
2. the foal may appear normal at birth but will develop leg and or joint problems at any stage up to three years of age, refer METABOLIC BONE DISORDERS.

PHASE 3 FOALING TO 120-150 DAYS WEANING

The mare, at foaling should be in good body weight condition, say SCORE 6-7 on the U.S. body scoring system and 3 to 3.5 on the Australian system, at a stage where the ribs are unable to be seen. This is the phase in the brood mare's reproductive cycle where her nutrient demands are increased considerably.

It is necessary to make adjustments to the ration of the mare immediately upon foaling, to cater for the increased nutrient demands of milk production. If the mare is fed the same ration after foaling as before, she will get only about 50% of the energy and protein she needs, and about 35% of the calcium and phosphorus that is required. The end result of all this will be a mare, rapidly losing body condition, reduction in milk yield and eventual cessation of milk production and a foal which is not growing as well as it should.

The milk production of the mare will be influenced by:-

1. her genetic ability to produce milk. Horses, generally are selected for every other feature, except milk production.
2. feed intake during the 90 days preceding foaling, especially the CALCIUM and PHOSPHORUS levels.
3. condition of mare at foaling, OVERFAT MARES can deposit fat in the udder tissues instead of milk secreting glands.
4. feed intake during the first 150 days after foaling.
5. daily water intake after foaling.

Feed nutrients are required for -

1. maintenance of the mare.
2. milk production
3. after service, growth of the new foetus.

By far the most pressing demands are for milk production.

The average mare will have a milk production output of about 3% body weight in the first 12 weeks of lactation and 2% of body weight in the period 13-24 weeks of lactation.

For a 450 kg (1000 lb) mare this equates to an average milk production level of 13.50 litres or kilograms (3 gallons) per day for the initial 12 weeks and 9.00 litres or kilograms (2 gallons) per day for weeks 13-24.

However milk production ability of mares is known to vary considerably. Studies have shown that mares, at the peak of lactation, can produce from 8 to 36 litres or kilograms per day with foal intake of milk being in the average range of 16 litres/day for the first 5 weeks after birth, rising to 18 litres/day thereafter.

MILK COMPOSITION

The average composition of the milk of cows and horses, in percentage terms, approximatesas follows:-

	COW	MARE	MARE
			DRY MATTER
WATER	87.00	90.00	0.00%
PROTEIN	3.40	2.00	22.00%
FAT	3.80	1.20	13.12%
SUGAR	4.90	5.90	61.50%
ASH	0.72	0.36	3.80%

TOTAL SOLIDS is the sum of all the constituents MINUS the water.

TOTAL SOLIDS	12.00	9.40

In relation to cow's milk, mares milk contains 41% less PROTEIN
60% less FAT
20% more SUGAR

There will be variations around these values dependent on breed of horse, milk producing ability and ration composition.

10 litres of mares milk contains 340 grams PROTEIN.
380 grams FAT.
490 grams SUGAR.

with an energy level of about 5.00 MCals. which will be provided by additional daily protein needs of 0.65-0.80 kg CRUDE PROTEIN. additional daily energy needs of 10.00-14.00 MCals. contained in about another 45-50% DRY MATTER.

In simple nutritional terms, the lactating mare will require about 4 kgs extra feed/day containing 17.5% CRUDE PROTEIN and 3.50 MCals energy, in order to produce 10 litres of milk.

There will also be an additional increase in daily water consumption of about 60%.

The increased feed requirements required by the lactating mare to allow satisfactory milk production are shown in the following table. Both PROTEIN and ENERGY levels per kilogram will remain the same, the number of kilograms supplied and the water intake will change.

DAILY MILK PRODUCTION LITRES	EXTRA D.M. REQUIRED	% INCREASE D.M. over 9kgs. 351	ADDITIONAL WATER	% INCREASE WATER over
7.5	3	33%	7.5	21%
10.00	4	44%	10.0	29%
12.50	5	55%	12.5	355
15.00	6	66%	15.0	43%
17.50	7	77%	17.5	50%
20.00	8	88%	20.0	58%

When consideration is taken of the MAINTENANCE NEEDS OF THE MARE and the MILK PRODUCTION NEEDS, the ration for a lactating mare has PROTEIN and ENERGY REQUIREMENTS as follows.

POOR MILKER 10 Litres/day

		PROTEIN	ENERGY
MAINTENANCE	9 kgs	10.0% C.P.= 900 grams	15 MCals
MILK PRODUCTION	4 kgs	17.5% C.P.= 700 grams	14 MCals
TOTAL NEEDS	13 kgs	1600 grams	29 MCals

GOOD MILKER 20 litres/day

MAINTENANCE	9 kgs	900 grams	15 MCals
MILK PRODUCTION	8 kgs	1400 grams	28 Mcals
TOTAL NEEDS	17 kgs	2300 grams	43 MCals

The mares' ration needs to contain at least 12.5% crude protein, and more likely 13.5% crude protein, commonly accepted as 14%, due to differences in protein quality, and 2.23 to 2.52 MCals of energy/kg of feed.

The most common ration to satisfy this need for PROTEIN and ENERGY will be mixed pasture and or mixed pasture hay. This mixed pasture and mixed pasture hay will also contain sufficient CALCIUM and PHOSPHORUS in the ration for milk production requirements.

IT is IMPORTANT to recognise that any lack of CALCIUM and or PHOSPHORUS in the diet of a lactating mare will be compensated for by the mare drawing upon her body reserves of both minerals. Once this maternal body reserve of both minerals is exhausted, and that will depend on previous feeding history, reductions then start to occur in levels of milk production.

The feeding of LUCERNE (ALFALFA) HAY to lactating brood mares needs to adopted with caution.

LUCERNE (ALFALFA) has a very high level of CALCIUM and a very low level of PHOSPHORUS and if it provides the complete diet and or supplementary feed to lactating mares, there is a very strong possibility that problems will occur in the future in the foals from lack of PHOSPHORUS and imbalance of CALCIUM and PHOSPHORUS in the diet. PHOSPHORUS deficiency in a brood mare is suspected of causing failure to come on heat and failure to ovulate.

The feeding of high levels of grain in any diet of brood mares MAY create two problems.

1. GRAINS contain reasonably high energy levels (3.20-3.80 MCals/kg) BUT will not contain enough PROTEIN (8-12%). This energy level is some 44%-70% more than the lactating mare requires on a per kilogram basis, and can lead to either a poor milking mare converting that excess energy into body fat or a good milking mare producing excessive levels of milk.

Lactating mares should be maintained at the same weight all the time from foaling to at least 6 months after foaling. Mares which gain weight in this period may, as with mares that also lose weight within the same period, take much longer to conceive than if a steady body weight is maintained, sometime sup to 30 or 45 days longer.

The production of excessive levels of milk production can lead to foals GROWING TOO FAST. This may appear to be a contradiction to some people but it is possible to push foal growth rates beyond the ability of the foal to maintain normal GROWTH RELATIONSHIPS between muscle and bone. EXCESSIVE GROWTH RATES will lead to more muscle being produced in relation to bone than should normally happen and eventually the bone is unable to take the weight and or the various forces created by this additional muscle. This then leads to the development of any of a number of problems which are collectively called METABOLIC BONE DISORDERS. These problems may occur during the suckling period or may not evolve until the horse is subject to physical exercise as in training.

Foal growth rate will be determined by a number of other important considerations including amount of milk available, however the average normal thoroughbred foal should be expected to have daily live weight increase of from 1.4 kgs/ day about 14 days after birth, steadily reducing to about 1.00 kg/day at 3 months of age and about 0.8 kg/day at 6 months of age.

The practice of weighing foals at frequent intervals is a very good way of double checking on the mare's milk production and foal growth. There is some evidence that foal growth, as an indirect measure of milk energy levels, is unaffected by the different energy levels in the mares' feed. The mares fed higher levels of energy in the ration tended to produce greater volumes of more dilute milk.

2 All grains are low in CALCIUM level and high in PHOSPHORUS level and some type of CALCIUM supplement needs to be fed to correct the imbalance.

SUCKLING FOAL PROBLEMS

It is possible that a foal will be born normally, behave and grow as expected for the first week or so and then suddenly start to develop various types of skeletal problems.

These can be due to:-

1. lack of milk production
2. excessive milk production
3. production of milk of abnormal quality.

REDUCED MILK PRODUCTION FROM THE MARE

Mares will produce less than desirable levels of milk production in any of the following situations:-

1. where she has insufficient total available feed or DRY MATTER to eat each day.
2. where the levels of either or both CALCIUM and or PHOSPHORUS in the mares' ration is incorrect.
3. where the diet lacks sufficient protein.

REDUCED MILK PRODUCTION by the BROOD MARE is extremely difficult, if not impossible to detect, unless the foals are being regularly weighed. Even so, this is determining the possible cause after the event. It is possible with ration analysis to detect this problem BEFORE IT HAPPENS, not after.

EXCESSIVE MILK PRODUCTION

This will probably occur in those mares who possess a genetic ability to be very efficient converters of feed into milk. The easiest way to correct this problem is to reduce the quality of the feed (protein and energy levels) but not the amount which the mare is receiving each day. This should have some effect on reducing the quantity of milk produced. Secondly, if milk production does not decrease, wean the foal, if before three months of age onto milk replacer and if after three months of age, onto creep feed.

ABNORMAL MILK PRODUCTION

Due to incorrect levels of CALCIUM and PHOSPHORUS in the milk. This is a genetic problem, cannot be changed and will occur each year in the same mare

SELENIUM SUPPLEMENTATION

This particular treatment will be necessary to mares before foaling and to newly born foals, in those specific areas where SELENIUM DEFICIENCY in the soil is known to affect the growth of young horses.

WEANING

At between 120 and 150 days after foaling, the ENERGY requirements of the foal exceed the ENERGY LEVELS in the milk produced by the average mare. WEANING should then take place at this time and the foal given access to pasture and supplementary feed.

WEANING SHOULD CONSIST OF:-

1 making the separation of mare and foal abrupt and final.

2 leaving the foal in the paddock where it has previously run and shifting the mare to another paddock, definitely reduces the stresses of weaning as the foal is still in familiar surroundings, knows where the fences and water are and usually has some mates still left behind.

3 wean mares over a period of days or weeks, at the start of the weaning taking some mares out but leaving some mares behind and repeating this procedure over a number of

days or weeks until al foals are weaned.

4 stop feeding any hay and or concentrate to the mare about one week before weaning is to take place, will assist to reduce milk production.

PHASE 4 MID PREGNANCY WEANING TO 90 DAYS PRE-FOALING

After weaning at 120-150 days, the mare should then be again fed exactly the same as a dry adult horse AT REST.

SUPPLEMENTARY FEEDING SUCKLING FOALS

The practice of providing creep or supplementary feeding facilities for FOALS up to weaning age but still suckling the mare is really not required, if the mare is fed the correct ration, producing adequate quantities of milk and the foal is growing at a satisfactory rate. The aim is to produce a foal where the growth and development of the bones and muscles are co-ordinated to-gether to produce a healthy horse.

Foals are often provided with a supplementary or creep feed as soon as they are capable of eating hard feed, generally about 30 days of age. Creep feed allows for less milk demand from the dam and greater opportunity for the foals to grow to their genetic potential. Creep fed foals are also less likely to suffer a setback when weaned from milk to hard feed and pasture as they are already used to hard feed.

Creep rations should have PROTEIN and ENERGY levels, at least equal to milk, to be effective as a milk replacement. If the creep feed, being supplied to a suckling foal IS NOT equivalent to the composition of mare's milk then the balance of the nutrients in the mares' milk will be upset and the foal will not grow as expected.

Such a CREEP FEED supplement, equivalent to mare's milk in composition will, on a DRY MATTER basis, contain a CRUDE PROTEIN level of 22% and an ENERGY level of at least 5.50 MCals. Feeding creep supplements to foals under 150 days of age with less PROTEIN and or ENERGY than these figures will be a waste of time and effort. FEEDS which contain these protein and energy levels are only obtainable in specially formulated rations, commonly called MILK REPLACERS etc.

Such CREEP FEEDS should not be fed AD LIB or the foal having unrestricted access. Foals can get too much creep feed or concentrate during the first 120-150 days of life, leading to the production of any one of the problems collectively known as METABOLIC BONE DISORDERS. CREEP FEED at the rate of 0.25 to 0.75 kgs of milk replacer/foal/day starting at 12 weeks (3 months) of age and increasing to 20 weeks (5 months) of age or until weaning.

GRAIN of any type, as a creep feed, for suckling foals is DEFINITELY OUT, if you are in any way interested in the long term health of the foal. Grain is TOO LOW in protein and TOO HIGH in energy to be of any value and whilst supplementary feeding suckling foals with grain will produce the slick, fat shiny foal which will probably win a show ring prize in a led foal class at halter, the grain will cause imbalances in PROTEIN and ENERGY to occur in the horse which will be seen at some stage in the future as some skeletal, joint and or tendon problem.

If the growth rate of the foal, suckling and with or without creep feeding at any stage up to 120-150 days of age, is NOT as required, it is probably better to wean the foal completely, from the mother and use some form of artificial feeding to replace and extend the previous milk intake. Such decisions can be made from birth when the foal may be left an ORPHAN to 150 days of age.

NOTE there is an increasing trend in some areas, to wean foals from the mare at 7 days of age. no matter how well the mare is milking, onto artificial milk replacer rations. This procedure is being adopted, not for the benefit of the foal, but to get the mare back in foal earlier, than if the foal was suckling. This procedure is full of problems, the most important one being that the mare's milk production has to be encouraged until 7 days of age, otherwise the growth of the foal suffers but as soon as the foal is weaned, the possibility of mastitis occurring is high. Further there appears to be some considerable problems with the foals adjusting to the artificial rations and current foal growth rates, after 7 days, leave much to be desired.

WEANING FOALS at one month of age, or thereabouts onto milk replacer, will produce foals which will always have slower growth in the first 12 months of age than if they were suckling the mare till 150 days, post foaling. However these early weaned foals will nearly always have an increased growth rate in the second year, known as COMPENSATORY GROWTH and both groups of foals will be a similar weight at the age of 24 months.

ORPHAN FOALS

The first and probably the most important point in the rearing of orphan foals is not to allow them to become too friendly with humans. Whilst one may have sympathy and feeling for an orphan foal, and wish to devote care and attention, well beyond normal limits, the orphan foal, spoilt when young, is without doubt the most difficult horse to break and train.

As young horses they develop an affinity with adults, instead of with horses, and this is satisfactory as long as the foal is young. However, as the foal gets older they do not forget the affinity and relationship that they have had with humans, and as a result when the time comes for education, i.e. tying up to posts, mouthing, riding, etc. the foal generally rebels. In fact, so essential does the human factor become in the orphan foals existence, that the foal relates the presence of a human to feed and then relates feed to a full stomach and then relates a full stomach to satisfaction and contentment. Unfortunately when the foal has grown up and is being handled, the human has to teach the foal to do and perform in a way by using methods which the foal will find as completely bewildering.

It is certainly in everyones interests not to spoil an orphan foal, no matter how sympathetic we feel for it and to let the foal be a horse rather than a human at every opportunity.

As soon as is practical, the orphan foal should be run with other horses to learn the basic herd instincts and other habits which are only learnt from the herd environment, sometimes called IMPRINTING. The worst foal or horse of all to handle and do anything with is the orphan foal which has grown up without contact with any other horse. Most times it would have been a lot better not to rear the foal as these types of horses generally get worse as they get older, and often may not be able to be educated with safety.

The second important point with the rearing of orphan foals is to ensure absolute cleanliness of all utensils and other items used in the feeding process. Digestive upsets and intestinal tract infections are easily caused by unclean feeding utensils. Cleanliness can be achieved by washing all utensils in the same solution used to clean and sterilise babies feeding bottles. By doing so after every feed and storing the buckets etc., in a clean place the chance of the foal getting some form of digestive upset can be reduced considerably.

IMPORTANCE OF COLOSTRUM

The ORPHAN FOAL must have access to colostrum. Colostrum is the stickly, yellow coloured milk produced in the first few hours or days after foaling. It is important for the early nutrition of the foal as it

1. contains antibodies or 'immunoglobulins" which confer "ready made" protection to the foal against disease - MOST IMPORTANT.
2. is a highly concentrated source of energy, protein, minerals and vitamins, especially Vitamin A.
3. is highly digestible
4. has a natural laxative effect to stimulate bowel movement.

The principal features of colostrum are Vitamin A content and the antibody content. The Vitamin A content is important as the foal is born with virtually no Vitamin A reserves. Likewise grazing generally does not commence until the animal is about three weeks of age. Hence if colostrum did not contain any Vitamin A, the young foal would have a three week period in which it would suffer a lack of Vitamin A. As Vitamin A is essential for all normal growth, a foal, without access to Vitamin A in the first three weeks of life, may not possibly survive that period of time.

The ANTIBODY content is important in that these confer to the foal the ability to resist and fight off infections and similar diseases. The foal is born without any antibodies in the body. Ingestion of antibodies is the time honoured system whereby the foal has been giving some protection for the first few months of its life before its own body is able to make the antibodies in sufficient amounts. The ability of the FOAL to absorb the ANTI-BODIES present in COLOSTRUM, starts to decrease immediately after birth and by 24 hours after birth, the foal no longer possesses the ability to absorb any antibodies present in any colostrum.

COLOSTRUM can be provided for the orphan foal in the following manner:-

1. FROZEN COLOSTRUM. Some studs and veterinary surgeons maintain a bank or supply of frozen colostrum taken from freshly foaled mares and this is the preferred method of getting colostrum into orphan foals. Provided the colostrum is collected in sterile containers and frozen immediately after collection, it will be suitable for feeding the orphan foals. There have, however, been some reports of illness and sometimes death in foals fed colostrum collected in less than ideal conditions and/or not frozen immediately on collection.
2. FRESH COLOSTRUM. Access to another mare which has foaled in the last 12 hours. The level of antibodies is reasonably high in the first 12 hours after foaling and then the antibody concentration will reduce considerably to almost nil at 24 hours.
3. ARTIFICIAL COLOSTRUM. If it is not possible to obtain fresh or frozen colostrum within a short period of time after birth, the following formula has proven satisfactory as an artificial colostrum - 1 litre cows milk, 1 thoroughly beaten egg, 2 tablespoons brown sugar, (white sugar will do), 20 ml cod liver oil and up to 20 ml paraffin. The paraffin level will need to be adjusted so as to

prevent the foal from scouring, but never more than 20 ml in the mixture - the least preferred method by far.

This mixture needs to be made daily and must be fresh when given to the foal.

This mixture does not contain the antibodies present in the normal colostrum but these can now be provided by one of two methods. As an injection from the veterinary surgeon, called IMMUNE GLOBULIN INJECTION and can be given to the foal the day after foaling or the veterinary surgeon MAY be able to obtain blood plasma from other mares which have just foaled and give this plasma, to the foal, via the jugular vein.

With all the above COLOSTRUM feeding methods, dose rate is 500 ml (about 1 pint) per feed, for at least two feeds, 2 hours apart.Once the foal has had a drink of colostrum the next problem is to find a way of feeding the orphan for the next 4-5 months.

FOSTER MOTHERING

The first, and least labour intensive, choice is to try and find a foster mother. As the orphan foal has had a drink of colostrum, the proposed foster mother could be any mare lactating but which has recently lost its own foal. The success of such foster rearing will depend on the maternal instincts of the mother and the patience of the foal owner. The sooner the orphaned foal is introduced to the foster mother, after her own foal has died, the better. Even so it may be necessary to mark or disguise the smell of the orphan foal from the mare. Smell of progeny is a very important aspect in the mothering process and each mare and foal combination appear to recognise each other, IMPRINTING, by the smell. As the orphan foal will undoubtedly have a different smell to the mares' previous foal, the following can be attempted to overcome the problem.

1. Get sample of mare's excreta, or that from the orphan foal. Rub a small quantity over the foal and also around the muzzle of the mare.
2. Use the scented pressure packs as sold for mothering up lambs, applying spray to the nose of the mare and the back and neck of the foal.
3. Use a bland strong smelling ointment such as 'Vicks' or something similar and apply to both mare and foal.
4. Some people have sometimes removed the fresh skin from the mares' dead foal and tied it onto the orphan so that the mare has the same scent as previously to relate to.

Even with the use of any one of these four methods, it will still be essential to place mare and orphan foal in a stable or yard and carefully observe for some period of time to ensure that the mare is not rejecting the foal completely, or physically abusing and kicking it. If foster mothering can be achieved, it is the most desirable way to raise an orphan foal, but a lot will depend on the mares temperament and mothering ability, and the owners' patience.

HAND REARING

If foster mothering is not successful or practical, then hand rearing, either individually by bucket or else by self feeding machine is the only choice. After the foal has had one or two feeds of colostrum, the feeding can then settle down to a pattern.

Initial liquid feeding may be done with a bottle and teat and most people find this the easiest way. Foals drink quickly compared to other young animals and can become physically exhausted drinking out of teats. The foal however can be readily taught to drink from a bucket by allowing the foal to suckle the middle finger with the palm of the hand pressed against the foals upper lip, and at the same time raising the bucket or feeding utensil so that the foals lips are covered by the liquid feed.

Possible feed formulations are -

1. 1 litre cows milk, 300 ml. limewater (1 teaspoon lime in a litre of cold boiled water, settle overnight and use the liquid portion), 60 grams (3 tablespoons) lactose or brown sugar.

2. Calf milk replacer with 60 grams or three tablespoons lactose added to each litre of prepared milk replacer.

3. Calf milk replacer at half recommended strength with 10 drops of vitamin mixture, 1 tablespoon calcium gluconate and one tablespoon honey per foal per day.

Start feeds at 150 ml per feed and at 2 hourly intervals for the first week. Ensure that all feeds are fed at 38-39 degrees C and all utensils are absolutely clean.

There is a some advantage in having the liquid milk replacer available to the foal all the time. Some U.S. work showed a decided preference to unrestricted feeding, with milk at room temperature. This technique may have advantages where any potential fly problem can be controlled, as with the liquid milk replacer being kept inside a fly proof building and where daytime temperatures do not get very high. However in any situation where flies are a potential problem and or daytime temperatures rise in the high 20's or 30's degrees Centigrade, causing the milk to "go off", this practice cannot be recommended.

In the second week, the feeds can be reduced to 4 hourly intervals, and the foal should be on about one litre of preparation per feed. By the end of the fourth week, the foal would be expected to be still on four hourly feeds but receiving and drinking about 2- 2.5 litres per feed. In the third or fourth week, the foal should have ready and continual access to hay and a possible concentrate mixture.

The volume of liquid should be slowly increased so that by the end of the fifth month the foal should be receiving 13-15 litres per day in four feeds. In the sixth month the foal should be able to exist on pasture alone, but there is nothing wrong with continuing liquid feeding if desired, but reducing the feeds to one or two per day.

Liquid intake needs to be carefully adjusted so that the foals appetite is satisfied. Adequate rest, hence contented and well grown foal will only follow full stomachs - without scours.

Another suitable schedule for ORPHAN FOAL feeding is as follows:-

DAY 1 COLOSTRUM	500ML or 1 pint/feed as desired.
DAY 2-7 FOAL MILK REPLACER	label instructions as desired introduce replacer pellets day 5
WEEK 1-3 FOAL MILK REPLACER	label instructions, change to bucket, pellets, hay, grain.
WEEK 3-5 PELLETED MILK REPLACER &/OR CREEP RATION	increase grain to 1kg/day plus liquid milk replacer, hay or grass AD LIB from now on.
WEEK 5-12 CREEP RATION	feed at 1% of body weight.
WEEK 13-16 75% CREEP RATION 25% ALFALFA HAY	feed at 3% body weight.
WEEK 17-24 65% CREEP RATION 35% HAY	feed at 2.5% body weight

WEEK 25-52 50% CREEP RATION
50% HAY feed at 2% body weight
WEEK 53 ON 45% CREEP RATION
55% HAY feed at 1.5-2.0% body weight.

NOTE CREEP FEED should contain 15-18% protein, 3.1 MCal/kg D.E., 0.85% CALCIUM and 0.60% phosphorus.

SCOURS

Scours can be a big problem in foals reared in the above manner. Nutritional scours will be caused by overfeeding, either too much milk or too much green feed, especially in the first 5-6 weeks after birth. NUTRITIONAL SCOURS are generally cream or brown in colour. If green feed is the cause, immediately reduce or eliminate this from the diet, if the cause is excessive milk intake immediately reduce the quantity of milk substitute given per feed. Treatment can be one of many ways. Junket tablets are worthwhile - they will expand inside the digestive tract and slow down the rate of food passage - generally the problem with nutritional scours. Human diarrhoea remedies may also be useful. Some success has also been had with the complete removal of the milk substitute and giving the foal the same quantity of water with 50 grams of glucose added per litre of water.

Bacterial scours are generally green and/or black in colour and are due to unclean buckets and/or mixing utensils.

Antibiotics and/or sulphadrugs are needed to control such bacterial scours, and as well attention should be paid to the cleanliness and cleaning up procedures of the feeding utensils otherwise the problem of bacterial scours will occur again.

STALLIONS

Contrary to some beliefs, sperm production by a stallion does not require any large increase in the composition or quality of the ration over and above that normally needed to maintain a dry adult horse of similar weight, in simple terms a gelding.

Any stallion should be able to be kept in reasonable condition by rations containing 10% protein and 2.80 MCals/kg energy. The biggest problem with stallions is the over-fat, under-exercised animal, which is more likely to have poor semen production and possibly lowered fertility, compared to well conditioned exercised horses. Chronic founder has also been diagnosed as a problem of considerable concern in overfed, underexercised stallions.

The composition of appropriate adult horse rations are detailed in earlier sections of this book.

The secrets with stallions are:-

1. EXERCISE. This is essential for stallions and the horse should, have a reasonably sized paddock available for day use. Riding and/or lungeing are also of value in providing the horse with the necessary exercise,if large day paddocks are not available.

2. The stallions should be at the ideal weight and condition at least two and possibly three months before the start of the season. Sperm takes about two months, from time of production in the testes before it is available for ejaculation at service. Hence sperm required for service in September will be produced in July. The stallion, therefore, needs to be in the peak of condition, and not over fat and underexercised in July to ensure suitable sperm for September matings.

Stallions should also not suffer any injury or setback during the breeding season. Such an event can render the stallion temporarily infertile for up to three months from the date of the setback or injury.

Stallions should be managed, fed and exercised not only to produce the ability to serve mares with fertile sperm in this season but also to ensure that the stallion will live as long as is possible, and continue to successfully perform in the following years.

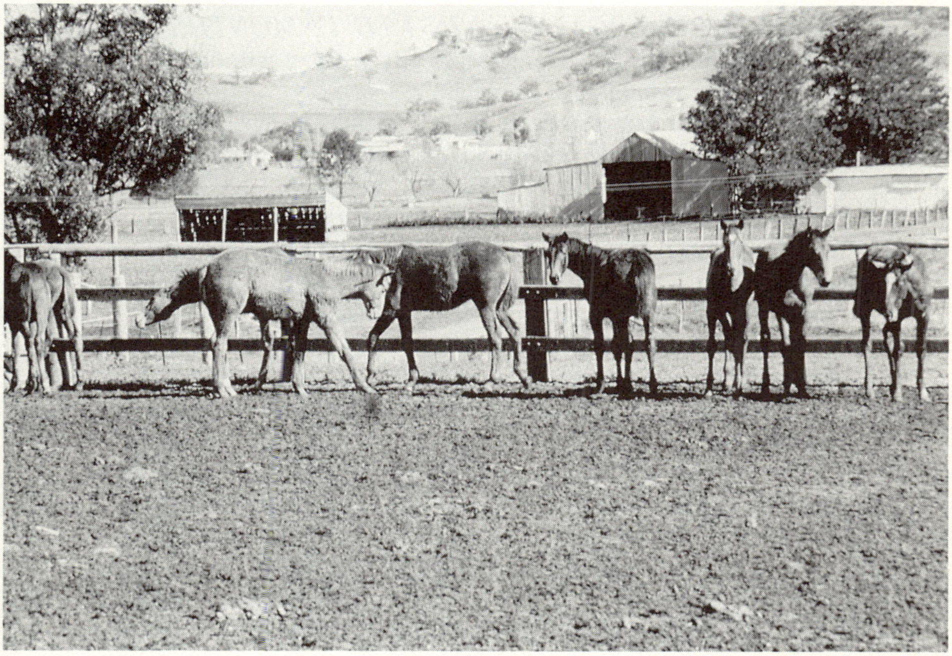

Thoroughbred weanlings

27. FEEDING HORSES WEANING TO 3 YEARS OF AGE.

This chapter is best divided into the following three reasonably distinct phases.

WEANLINGS FROM WEANING TO 12 MONTHS OF AGE
YEARLINGS 12 TO 24 MONTHS OF AGE
TWO YEAR OLD HORSES

Each of these growth stages are physiologically different and the horse will have differing nutritional needs, during each period.

WEANLINGS FROM WEANING TO 12 MONTHS OF AGE

At the age of 12 months, the average correctly fed foal will have attained a weight which should be 66% or two thirds of its mature weight.

During this period, from weaning at about 5 months of age, the daily expected live weight growth will slowly reduce from about 0.8 kgs/day at 6 months, to 0.65 kg/day at 9 months, to 0.55 kg/day at 12 months of age.

The WEANLING during this period requires feed nutrients which:-

1. supply enough BALANCED PROTEIN to allow the horse to grow at normal expected rates.
2. sufficient energy, in the ration, to allow expected rates of growth to occur but NOT EXCESSIVE levels of energy which may cause the development of any one of the many conditions, commonly called METABOLIC BONE DISORDERS.
3. CALCIUM and PHOSPHORUS present in the correct weights or amounts in the ration.
4. no imbalance of any description in the ration which will allow or encourage or cause any problem with EXCESSIVE LEVELS or DEFICIENT LEVELS of any feed nutrient.

RATION PROTEIN LEVELS

WEANLINGS require ration CRUDE PROTEIN levels of 18%-20%. More importantly, the protein has to be BALANCED or contain ALL THE 10 ESSENTIAL AMINO ACIDS. Horses of this age group have, in numerous experiments, showed positive response to the addition of the AMINO ACID LYSINE to most rations.

LYSINE CONTENT OF GROWING HORSE RATIONS IS THE MOST LIMITING FACTOR IN FOAL GROWTH, there should be at least 0.75% LYSINE in the total ration to ensure satisfactory growth. LYSINE requirements can also be expressed as 2.1 g LYSINE/ MCal of D.E./day.

The ONLY horse feeds which contain sufficient levels of LYSINE which is able to satisfy these requirements, are green growing mixed pasture and hays, lucerne (alfalfa) grazing and hay and two oilseed meals, soybean and canola. EVERY OTHER HORSE FEED HAS A LYSINE DEFICIENCY FOR GROWING HORSES.

FEEDING HORSES WEANING TO 3 YEARS OF AGE

RATION ENERGY LEVELS

WEANLINGS require sufficient energy to allow normal expected rates of growth to occur but certainly not EXCESSIVE ENERGY LEVELS that may cause nutritional disorders to occur or which may lead to joint, ligament and tendon problems, collectively termed METABOLIC BONE DISORDERS due to the possible effect of the excess energy on the reducing the thyroid hormone regulating effect on normal body growth.

Ration energy levels are related to DRY MATTER CONSUMPTION, which will be changing virtually every day as we have a young horse which should be growing fairly quickly. The following table will provide some idea of the possible DRY MATTER CONSUMPTION, for a thoroughbred type horse, expected to reach a mature weight of 450 kgs (1000 lb).

AGE	EXPECTED WEIGHT	EXPECTED L.W. GAIN/DAY	DRY MATTER AS % BODYWEIGHT	CONSUMPTION AS KGS FEED
6 MONTHS	200 kg	1.11 kgs	2.00-3.50	4.00-7.00
9 MONTHS	225 kg	0.94 kgs	2.00-3.25	4.50-7.30
12 MONTHS	305 kg	0.83 kgs	2.00-3.00	6.10-9.15

This projected DRY MATTER INTAKE has to be able to supply between 13 and 17 MCals of energy/day, the lower level being considered necessary for moderate rates of growth and the higher level being considered necessary for higher but satisfactory rates of growth.

AGE	ENERGY LEVEL MCal/D.E./day	D.M. INTAKE /DAY	DESIRABLE ENERGY LEVEL OF FEED/KG
6 MONTHS	13.00	4.00-7.00	3.25-1.85 MCals
	14.50	4.00-7.00	3.62-2.07MCals
9 MONTHS	14.25	4.50-7.30	3.16-1.95 MCals
	15.75	4.50-7.30	3.50-2.15 MCals
12 MONTHS	15.50	6.10-9.15	2.54-1.69 MCals
	17.00	6.10-9.15	2.78-1.85 MCals

As far as determining the ENERGY requirements of horses from WEANING to 12 months of age, these tables provide the following information.

1. Expected DRY MATTER consumption can vary tremendously, often up to 50%, dependent on whether the horse has a moderate growth rate or a rapid growth rate.
2. When ENERGY intake, in terms of MCals energy/kg of feed is considered, the variation is even greater, ranging from 3.62 MCals/kg, (the energy level of BARLEY and MAIZE) for rapidly growing 6 month old horses with low appetites to 1.85 MCals/kg (the energy level of average mixed pasture and or mixed pasture hay) for either moderate growing, big eating 6 month olds or fast growing big eating 12 months olds.
3. the average ration energy level is 2.54 MCals/kg with variations of minimum levels of down to 1.85 MCals or 27% drop and maximum levels of 3.62 MCals or 43% increase.

4. the overall variation range of energy levels amounts to 1.77 Mcals/kg or 70% of the average need.

This still does not let us work out the best energy feeds for the young growing horse, it is desirable, to get a little better than within 50% or so of energy needs.

EFFECT OF EXERCISE.

The ENERGY needs of the horse will be determined not only by the weight of the horse but also by the amount of exercise which the horse receives. As described earlier, in detail, in the chapter on FEEDING ADULT horses, EXERCISE INCREASES APPETITE, due tothe additional demands by the horse for extra feed nutrients to replace those feed nutrients used in the exercise activity.

EXERCISE was and still is important for the horse running free, after all flight is the horse's main form of defence, ever tried to catch horses in a large paddock ?

We can now develop some idea of ENERGY NEEDS of the young growing horse.

WITH PLENTY OF EXERCISE - LARGE PADDOCKS AND MOB SITUATION.

Appetite and hence dry matter consumption will be at the higher level of estimated feed intake, so energy levels in the feed will have to be in the range of 1.69 MCals to 2.15 MCals/kg.

WITH VERY RESTRICTED EXERCISE-SMALL PADDOCKS, ONE HORSE SITUATION

Appetite and hence dry matter consumption will be at the lower level of estimated feed intake, so energy levels in the feed will have to be in the range of 2.54 MCals to 3.62 MCals/kg.

CALCIUM AND PHOSPHORUS REQUIREMENTS

It is ABSOLUTELY ESSENTIAL that the amounts of CALCIUM and PHOSPHORUS in the rations of these young growing horses be correct. Any deficiency in either mineral WILL lead to bone development problems, possibly not developing until much later in life but nevertheless problems which will affect the ability of the horse to perform.

CALCIUM AND PHOSPHORUS REQUIREMENTS
YOUNG GROWING HORSES

expected mature weight 450 kg (1000 lb)

AGE	TOTAL DAILY REQUIREMENTS		DAILY REQUIREMENTS /KG FEED	
	CALCIUM	PHOSPHORUS	CALCIUM	PHOSPHORUS
6 MONTHS	27 g	15 g	0.675-0.385g	0.375-0.214g
9 MONTHS	27 g	15 g	0.600-0.369g	0.333-0.205g
12 MONTHS	26 g	15 g	0.426-0.284g	0.245-0.163g

The AMOUNTS of CALCIUM and PHOSPHORUS required by the young growing horse in this period on a PER HORSE PER DAY basis is reasonably constant, about 27 grams of CALCIUM and 15 grams of PHOSPHORUS in the ration Ca/P of 1.80/1.00.

SATISFYING TECHNICAL NUTRITIONAL REQUIREMENTS

There are many different types of management situations, which can be used for rearing young horses post weaning. Rather than attempt the impossible task of evaluating all such strategies, feeding regimes in two strategies only will be assessed and the reader can make any necessary adjustments using the information contained in this book.

PASTURE GRAZING – UNRESTRICTED EXERCISE

PROTEIN LEVEL REQUIRED	18%-20%
(must contain LYSINE)	
ENERGY LEVEL REQUIRED	1.69 MCals-2.15MCals
CALCIUM LEVEL REQUIRED	0.385g/kg
PHOSPHORUS LEVEL REQUIRED	0.314G/kg.

There is really only one type of horse feed that will fit these specifications and that is ACTIVELY GROWING MIXED PASTURE.

Provided the stocking rate of the pasture is such that the horse is able to obtain ALL its necessary DRY MATTER intake from that pasture, then any form of additional feeding is not required.

ADDITIONAL VITAMINS AND MINERALS

There will be no need for supplementation of any additional vitamins and or minerals on these pastures, all those necessary for the horse are present in natural correctly grown pasture.

Problems which may be encountered could be as follows:-

1 reduction in protein level as the pasture mature and go to seed.

2 increase in lignin level (indigestible fibre), leading to a slight reduction in energy level as the pasture matures.

3 excessive levels of CALCIUM and PHOSPHORUS, in pastures grown on some soil types. Will not be a problem provided the ratio of the two minerals are about 1.8/1. Problems will occur if there are excessive and or deficient levels of one mineral, compared with the other, as can happen in pastures grown on PHOSPHORUS DEFICIENT soils.

HAND FEEDING - RESTRICTED EXERCISE

PROTEIN LEVEL REQUIRED	18-22%
LYSINE supplementation has to be considered	
ENERGY LEVEL REQUIRED	2.54 MCals-3.62 MCals
CALCIUM LEVEL REQUIRED	0.675g/kg
PHOSPHORUS LEVEL REQUIRED	0.375g/kg

Compared to the nutrient needs of the young growing horse running freely on pasture, this horse has restricted exercise and so will have a reduced dry matter intake. This means that for satisfactory growth, additional ENERGY and CALCIUM and PHOSPHORUS has to be supplied in less total feed.

POSSIBLE FEEDS AVAILABLE

PASTURE HAY

PROTEIN level not high enough, generally about 14% for good mixed pasture, no need for LYSINE supplement.

ENERGY level too low, about 2.20 MCals/kg.

CALCIUM and PHOSPHORUS levels satisfactory.

NEEDS PROTEIN AND ENERGY SUPPLEMENTATION.

LUCERNE HAY

PROTEIN level generally about 16-20%, LYSINE level suitable, better quality lucerne hay can provide enough protein.

ENERGY level low at 2.30 MCals/kg.

CALCIUM level at about 1.37 g/kg about double daily needs

PHOSPHORUS level at about 0.24 g/kg, only about 60% of daily needs.

CALCIUM/PHOSPHORUS ratio about 5.5/1.

NEEDS ENERGY AND PHOSPHORUS SUPPLEMENTATION

GRAINS

PROTEIN level varies considerably, dependent on where and how grains are grown, generally in the order of 8%-12%, but always low in LYSINE.

ENERGY varies dependent on fibre level but in the range of 3.20 MCals/kg to 3.80 MCals/kg.

CALCIUM level varies with grains but in the order of 0.06g/kg, with a range of levels of 0.05 to 0.09.

PHOSPHORUS levels varies with grains but in the order of 0.34 g/kg, with a range of levels of 0.27 to 0.38.

CALCIUM/PHOSPHORUS ratio about 1/5.6

NEEDS PROTEIN SUPPLEMENTATION, LYSINE ADDITION and CORRECTION OF CALCIUM DEFICIENCY.

OILSEED MEALS

PROTEIN level varies considerably but on average about 41% with a crude protein range of 32%-46%

ENERGY level varies considerably but on average about 3.18 MCals/kg, with the range being from 2.80 MCals/kg to 3.60 MCals/kg.

CALCIUM level again varies, dependent on the oilseed meals, but on average is about 0.40 g/kg, with the range being 0.18 g/kg to 0.69 g/kg.

PHOSPHORUS level shows a similar variation as that of CALCIUM, average level being 1.06 g/kg with the range being from 0.71 g/kg to 1.30 g/kg.

CALCIUM/PHOSPHORUS RATIO average of 1/2.65, with a range of 1/6.77 to 1/1.88.

PROTEIN LEVEL TOO HIGH, LYSINE SUPPLEMENTATION NECESSARY, (except for SOYBEAN and CANOLA MEALS), CALCIUM LEVEL TOO LOW.

There is then NO ONE feed which can provide the necessary nutrient requirements for a fully hand fed, young growing horse in a situation of RESTRICTED EXERCISE. Each of the major feed groups detailed above have one or more problems in supplying the nutrient needs of these types of horses.

POSSIBLE MIXED RATIONS

In order to satisfy the hand feeding needs of these young growing horses a separate mixed ration has too be prepared, based on the following principles.

1. at least 50% of the weight must be roughage.
2. lucerne is the preferred form of roughage, due to high protein level and lysine availability but there is nothing wrong with good quality mixed pasture. Protein level may be a little low but this can be corrected by extra oilseed meal in the mix.
3. soybean and or canola meal are next favoured due to high protein level and lysine content, but palatability problems could arise if the amount of either of these meals exceeds 300 gram/day for this size horse.
4. the balance of the ration can be made up with grain.
5. the CALCIUM and PHOSPHORUS levels are then calculated and corrections made where necessary. In some rations, based on lucerne as the roughage, no corrections may be necessary as the high Ca/low P in the lucerne can be balanced by the low Ca/high P in the grains and oilseeds.
6. there should be no need for any other vitamin and or mineral supplement, except SELENIUM in specific areas.

Due to the variation in the feed nutrient contents of the many feeds, exact rations cannot be worked out until the feeds desired to be used are know as well as the costs of those feeds.

RESTRICTED EXERCISE FOR GROWING HORSES IS MOST UNDESIRABLE

refer chapters on ENERGY and NUTRITIONAL DISORDERS.

SUPPLEMENTARY HAND FEEDING GRAZING GROWING HORSES

There will be times, in the grazing situation, where the nutritional value of the pasture will decline at some season during the year. Any additional supplementary feed given to these young growing horses on pasture will be based on the principles outlined above for fully hand fed horses and rations calculated on the same principles.

GROWING HORSES 12 MONTHS TO 24 MONTHS OF AGE

RATION PROTEIN LEVELS

These horses are now growing at a much reduced daily live weight increase so the amount of protein required in the ration will be reduced compared to that of younger horses

Average CRUDE PROTEIN levels should be in the order of 13-15%.

RATION ENERGY LEVELS

These will increase, in general, as the larger horses exercise more, additional energy supplies are required for growth PLUS energy used in exercise PLUS additional heat requirements.

RATION ENERGY level needs to be about 2.87 MCals/kg of feed, certainly not lower and a little higher will not be any worry providing the horse is getting exercise. If the horse has limited exercise, be very careful in exceeding that energy level in the ration as the horse is unable to use any excess energy in exercise and activity.

CALCIUM AND PHOSPHORUS REQUIREMENTS

These levels are still CRITICAL in the ration.

CALCIUM requirements are of the order of 24 grams per day and PHOSPHORUS of the order of 14 grams per day.

FEATURES OF ABNORMAL GROWTH IN YOUNG HORSES

PROBLEM	POSSIBLE CAUSE	POSSIBLE CURE
Rapid growth	Too much energy in ration and restricted exercise	Decrease ration energy level and/or increase daily exercise

Note — the end result of this will prbab;y not occur until the horse is put into training when some form of breakdown or injury may occur.

PROBLEM	POSSIBLE CAUSE	POSSIBLE CURE
Restricted growth	Internal parasites (worms)	Drench
	External parasites (lice)	Treat
	Low protein level in ration	Increase ration protein level
	Amino acid imbalance	Correct amino-acid imbalance and or/change rations
	Ca/P/Vit D ration and/or daily amounts incorrect	Correct levels and/or ratios
	Vitamin A excess	Delete feed supplements containing Vitamin A
	Not drinking enough water	Add salt or electrolyte to ration
	Feeding excess iron	Cut iron supplements
	Feeding excess zinc	Cut out supplements containing zinc
	Feeding excess iodine	Do not feed supplements based on seaweed meal

NOTE:

1. The above are *NOT* definite diagnosis, only an indication of what the problem may be.
2. The horse may suffer more than one problem at the sametime.
3. Seek expert help rather than do something that may make the horse worse.

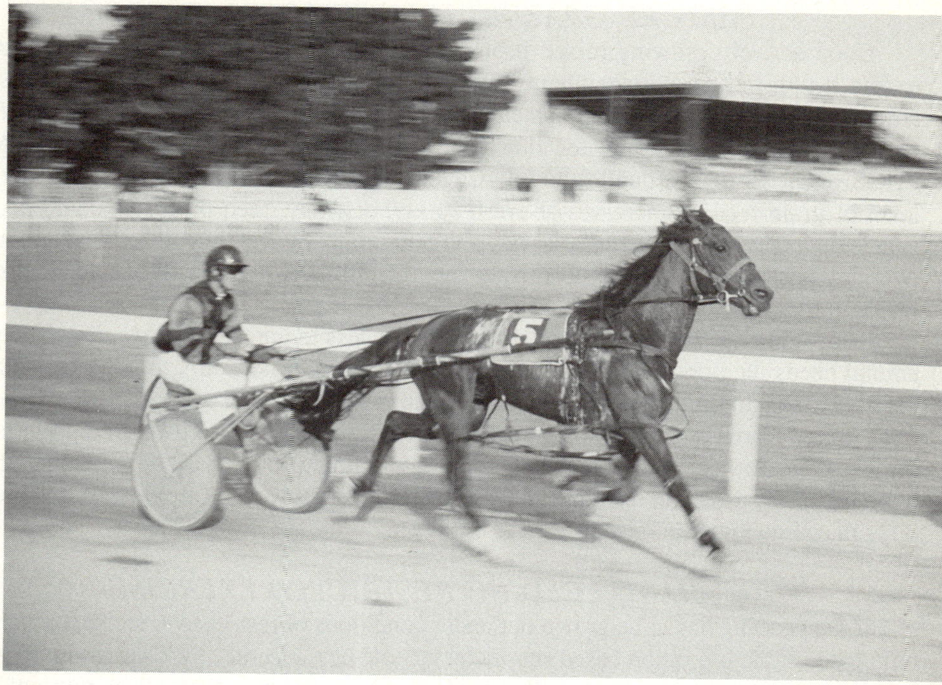

Two and three year old trotters are still growing and at the same time competing. Very careful attention needs to be made to the ration as well as the training programme to ensure the optimum results.

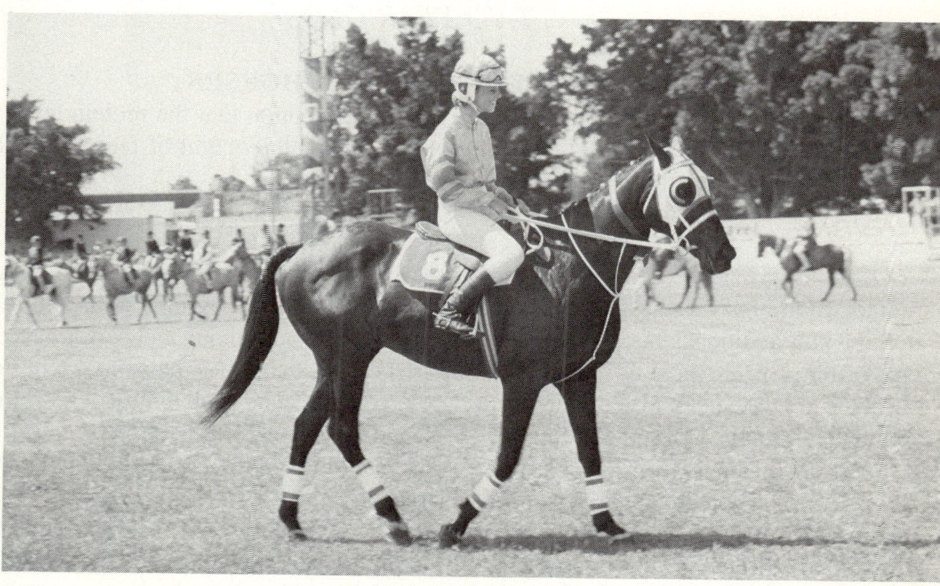

Young racehorses need special attention to their feeding rations. Ration has to allow growth as well as performance and there may be many individual horse variations.

PASTURE GRAZING UNRESTRICTED EXERCISE

Good actively growing mixed pasture will provide all the necessary feed nutrients, except it will be, on average about 25% too low in energy supplies. This can easily be corrected by feeding a grain supplement, about 0.20 kg oats/day/horse. At this level of grain feeding, there should be not too much of an imbalance created in the CALCIUM and PHOSPHORUS levels, due to the low Ca and high P levels in the grain. However if the level of grain feeding increases above 0.20 kg/horse/day, then problems could occur. A supplement of 50% lucerne (alfalfa) hay and 50% grain, by weight will be ideal and will get over any possible Ca and P problems, as the mineral level in one will balance the mineral levels in the other.

It is highly desirable that these horses have access to unrestricted exercise. The young animal needs the opportunity to exercise, at will, in order not only to grow satisfactorily but also to condition the tendons, ligaments and muscles as well as other parts of the body. Such horses reared under these conditions of UNRESTRICTED EXERCISE appear to have far less breakdowns and problems when put into training as opposed to the horse which is well fed but restricted in exercise to a stable and or small yard. Refer to earlier comments on high energy levels in feed.

HAND FEEDING RESTRICTED EXERCISE

If the yearling has to be grown out under conditions of restricted exercise, probably the only feed usable is a ration based simply on lucerne hay, lucerne chaff and grain. In general this ration, correctly compiled, will provide this type of horse with all its nutrient needs. The main problem will be to know the type of grain being considered and the maturity of the hay at cutting. Laboratory analysis can also provide these figures.

TWO YEAR OLDS

NON PERFORMANCE HORSES

Feed exactly as for yearlings, with the possible exception that the protein level in the ration may be decreased to 11-12%, only increase the daily weight of feed available, the horse is getting bigger so needs to eat more weight of feed/day.

PERFORMANCE HORSES

This age group, i.e. two year old racehorses and pacers or standardbreds in training, will require additional protein to replace the body tissues affected by the "wear and tear" of training plus additional energy to support the work load from training and performance. This type of horse is the most difficult to feed properly. Not only does the animal require feed nutrients to grow, but it also requires nutrients to perform at its peak physical performance. Extreme nutritional pressures are placed on this type of horse.

ALL FEED NUTRIENT DEMANDS of a 2 year old performance horse will increase by about 40% over and above the feed needs of the same horse at the same age which is not in training. DRY MATTER INTAKE will increase, as a result of exercise, from an expected level of 8.10 kg D.M. to about 12.00 kg D.M/day and this additional DRY MATTER intake may supply some of the additional feed nutrient requirements.

FEEDING HORSES WEANING TO 3 YEARS OF AGE

RATION PROTEIN LEVEL will need to rise to at least 17%. and MUST contain adequate levels of LYSINE.

RATION ENERGY LEVEL will need to rise to about 4.00 MCals/kg.

CALCIUM level will need to rise to 33 gram/day.

PHOSPHORUS level will need to rise to 20 grams/day.

The projected ration PROTEIN level of 17% is nearly equal to that protein level required by WEANLING FOALS.

The desired ration energy level of 4.0 MCals/kg exceeds the energy level of most common horse feeds, except the oilseed meals.

The levels of CALCIUM and PHOSPHORUS required are such that supplementation of the feed, by one or both minerals, may be necessary.

There are a number of other practical considerations which need to be considered when feeding 2 year old performance horses.

Correct electrolyte mixtures and supplementation can be just as important to the success of two year olds as can be the correct levels of the feed nutrients detailed above.

Be careful of the traditional "track sour" symptoms which develop in two year old in particular, especially when forced too hard early in the training preparation, often associated with high protein levels and or lack of LYSINE and the apparent inability of the young horse to utilise energy.

Two year olds reared as weanlings and yearlings, under conditions of unrestricted exercise, are always better conditioned to take the stresses of training as opposed to the two year olds grown under restricted exercise conditions, no matter what the feeding regime of the restricted exercise horse may have been.

Do not impose any hard training and or exercise on any two year old at all until the knees have "closed over".

Periods of long slow work, for two year olds, in the initial stages before fast work is attempted will be rewarded.

Increase energy level in the ration, with increases in the physical demands of the training programme.

If the horse at anytime shows evidence of shin soreness, or any other tendon and/or ligament problem, stop work immediately and rest the horse until he is fit again.

28. FEEDING PONIES

Ponies, in general, have the reputation for getting all sorts of nutritional problems which do not seem to occur in larger horses. Founder and colic in particular are often found in ponies and there is always the overfat pony in every district.

Horse lore generally has it that ponies have different feed needs to other horses, and pony owners sometimes go to great lengths to control their ponies rations.

Recent research work has shown that ponies possess a degree of insulin resistance in the muscles, not present in larger horses which allow them to be able to handle larger amounts of carbohydrate in the ration, without some of the problems which affect adult horses at the same intake level in relation to body weight. This appears to be as a result of the natural selection process of ponies, over any years, to survive under harsh grazing conditions.

This ability, of ponies, to handle larger amounts of CARBOHYDRATE energy, relative to body weight, than larger equines without problems, has allowed the pony to adapt to survival on unreliable feed supplies, often associated with reasonable levels of exercise, in the wild. However, the same ability to store excess levels of CARBOHYDRATE energy becomes a disadvantage when the domesticated pony has access to a consistent and reliable supply of good quality feed and little exercise.

The problem with ponies is simple. They are generally being fed rations which either contain too much energy for the ponies' work load, or are simply being fed too large a quantity of feed, with virtually the same result. The number of times that ponies, doing very little work, have been inspected and are being fed rations suitable for race horses, in training, continues to amaze.

The digestive tract of the pony and the method of operation is no different to any other horse. The pony does not possess any different digestive processes compared to the bigger horse, neither does the pony become affected by any of the feed components any more often PROVIDED that two golden rules are observed.

1. Never overfeed energy. Ponies can be considered as horses with low work loads, and, as such, the energy level of the ration should not exceed that required for maintenance and light work This basically means that grains and oilseed based products are not recommended for feeding ponies other than in token amounts. Details of the problems caused by overfeeding of energy are detailed elsewhere in this book.

2. Be careful with the weight of feed given per day. If a 450 kg. thoroughbred has a digestive tract capacity of 8 kgs of common horse feed or hay, the ponies feed intake will be proportionately reduced as the horse gets smaller.

As most ponies of about 14 hands generally weigh, in reasonable condition, about 350 kilos, animals of this size should on hand feeding receive no more than 6.2 kgs of dry matter per day, most of which should be good quality roughage in the form of pasture and or hay. If greater levels of feed are given, the pony may well eat in excess of its' actual needs.

Ponies have been known to get overfat and in fact to contract founder and/or colic on pasture alone. In a good or excellent season for pasture growth these conditions are not uncommon in ponies grazing improved pasture.

Ponies may well be over zealous eaters, in comparison to their body weight so it is important that the pony feeder is well aware of the problems stated above.

29. DONKEYS

The principles, outlined in the book for the feeding of horses, apply, in general, to the feeding of donkeys with the following important exceptions.

1. Donkeys are adapted, in nature, to survive in much harsher environments than the horse. The donkey will, for instance, survive on shrubs and similar forage which a horse will not eat. There is a small difference in the digestive tract of the donkey compared to the horse, which allows the donkey to satisfactorily digest and exist on much lower quality feeds (high in fibre) that a horse may well reject.

2. This slight difference in the digestive tract of the donkey means that, in practical circumstances, any pasture and/or roughage fed to donkeys should contain some stalks and/or other fibrous material. Clover or legume dominant pasture and or hay are definitely not recommended for the feeding of donkeys. The feeds are too soft and will pass too rapidly through the animal. Donkeys will generally exist happily on "rougher" hay than horses, and to feed such hay to donkeys is a correct management procedure, provided no mould or weeds are present.

3. Donkeys generally perform little work or exercise, when compared to some of the physical activities demanded of the horse. The energy needs of most donkeys can generally be satisfied by pasture and/or hay with a possible small supplement of grain. Grains are all high in energy and the overfeeding of grains, and therefore energy, to the donkey will generally produce a sick animal as in a horse. The principles of feeding energy in relation to work load applies equally to both the horse and the donkey.

Whilst in horses, the grain content of the ration can get as high as 1 kg per 60 kg of body weight, donkeys appear to have a maximum desirable grain intake of about 500 grams per 100 kg of body weight. A reasonably safe grain feeding level for donkeys is of the order of 1 kg of grain per 200 kg of body weight. This is approximately 60% less grain per 100 kg of body weight for the donkey than the horse.

4. Some donkeys appear to have cracking problems with the hoof walls, especially the donkeys which do not have access to rocky areas which tend to harden and condition the hooves. The new hoof treatments based on biotin may well be worthwhile as a feed additive for these animals.

5. Beware that donkeys may well develop a liking for some weed or favourite garden shrub which may well be toxic. Donkey's are not at all fussy about what they eat and certainly do not have the same acute senses of the horse in selecting growing plants for consumption. Every donkey owner should ensure that any pasture being grazed is free of any local plant which may be, in any way, toxic if ingested. As mentioned above, do not forget the possible toxic plants which may be in the garden as well, donkeys can stretch thier necks over the graden fence.

6 Donkeys also have a habit of eating paper, plastic, cardboard, aluminium foil etc. None of these are of any value whatsoever and, in fact, may lead to a sick or dead donkey. Always ensure that paddocks being grazed by donkeys do not contain any of the above, no matter how small the quantity.

30. ECONOMICS OF PROPRIETARY FEED SUPPLEMENTS

The horse owner is continually and persistently informed, advised and reminded that his or her horse needs to be fed any one of the proprietary feed supplements on the market.

One has only to walk into any produce store or saddlery to be immediately confronted by a number of boxes, tins and containers all containing the essential "extra" ingredients that will improve your horse.

To the person who does not understand the technical problems of horse feeding, the selection of a feed additive is often based on either:-

1. the pretty label
2. the easily remembered name
3. someone else's recommendation

Price of the pack or the actual cost per day and the level of active ingredient fed per day are often the last item that the average purchaser wants to know. Little regard is paid to the fact that:-

1. the animal may or may not need the product
2. that the component in the product may already be present in the feed being fed to the horse.
3. that by feeding the product, an excessive quantity of a component may be supplied, which by itself may be dangerous, or else, in combination with some other feed component, may also be dangerous.

For a detailed evaluation of these problems refer to the earlier appropriate sections of this book.

The following principles need to be adopted in determining whether in fact any feed supplement is of value in horse feeding:-

1. What is the work load of the horse?

   If the animal has a low level work load as described earlier in the book, it will probably be able to obtain all the necessary vitamins and minerals from the basic feeds. With very few exceptions, there is little advantage to the horse in feeding these animals with low work loads any feed supplements. Specific feed supplements may be of value for animals of medium to high work loads as detailed earlier in this book.
2. What is the vitamin and mineral content of the base feeds ? Remember all the base feeds fed to horses contain reasonable levels of most vitamins and minerals. These levels are often quite adequate to satisfy daily needs to most horses. Exceptions, of course, exist but these need to be carefully evaluated so that excess levels of certain vitamins and/or minerals are not fed so as to produce possible adverse reactions.
3. What is the actual daily cost of the supplement and the level of feed component supplied per day for that cost ?

The answer to section 1 and 2 are discussed elsewhere in this book. The approach to section 3 will be evaluated in the following paragraphs. The best approach to this problem is to look at some supplements available, for purchase, at the time of writing.

VITAMIN E

This vitamin is of value when used in performance horses and is one of the supplements which can be used at reasonably high levels, without the problem of toxic or undesirable problems occurring.

Four Vitamin E supplements were analysed for daily dose rate recommended by the manufacturers and the cost of such dose rates.

Supplement A supplied	1000 I.U. per day at	67 cents
B	3280 I.U.	52 cents
C	2220 I.U.	25 cents
D	2500 I.U.	15 cents

The following should be noted:-

A. The variation in daily does rates as recommended by different manufacturers is of the order of 228%

B. The cost per 1000 I.U. of Vitamin E varies from 6 cents to 67 cents

C. The product with the smallest recommended daily dose is the most expensive to use.

Reference to the section on Vitamins will show that the average horse is able to obtain sufficient Vitamin E from 2.2 kgs of average lucerne hay. E may be of value for performance horses and, if so, anyone using Vitamin E would be well advised to assess the cost effectiveness of the vitamin on the basis detailed above.

IRON SUPPLEMENTS

These are probably the most used and abused supplements fed to horses. There is a common idea that the more iron that is fed to a horse, the more red blood cells that will be produced. This is turn will allow more oxygen to be carried around the horses body and the animal will perform better. This approach is completely incorrect. For a detailed explanation on the problems of feeding iron to horses, the reader is referred to the chapter on minerals.

Five proprietary iron supplements were analysed for iron content based on manufacturer's recommendation and for daily feeding cost.

Supplement A supplied	0.110 grams Fe per day at	53 cents
B	0.600	37 cents
C	0.910	28 cents
D	0.640	80 cents
E	0.102	25 cents

Note the following:-

A. The variation in manufacturers recommended daily dose rates is nearly 800%.

B. The cost per 0.100 grams Fe varies from 3.1 cents to 48 cents.

C. The most common effective product would be supplement C

There is no consistency at all in the manufacturer's recommended dose rate or in the cost of the Fe fed.

The horses' optimum daily intake of iron is in the order of about 50 parts per million in the feed. A thoroughbred with a feed intake of about 8 kgs requires about 0.400 grams of iron per day. Reference to the section on minerals will show that most horse feeds contain more than adequate amounts of iron for all, but the horse with some specific iron problem. On this basis the feeding of iron for the normal horse is not technically justified.

However if iron must be fed, supplements A & E will only supply 25% of the horse's expected daily needs and are probably a waste of money. Supplements B and D will supply 150% the animals daily needs, supplement D however being at least twice as expensive as supplement B. Supplement C provides iron at the cheapest cost but at the highest daily dose rate. This would be the ideal supplement for use in anaemic horses, horses which have bled profusely, or in specific cases, where iron may be required.

CALCIUM SUPPLEMENTS

Calcium supplements are generally necessary in any ration which contains reasonable levels of grain and or grain by-product, all of which contain low levels of CALCIUM and high levels of PHOSPHORUS. At the same time, it is necessary that excessive administration of CALCIUM be avoided as problems can occur if the horse receives too much CALCIUM in the ration.

The following calcium supplements can be considered:-

MICRO-FINE LIMESTONE

This is limestone crushed as small as possible with most of the contaminants removed. It is available from most produce stores where its principal use is in the coating of inoculated clover and legume seeds. The limestone has to be pure so as not to destroy the bacteria that is placed on the seed in the inoculation process.

Micro-fine limestone contains 35% calcium and in order for a mature horse to receive 23 grams per day, the accepted daily requirement, 65 grams or about 2 tablespoons per day of micro-fine limestone, would be required.

At a cost of $5.10 per 25 kg bag, calcium would cost 2 cents per day.

DICALCIUM PHOSPHATE

This is frequently looked upon as a supplement of both calcium and phosphorous, containing 23% calcium and 19% phosphorous. D.C.P., as the product is commonly known, is of value in supplying calcium to those rations where the Ca/P ratio already has a range of 2/1 to 1/1. Such rations would principally consist of 50% lucerne and 50% grain. Any other ration would most likely have a Ca/P ration around 1/4 and the feeding of D.C.P. as a supplement to that type of ration would only increase the level of phosphorus in the feed and adversely offset the Ca/P ratio.

D.C.P. is available at about $3.00 per kg and 100 grams would be needed per day to supply the horse with 23 grams of calcium. The daily cost would be 7 cents.

COMMERCIAL SUPPLEMENTS

A number of these are available on the market and only one will be analysed as they all follow similar dose rates and recommendations. The product concerned contains 30% calcium, 3.6% phosphorous, plus magnesium, zinc, manganese, iron, Vitamin A and Vitamin D. The recommended daily dose rate is about 60 grams per day, supplying:-

18 grams of Ca	daily needs 23 grams	78% of daily needs
2.2 grams of P	14	15%

0.3 grams of Mg	6.5	5%
0.1 grams of Zn	18.0	0.55%
0.03 grams of Mn	not available	
0.1 grams of Fe	0.4	25%
18000 I.U. Vit.A	100,000 I.U.	18%
12000 I.U. Vit.D	3000 I.U.	400%

at a daily feeding cost of 31.2 cents.

As a calcium source, this is an expensive product, especially as 83% of the calcium is supplied by micro-fine limestone.

As can be seen from the balance of the analysis, the other components either supply very little of the horses' daily needs and the horse is probably getting these components from the normal feed anyway, or in the case of Vitamin D, is providing an amount well in excess of accepted daily needs. The figures for the daily expected availability of VITAMINS A and D probably do not exist in practice. It is most likely that both the vitamins are destroyed when mixed with the limestone and so will be ineffective in this type of mix.

The above figures clearly illustrate the need to clarify the effective cost of supplements. Calcium can cost from 2 cents to 31.2 cents per day for the same quantity of mineral, dependent on the source selected.

PHOSPHORUS SUPPLEMENTS

For horses which obtain most or all of their feed from grazing pasture, the easiest and cheapest way to provide a supplement of PHOSPHORUS, if needed is by application of superphosphate or a similar PHOSPHORUS containing fertiliser to the pasture.

If there is a need for a phosphorus supplement to be used in the hand feeding situation, it can be approached in the following ways:-

HOME MADE PHOSPHORUS SUPPLEMENT

Superphosphate is a common fertiliser used to correct the phosphorus deficiency existing in many soils.

Take 2 kgs superphosphate, not MO (molybdenised) superphosphate, and thoroughly mix in 4.5 litres or 1 gallon of water. Let stand for 24 hours and then pour of and retain the liquid. The residue in the bottom of the container must be thrown away as it contains, among other things, the fluoride portion of the superphosphate and must not, under any circumstances, be fed to the horses.

The liquid obtained will generally contain about 40 grams of phosphorus liquid per litre. As the horse generally needs about 14 grams of phosphorus per day, about 330 ml of the solution used to dampen the feed will provide the animal with its daily needs. Supplying the phosphorus by this method will cost about 3 cents per day.

DICALCIUM PHOSPHATE

This compound was discussed earlier in the chapter on MINERALS and is more a source of phosphorus, under present feeding conditions, than it is a source of calcium. The horses' daily PHOSPHORUS needs can be supplied by 70 grams D.C.P. at a daily cost of 5 cents. There is need to consider the excess calcium supplied by the D.C.P. as high levels of CALCIUM in the ration is not advisable.

OTHER PHOSPHORUS SUPPLEMENTS

In the U.S.A. there are a number of supplements used in horse feeding to supply phosphorus. Daily amounts necessary to supply 14 grams of phosphorus are detailed after each chemical.

Ammonium Polyphosphate	- 100 grams
Diammonium phosphate	- 70 grams
Monoammonium phosphate	- 61 grams
Monosodium phosphate	- 56 grams
Sodium tripolyphosphate	- 56 grams

MULTI-PURPOSE VITAMIN AND MINERAL SUPPLEMENTS

There are a number of these products on the market and they generally contain most of the vitamins and minerals considered necessary for horse feeding and often others which do not, in terms of present knowledge, have any value in the feeding of horses.

It is not the intention of this section to analyse all these feed supplements in detail, but rather to examine the principles and to indicate their value, if any, in the feeding of the horses.

These supplements can have the components broken down into various headings.

1. Protein - Often some form of protein source is present and is often used as the base for the thorough mixing of the other components. The label will detail the protein content at some value, say 16%, but when the actual amount of protein that the horse will receive each day is calculated, the amount is so small as to be useless. One such supplement supplied 1% of the horses daily protein needs when fed at label directions.
2. Energy - Often included in these compounds and generally in the form of fat and various sugars such as glucose fructose, dextrose and other compounds. In two mixes analysed, the energy provided, at recommended dose rates, amounted to 0.2% and 0.3% of the energy needs of a horse with a low work load.
3. Common Salt - Sodium Chloride. Generally in all mixtures and may be up to 36% of the weight. All horses need common salt but the salt can be fed much more cheaply as salt in the feed than as part of a vitamin mineral mix.
4. Vitamins, all are readily available in the common horse feeds, Vitamins A, B, C, E & K are all available to horses fed pasture, hay and common horse feeds and D comes at no cost from sunlight. These vitamins are present in all feeds in adequate amounts to supply any horse, at rest or only performing light work, with sufficient of each vitamin. There is generally no need to feed additional vitamins in these categories. In most instances the horse will not use the additional vitamin supplied.

   Vitamin D may be needed by horses which are stabled and/or rugged during the day. Rather than feed D in a vitamin and mineral mix, it is better to find a source of vitamin D alone, or else take the rugs off for two hours per day and let the horse out in the sunlight. Those people trying to attain a certain coat standard may well be surprised what a little sunflower seed in the ration and two hours in the sun each day will do for most horse coats.

   Vitamin B. Horses with medium to high work loads need B supplement but again it is better to be fed B as a separate supplement rather than in a mixture. The dose rate in mixtures are generally too low to be effective for performance horses.

Vitamin E may or may not be present in some of these mixes. The comments applicable to Vitamin B apply to Vitamin E.

5. Minerals - Calcium and Phosphorous - the rates which horses should receive, from these multi vitamin/mineral supplements, on recommended daily feeding are generally so small as to be of no value. In some supplements even the Ca/P ratios were incorrect. Iron - All mineral and vitamin supplements contain iron, often in large quantities, generally enough to provide the horse with levels which supply all the daily iron needs, or well in excess of the daily needs If iron has to be fed, for any specific reason, then the feeder should resort to a reasonable iron supplement with no other additives.

Most supplements contain one or more of up to seven additional minerals - potassium, copper, cobalt, manganese, magnesium, zinc, and iodine. All these minerals are present in normal feeds and there is no reason why they should be fed to any horse as a general supplement. If one of these minerals may be required, then it should only be fed under the direction of a qualified person as problems may occur. If the levels of these minerals fed on a daily basis, as per manufacturers recommendations, are calculated, it will be found in most instances that the daily level is so low as to be of no value.

1. Working Out Just What is in the Supplement - All proprietary feed supplements are required by law to carry on the label somewhere, the actual technical components of the product, and the concentration of those components.

   It looks very impressive to read down a list of 23 separate components on a label, but it is important to understand what they all mean.
2. Working Out the Daily Horse's Intake as Fed per Label Directions - It is important to be able to calculate the daily intake by the horse of each of the components on the label. The previous calculations on the iron and Vitamin E supplements are simple in that those products contain only one component, and in fact the component concentration in the examples used was shown on the label. However when a situation arises where the feed component is not specified on the label as the active ingredient, then access to a chemistry book and a calculator will be necessary to calculate the level of the component in the feed.

This can be clearly illustrated by trying to work out the iron level in one particular feed supplement.

Fe (iron) is present in three components. As red iron oxide, generally known as ferric oxide, but not stated as such on the labels, as ferrous sulphate heptahydrate and as part of a separate organic chelated mineral complex.

In order to work out the exact level of iron in the ration, it is necessary to know or have access to the chemical formula of the above chemicals and information that will tell you the percentage of iron in each chemical. Such data provides the following information.

Red iron oxide	70.0% iron	7.00 grams Fe/kg of supplement
Ferrous sulphate	20.0% iron	1.00 grams Fe/kg of supplement
Mineral complex	11.9% iron	1.34 grams Fe/kg of supplement
		TOTAL Fe 9.34 grams/kg.

Each kg of supplement contains 9.34 grams of iron and when fed at the recommended rate of 60 grams per horse per day, will provide the horse with 0.56 grams of iron, or 140% of the animals expected daily needs. This is in addition to the iron that the animal is already receiving from the normal feed and in practice the horse could be getting up to 200-300% of its daily iron needs if fed this supplement in conjunction with ordinary horse feeds.

This then means that the horse is receiving excessive levels of IRON, on a daily basis, greatly increasing the possibility of IRON toxicity occuring in the horse.

The daily feeding cost of most of these vitamin mineral supplements varied at the time of writing from about 45 to 105 cents per day, or on a weekly basis from $3.15 to $7.35.

Their technical ability to supply the horse with something that it is not already receiving from the normal feed is seriously questioned. Those vitamins and minerals that are supplied all appear, with the exception of iron, to be fed at recommended levels so small as to be of little or no value to the horse.

The iron level of most of these products is in fact too high, and separate feeding of iron is recommended.

If the horse must have some form of supplement, consider what the horse is receiving in its feed, remember all feeds contain some or all of the vitamins and minerals, and then select a specific product if available to do the job.

31. PRACTICAL HORSE NUTRITION GUIDELINES

1. Correct horse feeding is based on supplying feed in relation to your horse's needs. This is best done on a weight basis as it is possible to measure both feed and horses in terms of weight and, therefore, have a common basis of comparison.

2. Think of feed in weight, not leaves of hay or quarts or saucepans of this and that. Weigh your normal feed containers, full of the different feeds on the kitchen scales, and write the details down for future reference, you will be surprised as to the weight/volume of the feeds, known as ENERGY DENSITY.

3. Get some idea of the weight of your horse, on a vehicle weighbridge is best, weight tapes have about a 20% error or, at worst, use one of the many tables commonly available.

4. BODY CONDITION SCORING is an excellent way of assessing your horses' condition. If you do not wish to use either one of these systems, the ideal condition for most horse is when you can feel the ribs but cannot see them.

5. Ensure that the horse is continually and thoroughly drenched to remove all internal parasites or WORMS, you cannot feed horses and worms at the same time.

6. Mixed pasture, with both a grass and legume (clover) component, will be sufficient for most pleasure horse's daily feed needs, if the animals are grazed at a reasonable stocking rate.

7. If supplementary feeding horses, which also have access to pasture grazing, make sure the horse is not using the pasture as a PARKING LOT. There are very valuable feed components in that pasture which the horse should eat and at a much cheaper cost than in grain and concentrates. If you offer the horse HARD FEED, they are like children in a candy shop, they will eat the "candy" first and leave the decent food until later.

8. Always ensure clean feed and water containers.

9. Make sure the horse's teeth are not sharp, cutting into the tongue and or gums, affecting feed intake.

10 Always ensure that the horse has enough weight of feed to satisfy its daily appetite, the horse cannot digest feed and perform properly, with air, in the digestive tract.

11. When horses are stabled and fully hand fed, feed at least three times a day and ALWAYS leave some hay in the hay net. When grazing the horse can spend from 16 to 20 hours/day eating.

12. Avoid mouldy, dusty and or weed infested feeds.

13. Crushed or Crimped grain is the best if you do not want to feed whole grain. All other methods of grain treatment, Cracking, Rolling etc. can cause loss of feed nutrients, due to attack by oxygen, whilst some other methods of feed preparation use bad quality grain combined with added water and make a lot of profit out of selling water.

14. Be careful when buying lucerne chaff that the green colour is not artificially added. Place a small quantity of chaff in a glass of water, if green dye is present, it will colour the water in about half an hour.

15. Chaff should be fed in limited quantities, sufficient to get any additives and or grain into the horse. Too much chaff can increase teeth problems, cause digestive problems and cost extra money.

16. WHEATEN and OATEN CHAFF are very low in protein, lacking in amino acids, low in energy, high in fibre and hence most indigestible, low in CALCIUM and deficient in VITAMIN A. Lucerne or mixed pasture chaff is by far the preferred chaff with none of the above problems.

17. Lucerne chaff DOES NOT contain any more dust than Oaten or Wheaten chaff, the problem of HEAVES or decreased lung function is not only a dust problem but a problem caused by six or seven factors, the most important of which is stable ventilation.

18. Note any change in the daily feed consumption, a sure indicator that something has or is about to go wrong.

19. Know your horse's expected daily intake of water, any large variations in daily intake will need investigating, and will be an indicator of something about to go wrong with the horse. Adequate water should be available at all times and the horse should be encouraged to drink whenever possible. Partial dehydration, which you cannot detect or measure, can be a problem with performance horses.

20. Do not allow a hot horse to drink too much water, allow just enough to satisfy initial thirst and the balance when the horse has cooled down

21. Do not give any type of concentrate or hard feed to a hot horse, roughage only for at least 45 minutes, until the horse has cooled down, known as "R and R", or REST and ROUGHAGE.

22. Avoid sudden feed changes in an active horse, take at least 3 weeks making gradual changes in any ration.

23. If letting a horse down, going from mainly hard feed to pasture and or hay, do so slowly over a number of days and not overnight.

24. Become an expert in FAECAL (dung or excreta) assessment, the colour, texture and frequency of faecal production can tell you a lot about the health and well being of your horse.

25. INCORRECT FEEDING of ENERGY is the most important common problem of practical horse feeding.

26. ENERGY levels in the ration are directly related to the amount of exercise the horse gets.

27. Be careful of the ENERGY DENSITY of grains, the relationship of volume weight and energy content. The same volume of corn (maize) contains about 80% more energy than oats.

28. For horses on complete hand feeding, ensure that at least 50%, by weight, of the daily ration is roughage.

29. The average pleasure horse gets enough energy from hay and other roughages and grazing to provide all the energy required. Grain or CONCENTRATES, to these types of horses, in any quantity, can only cause problems.

30. If you must feed grain to the pleasure horse, no more than 0.5 kg/day for the average pony and no more than 1.0 kg/day for the average big horse.

31 Ponies are able to handle lower energy levels in the ration, compared to bigger horses, DO NOT OVERFEED ENERGY TO PONIES.

32. The weight of roughage in the ration, hay, chaff, pasture etc., should ALWAYS exceed the weight of the concentrate or hard feed portion, EXCEPT in exceptional circumstances with performance horses where full technical evaluation of the feeding and training is continually being carried out.

33. Energy content of rations for performance horses needs to be increased in line with increasing work loads.

34. Exercise improves appetite and general health.

35. OVERFEEDING and or INSUFFICIENT EXERCISING of young growing horses upsets or alters the natural body growth patterns and balances between BONES and MUSCLES and causes MUSCLES to be developed at a faster rate than BONES and JOINTS, leading to breakdowns when these rapidly grown horses are put into training.

36. OVER FEEDING OF ENERGY, in relation to the amount of exercise the horse gets, CAN CAUSE HORSES TO BECOME DIFFICULT TO CONTROL AND TO MISBEHAVE, and various other possible problems such as COLIC, FOUNDER, TYING UP, THUMPS, and numerous other conditions.

37. Fat or oil based feeds are a reasonable technical source of energy but are only desirable for any horse which is really working hard and certainly not of value for the average pleasure horse or the horse which does not do much work. Palatability problems may result with FATS in the ration, and the energy can often be obtained at a better price from other energy sources.

38. There is no such thing as HOT FEEDS. Some feeds contain more energy and less fibre than others and the term HOT FEEDS is, generally, incorrectly referred to a high energy feed which is being fed to a horse, at weights well above the horse's daily needs. The horse gets far too much energy in its ration compared to its daily needs, and the first sign of TOO MUCH ENERGY in a ration is a horse which misbehaves, plays up and is hard to handle. The solution to HOT FEEDS is to reduce the grain content of the ration, the problem is a human problem, not a horse problem.

39. The second most important practical horse feeding problem is insufficient CALCIUM in the ration. CALCIUM in conjunction with PHOSPHORUS is responsible for many things in the horse, the most important being BONE formation and maintenance. Lack of CALCIUM in the ration does lead to bone and muscle problems.

40. The third most important practical horse feeding problem involves PROTEIN, which builds and maintains all body tissues. Lack of insufficient PROTEIN in the ration affects many things but the two most important are restricted growth in young horses and reduced performance in older horses.

41. PROTEIN QUALITY is as important as level of PROTEIN in a horse ration. Proteins contain a number of AMINO ACIDS, 10 of which are essential for the horse and need to be in every ration. Very few horse feeds contain the 10 ESSENTIAL AMINO ACIDS.

42. The availability of ELECTROLYTES are the next most important practical horse feeding problem. The average pleasure horse does not sweat enough to need electrolyte supplementation, that horse can get all its electrolytes from the normal feeds.

43. Any performance horse needs to be on continual daily electrolyte supplementation whist in training and competing. JUGGING and other methods of giving large electrolyte doses are mostly excreted in the urine, so are of no value.

44. Most horses on grazing or a mixed ration of hay and grain DO NOT NEED any vitamin or mineral supplement. Those VITAMINS and MINERALS are already in the natural feeds.

45. The exception to this rule is common salt. All horses require a daily supplementation.

46. SPECIFIC VITAMIN and MINERAL supplements may be advisable for some performance horses but these need to be evaluated for each individual horse.

47. VITAMINS and MINERALS can interact with other feed components and can be dangerous causing very sick horses and sometimes death.

48. If feeding supplements, LEARN TO READ A LABEL AND UNDERSTAND WHAT IS IN THE SUPPLEMENT AND WHY?. Carefully evaluate the contents of such supplements. Is the supplement duplicating what is already available in the common feeds? Are the components in the supplement stable when mixed or have they disappeared between mixing and feeding? Is the supplement cost effective?

49. Complete feeds,- everything in the one bag - , from reputable suppliers, are suitable for the pleasure horse, IF SUPPLEMENTED WITH HAY which is freely available. There are much better ways of feeding performance horses however.

50. Feed horses as individuals, learn their individual likes and dislikes.

51. Every horse has individual feed preferences, the same as humans. Feed the horse what it will eat, NOT WHAT YOU WANT THE HORSE TO EAT.

52. Some horses will not eat SWEET FEED, containing reasonably high levels of MOLASSES, they just do not like it.

53. Do not be fooled by the palatability of some prepared horse feeds. With current commercial flavourings, it is possible to get a horse to eat sawdust but it does not do him much good.

54. Recognise the signs of a well fed healthy horse, contentment, alertness, healthy appetite, sleek coat, normal temperature, pulse and respiration.

55. It is impossible to feed beyond genetic capacity, there will always be thin horse and fat horses, exactly the same as there are thin people and fat people, body condition is initially determined by genetic or breeding, feeding only allows that genetic factor to be realised.

56. FEEDING WILL NOT SUBSTITUTE FOR TRAINING. If the horse's organs and muscles are not conditioned, by training, to use the extra feed, you are wasting your time.

57. PERFORMANCE ABILITY is also genetically determined. All the feeding and training in the world will not improve a horse whose genetic make up restricts its capacity to perform.

32. THE PEARSON SQUARE

The Pearson Square is a method of calculating horse rations and is frequently reported in American literature.

The Pearson Square is based on the differences in the nutrient levels of individual feeds. Using energy as an example the principles involved are as follows:

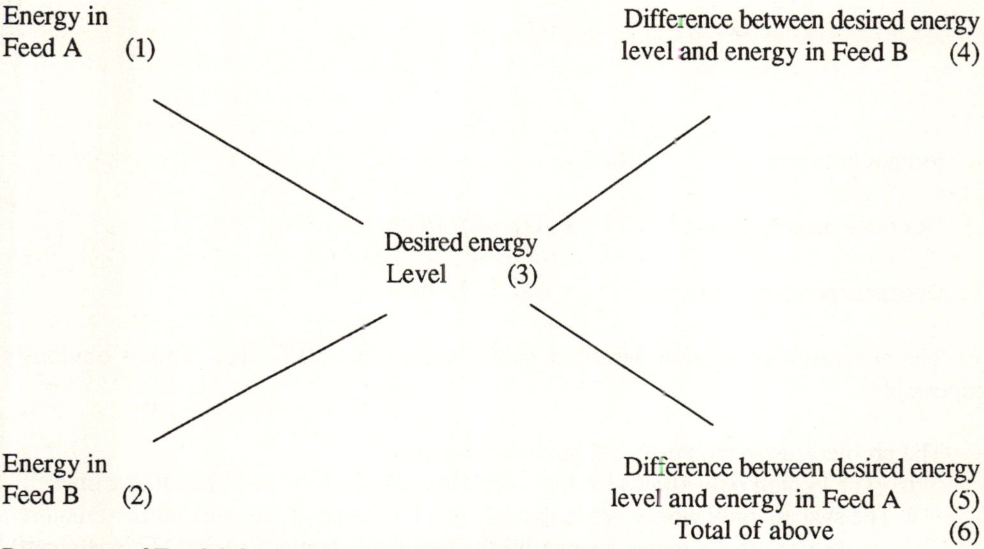

Percentage of Feed A in the ration = $\frac{(4)}{(6)}$ x 100 as percentages

Percentage of Feed B in the ration = $\frac{(5)}{(6)}$ x 100 as percentages

Relating this method to an actual ration, the ultimate is a ration of 14% protein and 55% energy using oats and lucerne as the base feeds. Calculating the energy content is the first step.

Energy in oats

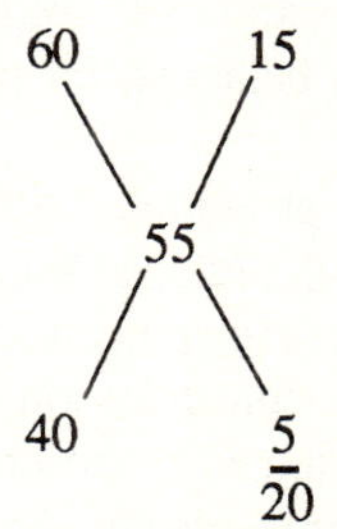

Energy in lucerne

Desirable grain percentage $\frac{15}{20}$ x 100 = 75%

Desirable lucerne percentage $\frac{5}{20}$ x 100 = 25%

To get a ration of the two feeds with a combined energy level of 55% will need a mix of 7.5 kgs of oats and 2.5 kgs of lucerne.

In this calculation the method works satisfactorily, especially as the energy levels of the two feeds are above and below the desired energy level of the final product.

The same ration needs a protein level of 16% so the respective values for protein rather than energy are substituted in the calculation as follows:-

Protein in oats 10% 2

16%

Protein in lucerne 14% $\frac{6}{4}$

Desirable percentage oats $\frac{2}{4} \times 100 = 50\%$

Desirable percentage lucerne $\frac{6}{4} \times 100 = 150\%$

The end result is a ration based on 150% lucerne and 50% oats. This is obviously impossible.

The problems with the Pearson Square are is follows:

1. The system only allows for the calculation on one food component at a time.
2. The system only works when the desired percentage of the one nutrient required is between those values shown by the two feeds being assessed. This is clearly shown in this example where the energy level can be calculated as the respective energy level of oats and lucerne are above and below the desired energy level of the final feed. However in the calculation re protein, the desired protein level is not between the protein levels of oats and lucerne and accordingly an obvious incorrect result is obtained.
3. The method is only of value if one nutrient is being sought in a ration. Even if the desired protein level is the above example was 12%, the Pearson Square method would produce a ration balanced for protein consisting of 50% oats and 50% lucerne.

Our desired ration containing 12% protein and 55% energy will therefore consist of 50% oats and lucerne to give the required protein percentage and 75% oats and 25% lucerne to give the desired energy percentage.

4. The system does not allow for the consideration of the cost of differing horse feeds.
5. If more than one feed component is to be considered, the Pearson Square as demonstrated, will produce incorrect results.

REFERENCES

BOOKS

1. AUSTRALIAN FEED COMPOSITION TABLES, NATIONAL COLLECTION (1970-1987) A.F.I.C.-C.S.I.R.O.
2. HORSE AND PONY NUTRITION Anderson E.A. & J.R. R.M. Williams.
3. FEEDS AND FEEDING Morrison F.B. The Morrison Publishing Company.
4. FEEDING FARM ANIMALS Hewitt A.C.T. Angus & Robertson.
5. FEEDING THE HORSE The Blood Horse Library U.S.A.
6. HORSE NUTRITION Hintz H.F. Arco Publishing Inc.
7. EQUINE NUTRITION Leighton Hardman A.C. Pelham Books.
8. FEEDING AND CARING OF THE HORSE Lewis L.D. Lea & Febiger.
9. EQUINE NUTRITION & FEEDING Frape D. Longman.
10. ANIMAL NUTRITION 4th ED. Mcdonald P.,Edwards R.A., Greenhalgh J.F.D.,Longman.
11. BASIC NUTRITION & FEEDING 3rd ED. Church D.C., Pond W.G. Wiley.
12. NUTRIENT REQUIREMENTS OF HORSES 5th ED 1989 National Academy of Sciences Washington D.C. U.S.A.

SCIENTIFIC CONFERENCE PROCEEDINGS

13. POST GRADUATE COMMITTEE IN VETERINARY SCIENCE PROCEEDINGS NO 63 NUTRITION 1983 SYDNEY UNIVERSITY.
14. POST GRADUATE COMMITTEE IN VETERINARY SCIENCE DIETARY MANAGEMENT IN DOG, CAT & HORSE PRACTICE 1988 SYDNEY UNIVERSITY
15. THE HORSE A Seminar to aid Research SYDNEY UNIVERSITY 1982
16. EQUINE NUTRITION Proc of Fourth Bain-Fallon Memorial Lectures. A.E.V.A. 1982.

SCIENTIFIC JOURNALS

Some 157 scientific papers, relating to experiments on the feeding of the horse and appearing in the following scientific journals, up to March 1989, were researched.

A. AMERICAN JOURNAL OF VETERINARY RESEARCH.
B. VETERINARY RECORD.
C. THERIOGENOLGY.
D. EQUINE PRACTITIONER.
E. MODERN VETERINARY PRACTICE.
F. JOURNAL OF NUTRITION.
G. CORNELL VETERINARY JOURNAL.
H. JOURNAL AMERICAN VETERINARY MEDICAL ASSOCIATION.
I. EQUINE VETERINARY JOURNAL.
J. PROCEEDINGS AMERICAN ASSOCIATION EQUINE PRACTITIONERS.
K. JOURNAL ANIMAL SCIENCE.
L. AUSTRALIAN VETERINARY JOURNAL.
M. JOURNAL EQUINE VETERINARY SCIENCE.
N. NEW ZEALAND VETERINARY JOURNAL

INDEX